FITNESS IS FUN

DAVE PROWSE
with John Parker

W.H. ALLEN · LONDON
A HOWARD & WYNDHAM COMPANY
1979

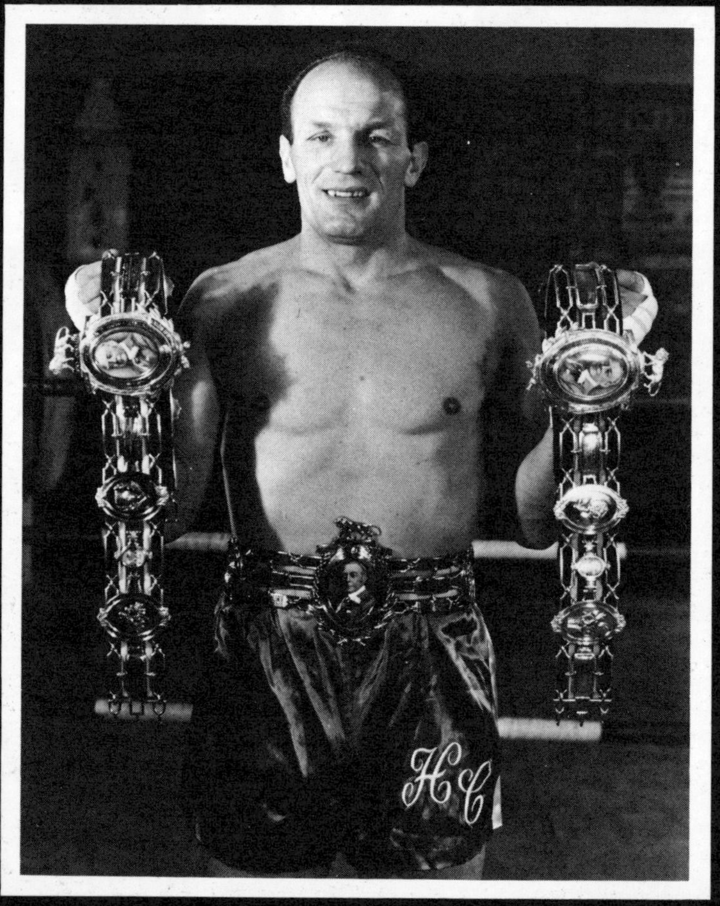

Introduction by Henry Cooper, former British and Empire Heavyweight Boxing Champion:

I have always kept myself fit. Of course, it is self-obvious that I must have been fit to be a boxer, but more than that I have always taken a keen interest in keeping my body in tip-top shape for ordinary living. So I've been exercising for more years than I care to remember—when I was a boy, through my years as an amateur in the ring and right through to when I held the British and Empire Heavyweight titles and had a shot at the world title too. Now I've retired from boxing I still exercise regularly to keep myself physically and mentally on top form.

I've known Dave Prowse for more than ten years now and you can take it from me that he's a real expert in the business. He has made a deep study of this whole art of exercise and from his own experience has devised the series of programmes he's laid out in his book. And he's no mere muscle-man either. Anyone who can lift seven hundredweight, play Shakespeare and Darth Vader, and teach road safety to countless thousands of kids, has to be quite a remarkable man.

The principles I've trained on are very similar to those which Dave Prowse lays out so clearly in his book. A boxer trains to a peak for his bouts, but in general he is seeking strength, stamina and coordination. What Dave Prowse has done is to evolve a system of exercising and put it together in such a way as to make the whole business of keeping fit full of pleasure and fun.

Henry Cooper

Book Design by Bob Hook, Photography by Graham Miller

Printed and bound in Great Britain by Butler & Tanner Ltd, Frome and London
W. H. Allen & Co Ltd, 44 Hill Street, London W1X 8LB ISBN 0 491 02356 1

Contents

I admire talent, and I admire success; and both come in a variety of different ways. Piano artistry, success in business, athletic brilliance, academic prowess; all these command my admiration and hold my attention. In particular, I feel that anyone who makes the most of the attributes he is given at birth is worthy of admiration.

I have always been a big guy. That was part of what I was given. And at school I was like greased lighting. I could out-run and out-jump anybody even though I was competing with boys much older than myself. I had two ambitions. I was going to be an international athlete, and I was going to play rugby football for England.

The fact that at thirteen I fell ill and spent the next four years in hospital and in a leg-iron was quite irrelevant to this ambition. There was no doubt in my own mind that I would recover and would be as fast as I ever had been. Long before the doctors released me, having discovered that I did not have tuberculosis after all, I was sneaking off to the swimming bath, getting out of my leg-iron, and plunging in.

There was no doubt in my mind that I would take up where I had left off. I was not interested in any of the career lectures, I didn't care that my academic progress was not as good as it might have been. I knew that everything would fall into place when I was fit again. Subsequently I've discovered that I'm quite good at drawing the line, standing outside myself and taking a good look at what's happening to me. I suppose that the first time I really did this was after I had tried to play rugby football again.

It was a rude awakening. All I remembered was that I used to be the biggest, fastest guy on the field, and no-one could stop me. Now I was the slowest, tallest, skinniest individual and, it seemed, the natural target for all the tough guys on the other side. Whereas before I had left them all standing, or if they had got near enough, I had been able to fend them off, now I spent most of the game face down in the mud. I was forced to realise that I was not going to be an international athlete, or play rugby for England. I had to find something else.

I found it through my body. At first, exercising was just a means to an end – to restore my wasted muscles to health and to get the girls to look at me. I turned out to be good at it, and I was soon able to sublimate my ambition to become an athlete into becoming a body-builder; and just as I had had no problem before in knowing what I wanted to do, now there was no doubt in my mind but that I was going to enter the Mr Universe competition.

From these simple beginnings I entered competitions against some of the greatest physiques in the world; later I judged those same physiques and I became heavyweight weightlifting champion of Britain and represented my country at a world championship and at the Empire and Commonwealth Games. I was privileged to meet and talk to many people who had formative influences on me, who passed on their accumulated knowledge to me. I have met the top athletes, the top coaches, the top dieticians and sporting doctors and the top administrators from all forms of sporting endeavour.

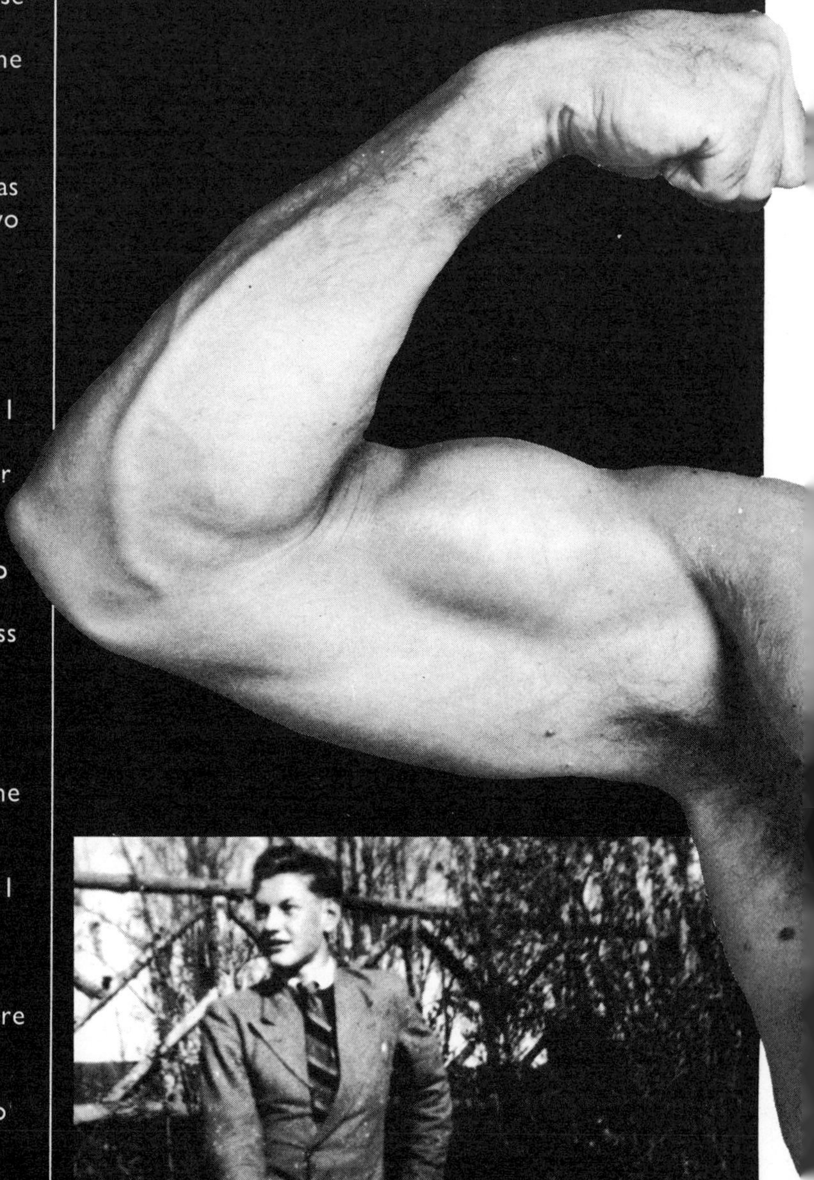

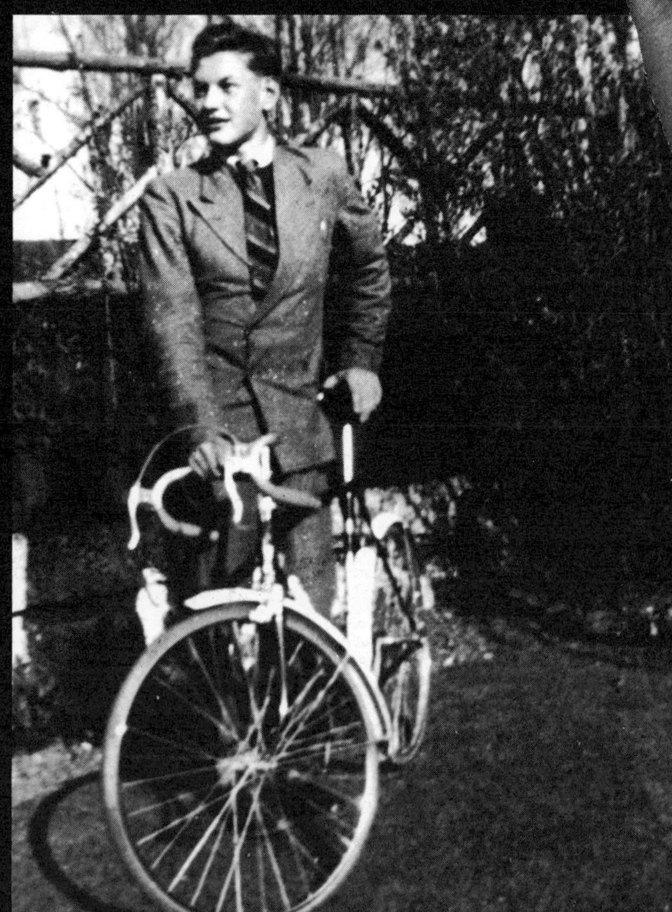

ABOVE: WITH MY FIRST BICYCLE, BEFORE I ENTERED HOSPITAL.
OPPOSITE: WITH MY SISTER JEAN.

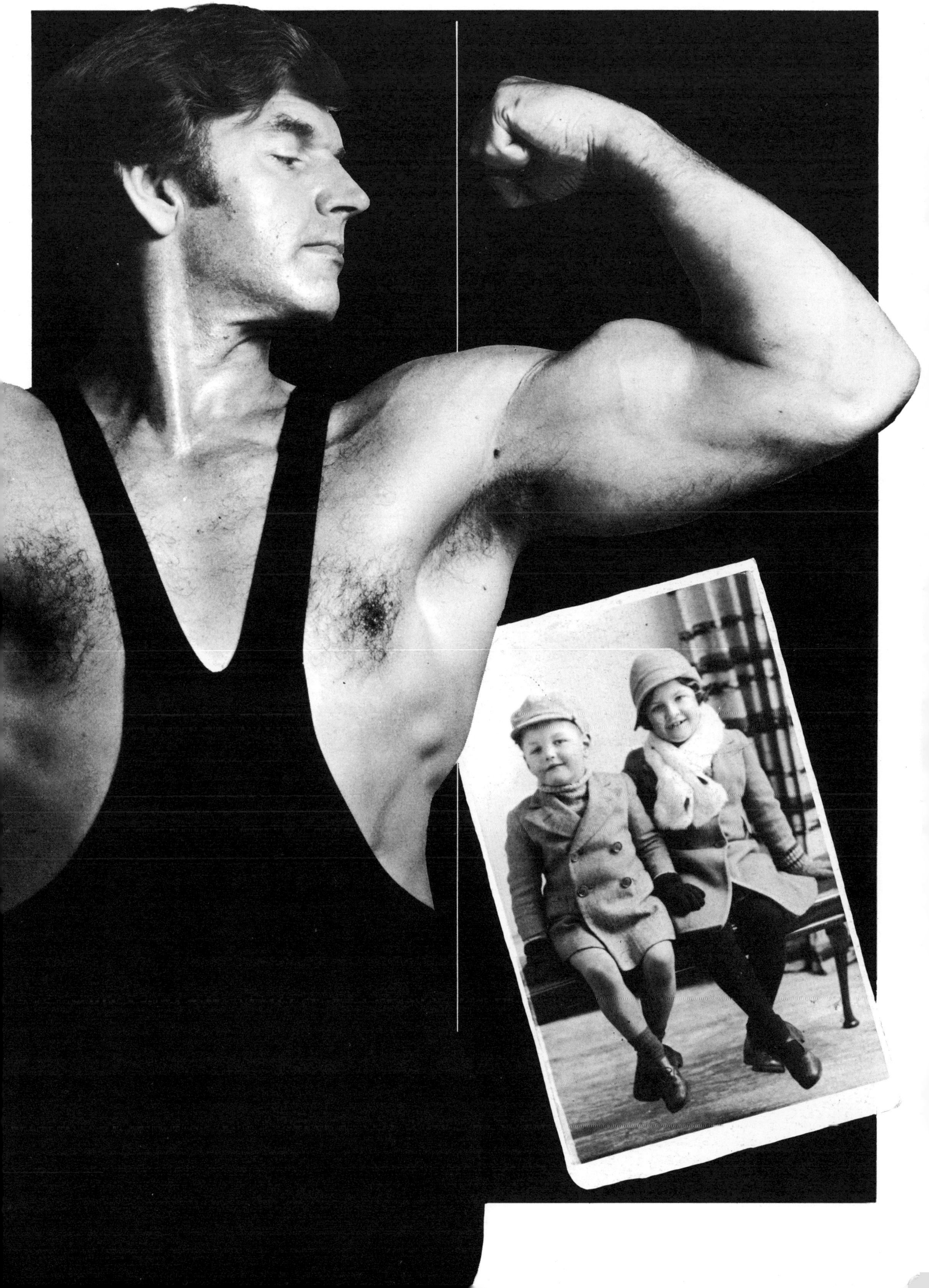

From these contacts and from the trial and error of my own experience, I have developed my own techniques which I pass on to others through my own health studio; and now I would like to extend my audience through this book. Let me give you an example of what I mean. Later in the book I talk about muscle ranges, a basic knowledge of these is essential for anyone who wants to know how to exercise his muscles correctly. On a recent trip to the United States I was training in one of the world's top gyms when I met a body-builder with a marvellous physique and above all superb biceps. I was asked, as Darth Vader, to pose for pictures with him. He took about an hour to warm up. When he eventually came out I asked him, in some admiration, which exercises he had used to develop his biceps to such a peak. 'Preacher curls,' he answered. I didn't say a thing, but in fact that particular lift has nothing to do with peaking the biceps.

Nothing annoys me more than people who say to me: 'You are lucky.' Indeed, I was lucky to be born a big chap with the determination to develop my physique. But it was not luck that put me in hospital for four years and turned me into a beanpole weakling. Nor was it luck that turned me into the British heavyweight weightlifting champion. It has taken 25 years of hard work to develop the physique I now possess and the know-how to go with it.

When I was a youngster, my relations – even my mother – would say to me, 'You're wasting your time. Why don't you settle down and get a regular job?' Or they would ask if I didn't think I ought to be in an apprenticeship, or something similar. I would reply, 'I think I know what I'm doing, thanks very much,' and they went away shaking their heads. Then, when I had started getting somewhere, these same people would come up to me and say, 'Always knew you'd do it, Dave. I always knew you'd get there.' All I could think was, 'Oh yes . . . ?'

I have always found that the really successful people are fit both physically and mentally; and usually, the more successful they are, the more concerned they are about their own physical fitness. The successful businessman for instance, realises that he has to eat too much, drink too much and do without sleep or relaxation too often; but he will deliberately set aside periods of the day when he does in fact train. I have several clients who do just this. Major businesses are aware of the importance of keeping fit, and now provide superb sporting amenities not only for their top executives but for the whole of their staff.

If I could summarise what I want to say in a sentence, it's this: get fit first. Whatever you do, you will do it better if you are fit. And you don't have to be lucky to be fit. It's up to you.

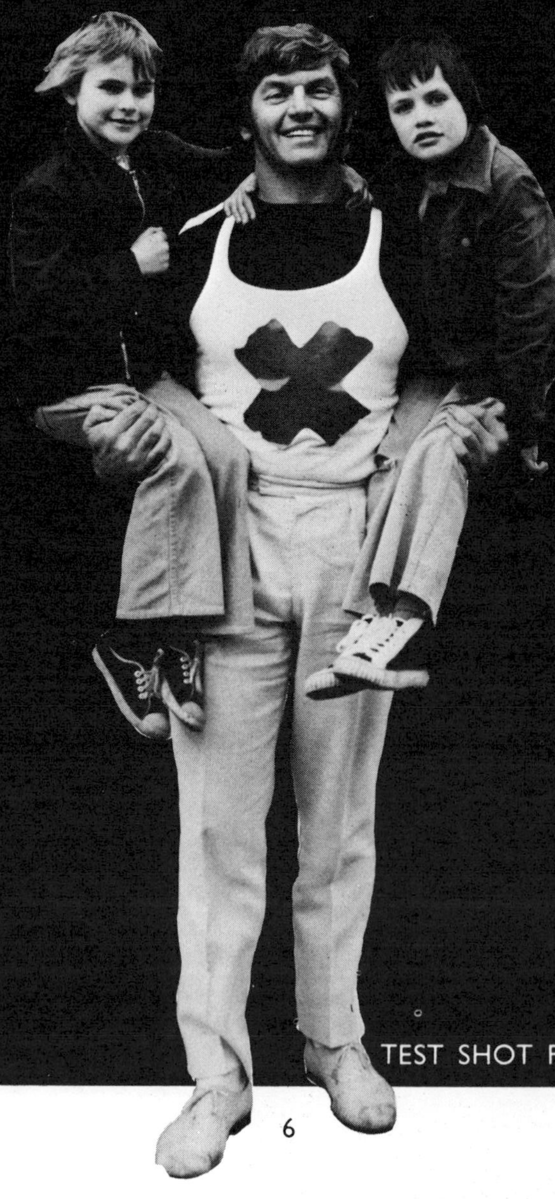

TEST SHOT FOR THE GREEN CROSS CODE.

Chapter I

SUCCESS THROUGH MY BODY

My father died when I was five years old, in 1941. He was a great drinker, my father, and when he was forty-one he had a duodenal ulcer which burst, so he was rushed into hospital for an operation. It was successful and he was stitched up, but the stitches burst and he died within a few hours.

My father was quite a small man, only five feet eight inches or so. But he had been a very good athlete, and he might have been a professional footballer had he not turned up drunk when he was given a trial by Bristol Rovers. I don't think he even saw the ball, let alone kicked it. But I've often wondered what the course of my life would have been if I had had a father to guide me. Mother did her best, of course, and whenever I got into a bit of difficulty that she could not handle – when I was finding out about sex, for example – she would ask the next-door neighbour to come over and have a chat with me. It did not help very much and really I grew up making all my own decisions – at least after the doctors had finished with me.

I don't know where I got my size from – now I'm six foot seven and usually weigh around 19 stone. Both my sister and my brother are normal-sized people – in fact my sister is quite petite, and although my mother was well-built, she only really put on weight after she began to have children. But I do remember always having a tremendous appetite. I'd come home from Fonthill Secondary Modern School, where I started my education, and think nothing of cutting a loaf in half and eating both halves, spread thickly with butter and marmalade. Then I'd have my own tea, and when the lodgers came in for their evening meal I'd sit down and eat with them. When they had finished I'd clean up all the left-overs and then go down the road to a friend's house and do the same there. I was always hungry.

At Fonthill I made quite a name for myself as an athlete. I was big for my age and I cleaned up all the sprint races in the Bristol area – the 100 yards and the 220. I was really fast. I was supposed to be fairly bright then but when they put me in for the eleven-plus examination, to go to grammar school, I failed. Or at any rate I was a borderline case, so I went for an interview. They asked me what I wanted to be when I grew up, and I said, 'A jockey.' That was enough to put anybody off, for even then I was five foot nine inches tall and well-built, so needless to say they failed me. They put me in the secondary modern after all, and I came top of the form in the first year. So they gave me another shot at the eleven-plus, and this time I passed, so I went to the Bristol Grammar School after all.

Really this turned out not to be a good idea in the end. I had made a big reputation at Fonthill, particularly as an athlete, and I went from the top there to the bottom at Bristol Grammar School, where they were not so fond of sport. They were keener on the academic side of things. So I had to struggle merely to keep up in class, and my athletics and rugby didn't do me much good. Rugby was the only ball game I was ever really interested in. I used to play lock, or in the second row, and then they put me on the wing because of my speed. I wasn't keen on soccer, and I hated cricket. In class about the only subject I really liked was art. I was interested in geography and history, but I wasn't much good at either of them. Maths I hated, although in the finish I surprised everyone by getting GCE. In any case, I only had two years at the Grammar School before I went into hospital with knee trouble.

I was spending most of my time training for sprinting, and one day, when I was about thirteen, I suddenly noticed that my left knee was swollen up, and I couldn't straighten it properly. It was affecting my speed, and that was what I was concerned about. It didn't hurt me, but I just couldn't understand why it was slowing me down. Eventually I went to my mother and she sent me to the doctor. He gave me a note and got me an immediate appointment to see a specialist, and within days they had rushed me into a tuberculosis sanatorium, Winford Orthopaedic Hospital, with a suspect TB knee. They then proceeded to do all sorts of tests, to try to prove I had TB, but all proved negative. There was never any reaction at all to the tests, but the doctors were convinced that I had all the symptoms, and as a result they didn't really want to let me out until they'd proved it either way. Eventually they decided to immobilise the knee. They put me into a 'Thomas's splint', like a leg-iron which goes from your groin down to your ankle, suspended on a T-piece at the end of the bed. Your leg goes up in the air, and you're immobile, tied in to the end of the bed. It also tends to stretch the knee, as it's on a sort of turnkey, and you're fastened down by a lot of plaster. After nearly twelve months altogether, they sent me home, with the left leg in a leg-iron, and I had to report back to the hospital every so often.

Of course, this was a TB hospital, and also a cardiac unit for kids, and we were fed on the best of everything – all the milk you wanted to drink and super food. So it was not surprising, I suppose, that I started to grow – as I was eating like a horse and totally inactive in bed. When I went in I was five foot nine; when I came out I was six foot three.

That year in hospital really played havoc with my schooling. If I'd been behind before, now I was virtually out of sight. We did get some teaching in the hospital, but there was no comparison between that and the educational standard they provided at Bristol Grammar School. In that year I'd missed out on so much of basic knowledge. To this day I don't know a thing about logarithms, or calculus. I missed out even on sex education, but I caught up on that on my own later . . . but I must admit that I never really liked school anyway.

I wasn't in the least interested in girls until I was about 17, when I really got interested in the church. I met my first girl friend at the youth club and went out with her for about three years. She was the love of my life, and we got engaged; but she went on a hairdressing course to London and when she came back she had had a good time and met a boy she liked. She asked me if I minded her writing to him, which I resented, of course, and that was the beginning of the end of my first romance. But it took about three months to die.

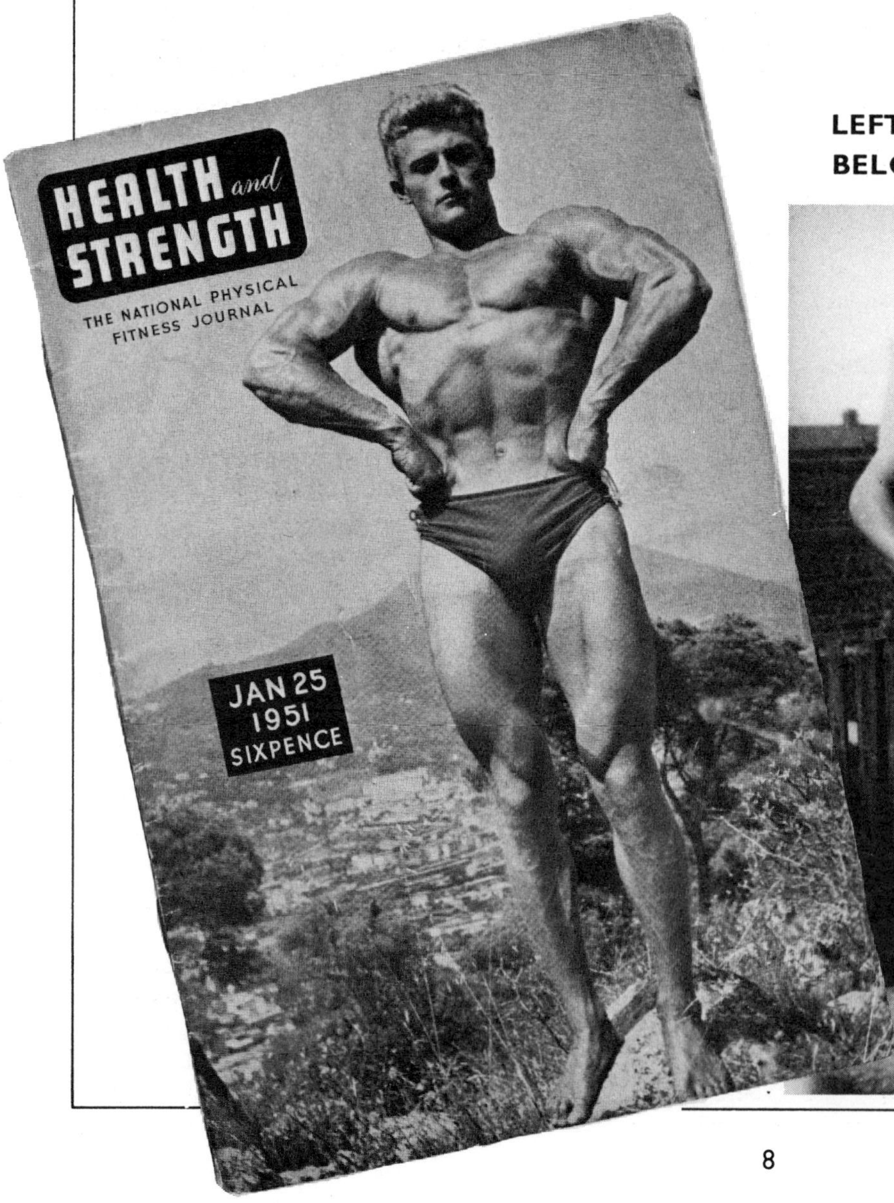

LEFT: THE COVER THAT STARTED IT ALL.
BELOW: MY FIRST BODY-BUILDING POSE.

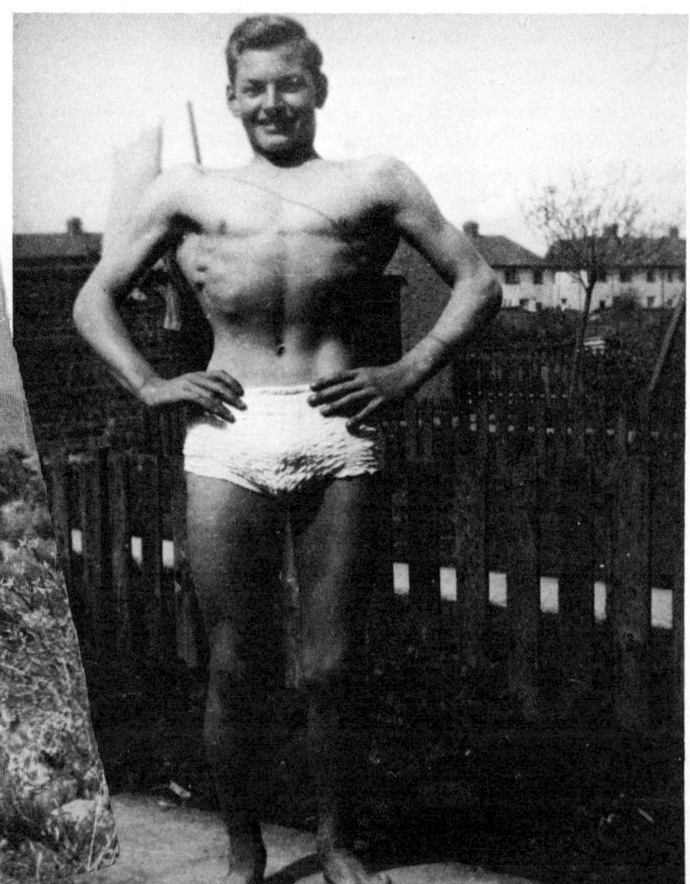

When I was 17 the doctors told me I could take the leg-iron off. They had eventually decided that I didn't have TB after all, and all the past four years had been for nothing. By this time my right knee had been swelling up too, but the doctors did not take much notice of that. They told me that they had decided that the swelling was really the body reacting to my rapid growth. So there I was, a gangling youth of 6ft 5ins, weighing eleven stone, with my left leg about half the size of my right, because the muscles had not been used for four years. There was no mobility in my knee, and I was told to go for physiotherapy treatment and to do some exercise to strengthen it. So I did this, and started going swimming and exercising.

It was funny taking that leg-iron off. Of course I was glad to see it go, but it was almost as if I had thrown away an essential part of me. I tended to use the leg-iron as a crutch, not only for myself but for the world at large. If I was hurrying for a bus, for example, the driver would see this long streak hobbling along swinging the leg-iron and he would stop and wait for me. Now no-one could see I had been ill, and no matter how oddly I ran, the bus driver now did not wait – I was just another mug who had missed the bus. So it took some time to adjust.

One day I was walking down a street in Bristol and the cover of a magazine *Health and Strength* caught my eye with this fantastic sort of blond god portrayed on it, and I went in and bought it. Actually I've still got that cover. The magazine contained several articles about these guys and how they trained, and what it had done for them, and I started to think seriously about proper exercising. I had nothing particular in mind; primarily I saw exercising as a means of improving my physique. My brother-in-law was living with us at the time, and he got interested and sent away for a Charles Atlas course. We started doing all the exercises in the bedroom and I began to show very quick results. After a few weeks a lump came up on my forearm, which looked almost like a growth, but in fact was the first muscle I'd ever seen. Then my brother-in-law split up from my sister and left home. But he left the Charles Atlas course behind him and I carried on on my own.

I also continued to buy *Health and Strength* (it was fortnightly then – now it is monthly) and one day I read in it that the area organiser for the Health and Strength League lived in Bristol, so I thought I would pay him a visit.

My mother took a hand then, She had been worried about my buying the magazine, with all these pictures of male physiques in it. It was the time when posing straps and posing pouches were in vogue, rather than chaps posing in swimming trunks, and she thought I was going queer. So she insisted that if I was to go and see this man, I must take my brother with me as protection. He was three years younger and still quite small, and the idea of him as a chaperon was quite something. As a matter of fact, in all the years I've been in the body-building business, I've come across very few homosexuals. Of course there are some, as in every walk of life, but they have never bothered me and no-one has ever made any advances.

So we trotted up together to see John Irwin, the organiser. I'll always remember him. He was weight training when we arrived – and I had never seen a barbell before. (See Chapter Eight for a description of weights and equipment.) The Charles Atlas course was all free exercises. John had quite a good physique, but obviously nothing like the standard I was going to encounter later on. His arm measured 14 inches around the biceps, and at that time mine measured on average 11 inches. I had a 36 inch chest, and John's measured 38 inches, expanding to about 40. He would do his training and then pose in front of a mirror, and I'd look at his arm and think, 'Enormous!' My one ambition was to develop a 14 inch arm. John Irwin was my original encouragement. He asked me up to his house to train, and we would work out together in his kitchen with a couple of other fellows. One of them was the junior Mr West Britain, Peter Nicholls. John had a whole variety of weightlifting paraphernalia which he used – not only in his kitchen but in the garden as well. The exercises we embarked upon were all basic beginner's stuff, almost exactly the same as those I describe later in this book, exercises like the standing press, bench press, bent-over rowing, dead lift, and so on. In fact, in spite of the new techniques that come along from time to time – new fads you might call them – there's very little new under the sun in weight training. The basic standard exercises remain the same. The exercises which I did 25 years ago when I was starting are exactly the same as those which I teach today to beginners in my gymnasium. Going even further back, to around the turn of the century, William Pullum, who is regarded as the 'father of British weightlifting' used to have a training system in which he prescribed the 42 lifts recognised by the British Amateur Weightlifting Association which started at number one and went through to number 42. It took about a fortnight to complete the course. . . . But the majority of those lifts still exist today. It's the way the exercises are performed now, and the way they are put together to form a schedule that is different.

It was encouraging to me that I made relatively easy progress at the start. The muscles tended to come very easily for the first six months. It was only later that my progress tended to slow up and I began to fight like mad for every eighth of an inch. The body becomes accustomed to a work-load very quickly, and then one has to vary the load, and the training system in order to place an additional work-load on the part of the body you're trying to improve.

As I had spent the best part of four years doing absolutely nothing, obviously my body was absolutely ripe for exercise and improvement. I just lapped it up.

But I was the clown of this group, and I was always telling jokes and making them laugh, and eventually they told me to get the hell out of it, as I didn't take things seriously enough.

However, I was really hooked by now, and I found somebody who had a fiddle with one of the steel companies, and bought my first barbell set, for about £2.50p and carried on on my own. I grew really fanatical about body-building. It affected my schoolwork – I was training when I should have been doing my homework – and I had only one topic of conversation. The only thing I was any good at was art, and most of my form who went in for the GCE in art 'borrowed' my pictures for their entries. We had to build up a 'portfolio' during the year's work and I used to be able to draw or paint with a great deal of facility, so it would only take me an hour or two to paint what would take the others days.

My fascination with body-building was so overriding that it also affected my choice of jobs. I had to get a job that would allow me the time and the money to carry on my training. I managed to join an aircraft company in their material accounts office as a trainee costs and works accountant. I stuck it for about a year and hated every minute of it. I would train at least four days a week in the evening at home, spending three or four hours each night just lifting weights. By now I was putting on weight fast, and I wanted to enter physique competitions. I was still eating prodigious quantities of food and was always hungry. I've never had to diet – in fact even now my problem is that if I don't eat properly and train as well I can't keep my weight up.

As a few examples of how I started. . . . I can remember on the bench press lifting a total of 90 pounds in one almighty all-out effort. Recently (around 25 years later) I lifted 490 pounds; which might give you some idea of the progress that can be made if you are really dedicated. I used to do curls with about 60 pounds; Later I became British record holder on the curl, lifting 202 pounds. When I started, I did straight-arm pull-overs with just the empty bar weighing about fifteen pounds. I couldn't manage any more. I eventually became the British record holder with 160½ pounds. And on the two hands dead lift, the heaviest I could manage was 250 pounds after training with John Irwin. Eventually my British record was 678¾ pounds; and I went to Scotland and lifted the Dinnie Stones which weighed 780 pounds altogether, but I could never formally claim that as I wore wrist straps. . . .

I began to learn the techniques of lifting, the secret of breathing, and how important it is to breathe at the right moment. I learnt, for example, that if you hold your breath too long under pressure you use up all the oxygen and black out. I've always said that the physiologically correct way to breath is to inhale at the start of the major effort, so you have a lung full of air when the weight is at its heaviest. On the bench press, for example, you inhale either at the beginning or as the weight comes down to your chest. You hold your breath as you push it upwards and exhale as you lock it out. Some people even have to learn how to breath out to prevent the blacking out I've just mentioned. All you have to do is to count, out loud. If you are speaking you are actually exhaling – passing air over your vocal chords; so you will not hang on to your breath and let it out in a great gasp at the end.

I didn't do too well in those early competitions, because although I was improving and gaining weight

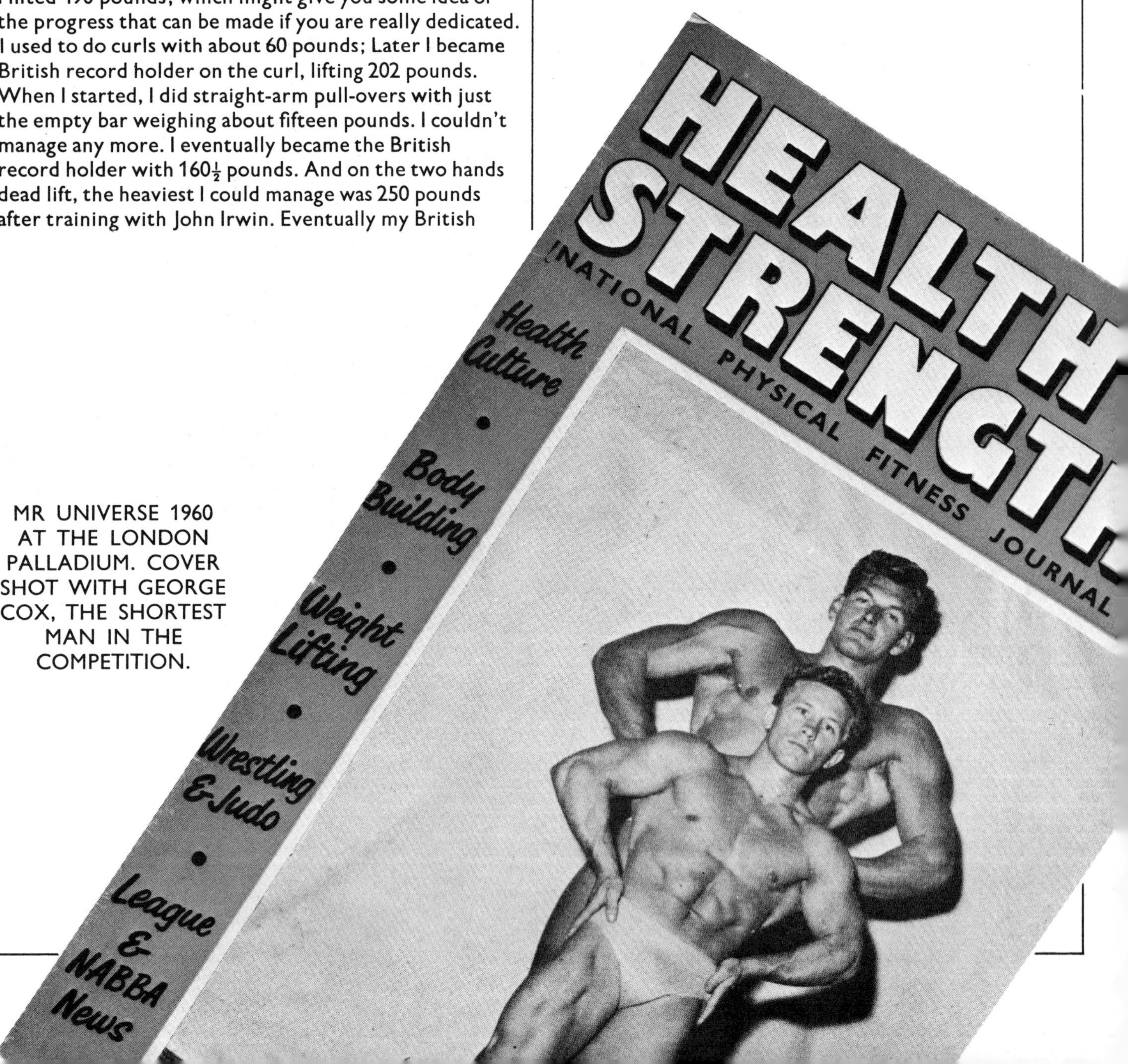

MR UNIVERSE 1960 AT THE LONDON PALLADIUM. COVER SHOT WITH GEORGE COX, THE SHORTEST MAN IN THE COMPETITION.

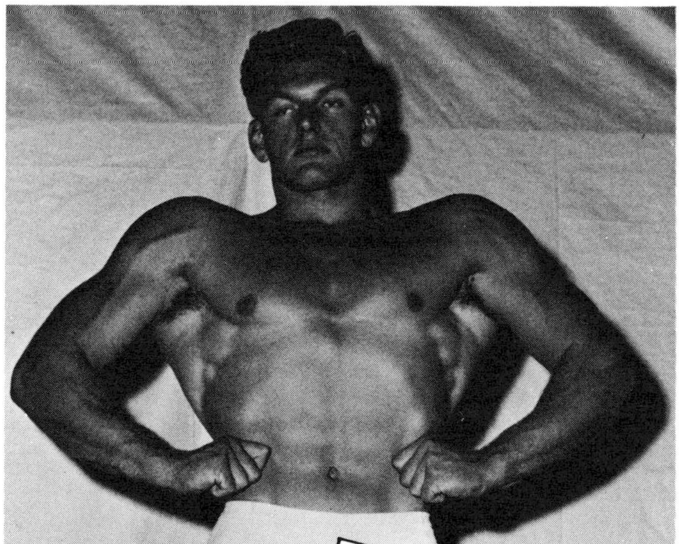

fast, it took a long time to show. A stone on a man of average height is noticed immediately; on one of 6ft 5ins, as I was, it was nothing. I could never win, because in those days there were two other blokes who seemed to enter the same competitions, and one or other of them always beat me. They were Graham Price and Ron Thomas.

They were very nice guys, and gave me plenty of tips. Ron is still in training – he's with the fire service in Bristol. He recently won the senior Mr Britain title for the over-forties. Graham emigrated to Australia or New Zealand, and I've lost touch with him.

When I started exercising, there was no doubt that I wanted to be big and muscular. There were plenty of reasons for this – I wanted to be attractive to girls, to have people stop and stare at me when I walked onto a beach, and that sort of thing. But as soon as you go into a body-building programme it becomes patently obvious that you only make body-building gains through two

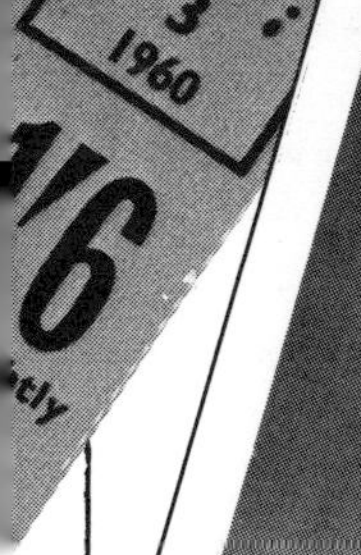

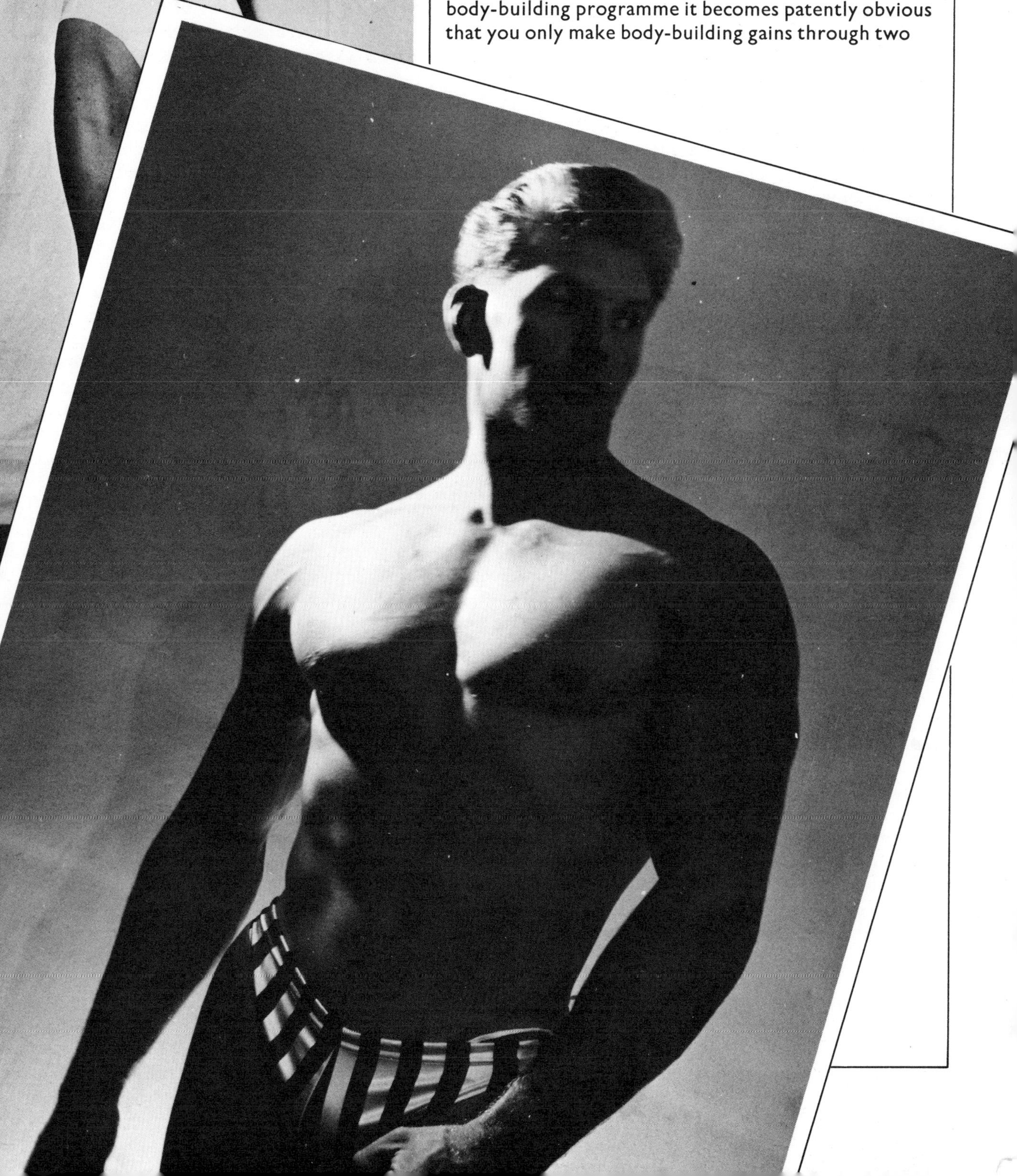

things – training and dieting. The reason you put on weight is that you force feed – just like fattening up turkeys for Christmas, if you like – but you control the weight gain by your training. You pick up tips as you go. At first, of course, you are learning from people who know only a fraction more than you do and you have to distinguish between good advice and bad advice, and sort out what suits you. I went to as many Mr Universe competitions as I could, to talk to the big guys and persuade them to tell me about their training techniques. Although I was by nature quite a reticent young man, when I wanted something I could be quite tenacious, and many a champion body-builder has sat down for ten minutes and given me his secrets. It certainly used to be like that, 25 years ago; but big money and commercialism have got in and nothing is as friendly as it used to be. Now there is too much competition.

I started going to the Mecca Dance Hall in Bristol, which was called The Glen. It was the place where all the youngsters got together. Rock 'n' roll was just starting and two nights a week the hall was full of Teddy boys, and there were nothing but punch-ups. I used to go there on the more respectable nights. By this time the 14 inch arm had come and been left a long way behind, and I was beginning to get publicity for myself in local body-building contests. With my size I obviously caught the eye, and the manager of the ballroom got to know me quite well. One day he asked me if I could help him out, part-time, to keep order on Mondays and Saturdays, the rock 'n' roll nights. We were called ballroom supervisors, but we were really bouncers. We used to get loads of scraps and plenty of aggro, but probably because of my size, the other blokes always used to leave it to me to sort things out. I developed quite a reputation in Bristol.

I've never actually been challenged to a fight by anyone – probably because I am so much bigger than the average guy, so perhaps they think twice about it. One night during one of the punch-ups, a bloke hit me over the head with a chair, but I didn't feel it and only knew I'd been hit when afterwards I found blood running from my head. I developed a technique as a bouncer. If ever there was a scrap, 99 times out of a hundred it would be between two guys, and the thing to do was to get rid of the man who was getting the wrong end of the stick. In the first place he was grateful for being saved from a beating-up, and secondly it left nobody for the other man to fight. You'd take the loser off the dance floor and go back for the other chap a bit later, when it was convenient.

My reputation spread through the Mecca circuit, and other ballrooms round the country would telephone and ask for my services, but I never went anywhere else. We cleared up Monday and Saturday nights completely by this method, and then the manager, who became a good friend, offered me my first real break. He said he would pay me £12 a week to work as a bouncer, evenings only, which would release me to do my body-building training all day and every day. It was great.

I found a friend, a car dealer named Bob Osborne, to train with and we turned out every day. You need a partner to go in for body-building. It's a lonely life anyway, and you must have someone on hand in case anything goes wrong, when you're handling heavy weights. There's always the possibility of getting stuck with three or four hundred pounds across your chest.

I stayed with Mecca for four years, and in that time became well-known in local physique contests, gaining a high place in the Mr West Britain competition. As a result, I was invited to enter the Mr Universe competition, which was held at the Palladium in London. I was the biggest and tallest man ever to enter for Mr Universe, but obviously I came nowhere. I'm too tall, at 6 feet 7 inches, for physique contests. In fact, George Cox, the smallest guy at 5 feet 1 inch, and I got more publicity for the contest than Mr Universe himself.

For the uninitiated, let me explain that in a physique contest the contestant is actually judged for only a minute or two, at the most. In that time he has to adopt a series of poses designed to present his body in its best light to a number of judges. He will have spent months, possibly years, getting all this right, showing off his good points, disguising his not-so-good ones. My best feature was my chest, followed by my back. My worst was my left leg (the bad one) and I spent long hours devising poses that would present my right leg in front of my left. Of course it was all up to the judges, who could condemn you at a whim.

I remember on one occasion when I was a judge myself at a Mr Universe competition. Four of the physiques were outstanding, including probably the most muscled man I have ever seen. His name was Serge Oliva, a Cuban who defected to America, and he developed one of the biggest physiques ever seen. He was truly massive, bigger even than the world champion Arnold Schwarznegger. He was so big that his biceps measured 23 inches – as big as a girl's waist. He used to have to slit the arms of his T-shirts to be able to wear them.

Well, we were looking at these four finalists when one of the judges leaned across to me and said, 'Do you notice anything out of the ordinary with Oliva?' 'No,' I answered, 'Except that he's enormous.' 'What about his head? Don't you think it's small?'

'Well, now you mention it, I suppose it is a bit small.'

'Well,' said my fellow judge. 'He must want a head like a pin to develop a physique like that.'

I must say I felt sick. Oliva, and the others for that matter, had been training for all those years, just for some competition judge to dismiss him with a snide remark like that.

In fact, it was at the Palladium that it suddenly dawned on me that this was all wrong. I was actually posing on stage when I began to think that I was wasting my life. All this taking on jobs so that I could train was not getting me anywhere. There must be something that was better in life than just to stand in front of a thousand or so admiring people and flex my muscles. I still wanted to train, but I knew now that there must be a more worth-while object to it. And it was time I settled down, and got myself a career.

When I was about 25 I decided it was time I left home. My mother, who was very religious, disapproved of my going out at the time with a divorcee. She was a super girl, but this was all wrong for my mother, so I decided to leave. I found a flat just round the corner from the dance hall. What could be better? There I was, complete with my own establishment right on the doorstep. That's what it became, of course, my own seduction parlour, the biggest den of iniquity you could hope to find. It was so successful, in fact, that in three months I was so physically run down I had to go to hospital to recover. My knees swelled up again, my weight dropped off and what happened to the weight training I can't remember. It was a real physical breakdown. I never returned to the flat – I sent someone round to fumigate it, I suppose, and went back to mother.

For a couple of seasons I worked at the Henleaze Lake a big swimming club, during the day, while I was still bouncing at night. I was probably the worst swimmer there, but they wanted someone to superintend the swimming pool, clean the place out, and train the members. It was ideal, spending all day beside the pool and getting paid for it. It also coincided with my disillusion with body-building for its own sake, and I decided to take up powerlifting, or, as it is known, strength-set lifting.

Although this now has international recognition as a branch of the sport on its own, at that time it was regarded as the poor relation, more a step on the road to 'proper' Olympic weightlifting. There are three lifts in strength-set. They're the basic lifts a body-builder does in his training.

1. The two hands curl; where the weight is lifted with the hands underneath, and then brought to the chin by using the biceps only;

2. The two hands dead lift; where you just pick up as much as you can off the floor and stand up straight with it hanging at the full stretch of your arms; and

3. The knee bend, or the squat.

Strength-set was seen as a means to allow body-builders, who obviously had potential, to progress towards becoming Olympic weightlifters. It fitted my new ideas, formulated at the Mr Universe competition, admirably. I'd gone through the alternatives. I'd been to the local wrestling club and fought a draw with the Metropolitan Police Heavyweight Champion, but the groan and grunt game didn't appeal to me. I went down one night to the local boxing club, but the spectacle of blokes beating the hell out of each other was definitely not for me. I tried shot-putting and discus-throwing at the athletics club, but I found that I just didn't have the

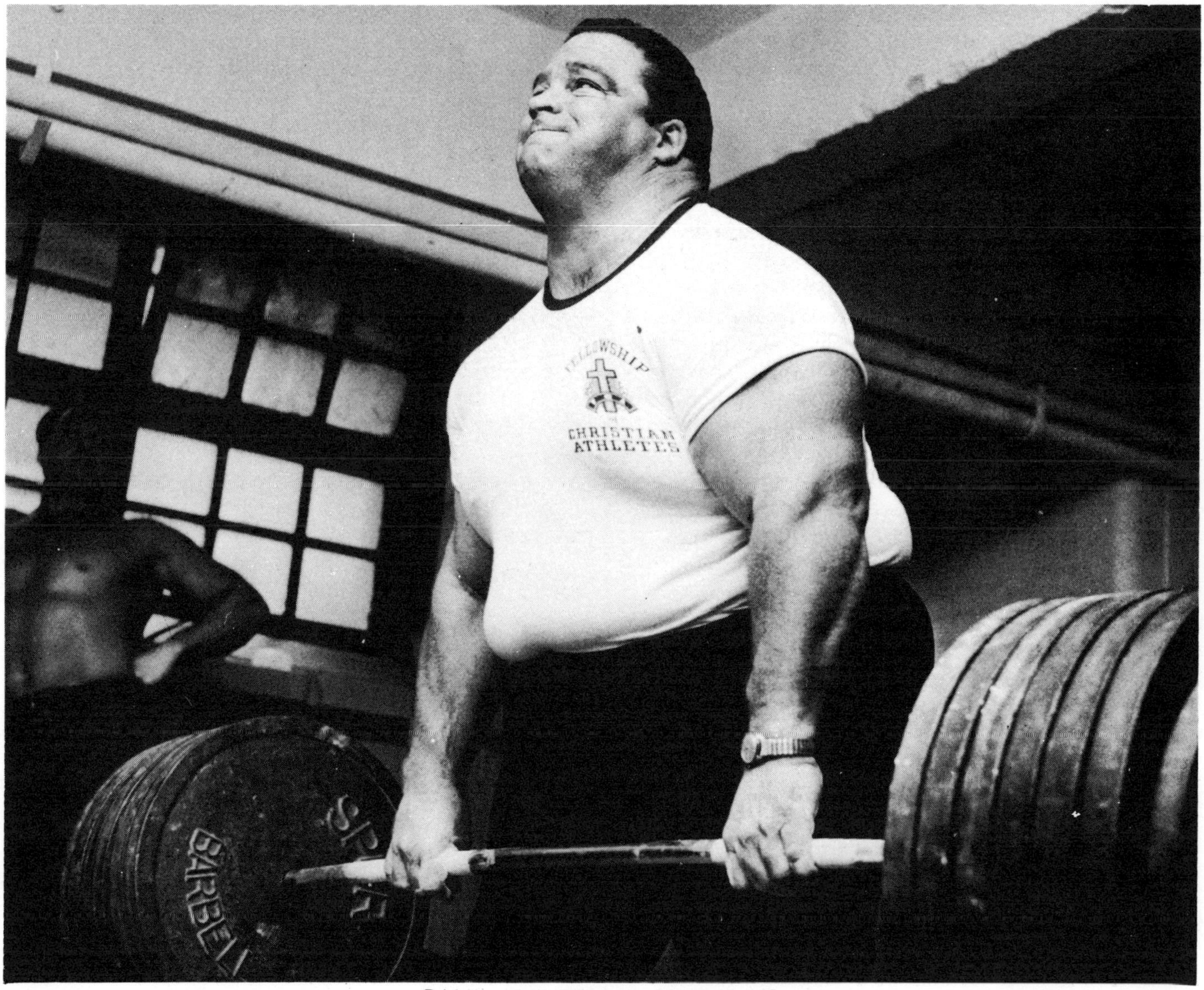

PAUL ANDERSON OF THE US.

speed. That may sound surprising, but it's true. My years in hospital had taken all my speed from me. Shot-putting particularly is very much a speed event. Parry O'Brien, the first ever 64 foot shot-putter, only took up the sport because he couldn't get into his college 100 yards team with a speed of 9.9 seconds. You have to 'explode' from nothing to flat out in seven feet. That's real speed. I just didn't have the athletic ability to be top-class, even though I had the strength – by now I weighed nineteen stone – and if I was going to do anything it had to be in the top class.

If you are interested in my own weight/fitness ratio let me say I began training in 1951 when I was 6 feet 5 inches tall and weighed 11 stone (165 pounds). In 1960, when I entered the Mr Universe contest, I was 17 stone 3 pounds (241 pounds). In 1962, when I weighed in for the World Championships in Budapest I weighed 17 stone 13 pounds (251 pounds) and when I went to the Commonwealth and Empire Games in Australia a few months later I weighed 18 stone 4 pounds (256 pounds). When I turned professional in 1964 I was at my peak, about 19 stone 10 pounds (276 pounds). My current weight is 18 stone 7 pounds (259 pounds) and I find that if I don't diet properly and exercise I tend to lose weight.

I built a little 'cage' for myself at the lake, and Bob Osborne, mentioned before, came along to train with me, and I began to break all the local records at strength-set lifting. Eventually I held several British records. On the dead lift, I lifted 678¾ pounds, which was equivalent to lifting a grand piano. On the two hands curl I held the British record at 197 pounds (I also held the Western Counties record at 202 pounds, but there were not enough judges present for it to be classed as a British record). On the straight-arm pull-over, where you lie down and bring the weight from the floor at full stretch behind you with arms straight to the over-chest position, I lifted a British record of 160½ pounds.

The major step forward for me in weightlifting came when I was competing in a strength-set competition in Bristol in 1960. The current British Olympic heavyweight weightlifting champion, Dennis Hillman, who came from Horsham, was the referee, and after the competition he told me that I was a bloody fool.

'I think you've got a lot of potential as an Olympic lifter,' he said. 'You're wasting your time with all this rubbish. You'll never get anything out of it because it's not recognised as an international sport.' (Now, of course, it is recognised.)

He challenged me to a match after the competition. He was to do the two hands press, the first of the three Olympic lifts. You pull the weights up to the shoulders and then, keeping your legs straight, just press the weight above your head to arm's length. I was to do the press behind neck, the usual method used by body-builders, in which instead of pressing from the front of the shoulders, you press the weight from the back of the neck. I think he knew that he was on to a good thing, because, although I didn't realise it at the time, the two hands front press is a lot easier to do. Anyway, I took him on, and I pressed 270 lbs, quite a commendable press; and Dennis pressed about 310 lbs and beat me by 40 lbs. Afterwards he said that he was convinced that if I trained for the Olympic weights I could be very good.

This was the first real encouragement I had ever had, and I determined to try to do my best. I found out that the Amateur Weightlifting Association ran courses at Bisham Abbey and Lillieshall, and I went on a couple of them basically to learn the new techniques from the national coach, Al Murray.

In those days there were three Olympic lifts, now there are two. The first was the two hands press, described above, which is no longer included; then there was the two hands snatch, in which the bar has to come from the floor to arm's length in one movement. And thirdly the clean and jerk, where you lift the bar to your shoulders and then jerk it to arm's length, bending your knees as you do so.

Al Murray taught me a lot, but I learnt even more from Bill Miller, who coached Louis Martin, the world champion at mid-heavyweight (up to 14 st 2¼ lbs, or 90 kilos). In 1961 I received an invitation to compete in the British Olympic Championships and was placed third, behind Dennis Hillman and another very well-known lifter, Ted Morton. Ted was a great chap, but the perennial runner-up. Denis totalled 880 lbs and I did 835 lbs. In 1962, I beat Dennis and became British Heavyweight Champion. That year I totalled 915 lbs to Dennis's 880 and I continued to beat him thereafter. Dennis was a really nice man and very well educated with it. He eventually became Army Pistol Champion as well, and you can imagine this 22 stone soldier holding the pistol like a toy in his massive fist. I kept meeting him in various competitions, and we always had a psychological battle of wits. He would come up to me in the dressing room and the conversation would go something like this.

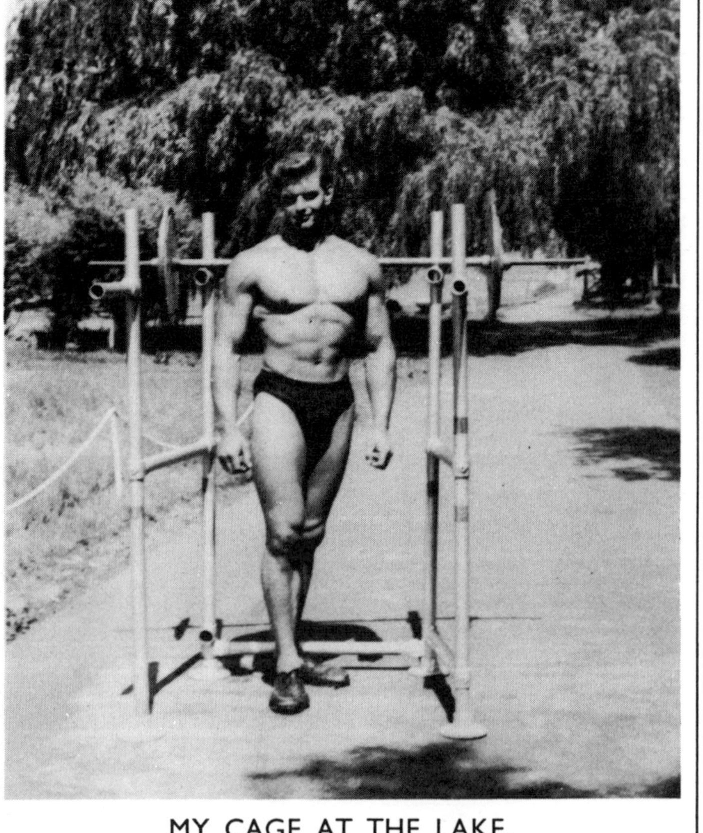

MY CAGE AT THE LAKE.

Me: How's the lifting going, then Denis?
DH: Fantastic . . . at least it was till last week.
Me: How's that then?
DH: D'you know, I had 360 at arm's length . . .
Me: (With sinking heart, because my best press was about 40 lbs below that) Well, what's gone wrong then?
DH: Oh, I've got a terrible shoulder injury. Can't lift a thing.
Me: (Insincerely) Hard luck. Well I've been pressing about 340 . . .

I don't know whether he had any shoulder injuries or not, but anyway I used to end up beating him and I often wonder if he regretted the day he urged me to turn 'legit' as it were. Denis was a great presser, but not especially good on the snatch and the clean and jerk, you never knew whether the bar was going to go straight up, or Denis would go straight down, and I think this shortcoming in technique stopped Denis from becoming a very great lifter indeed.

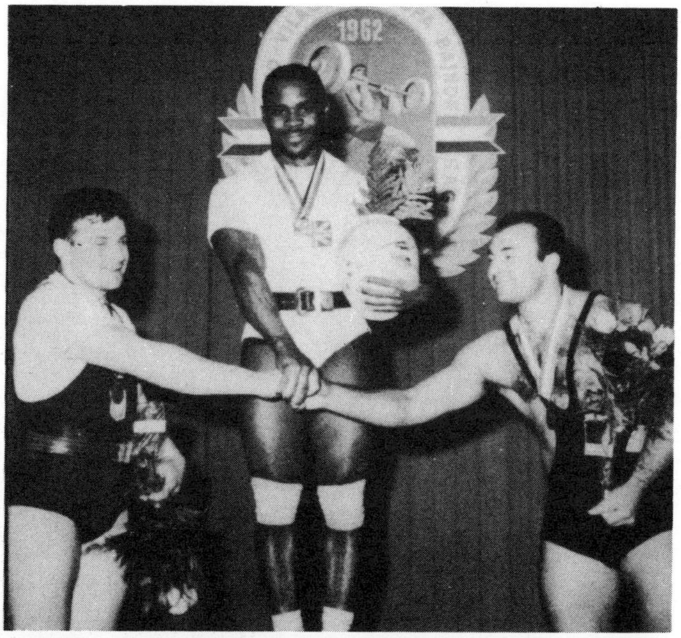

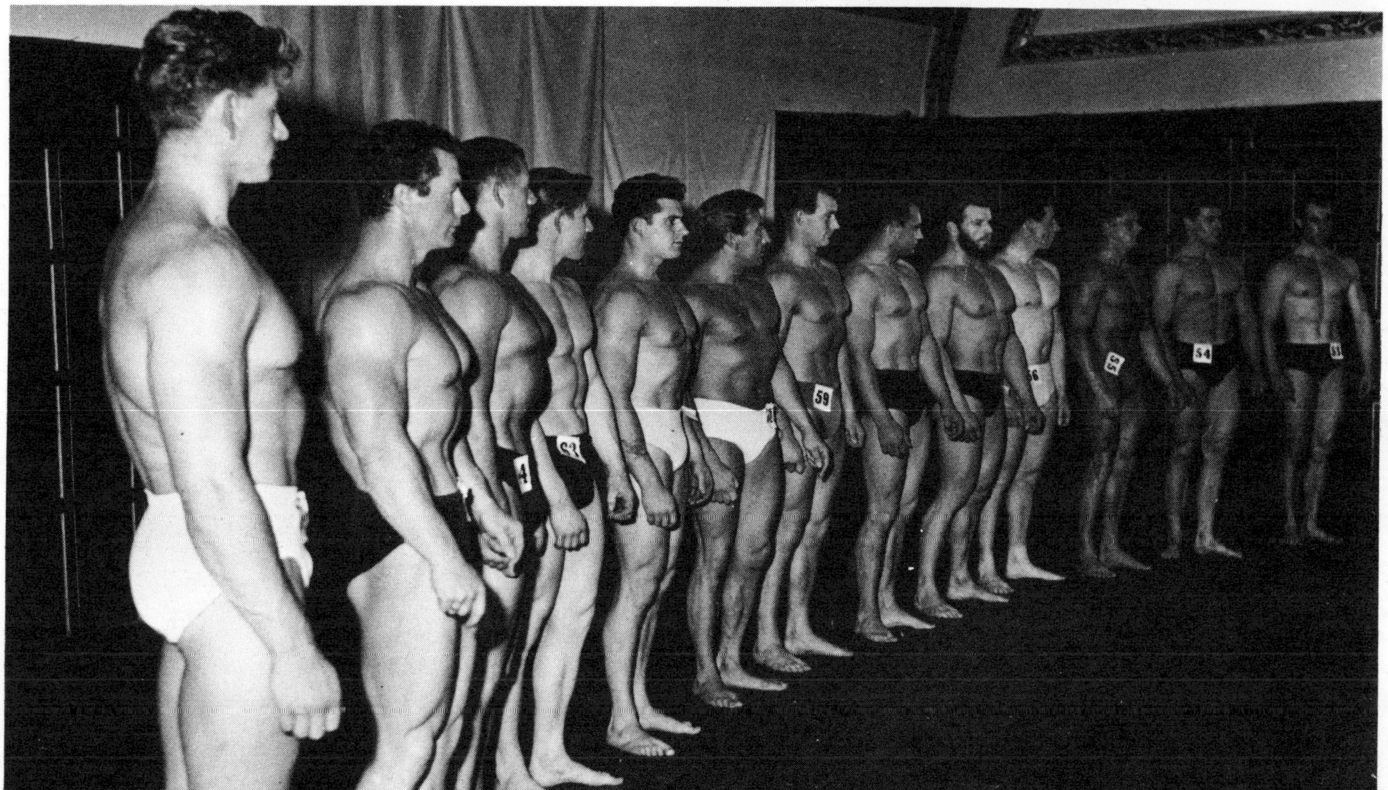

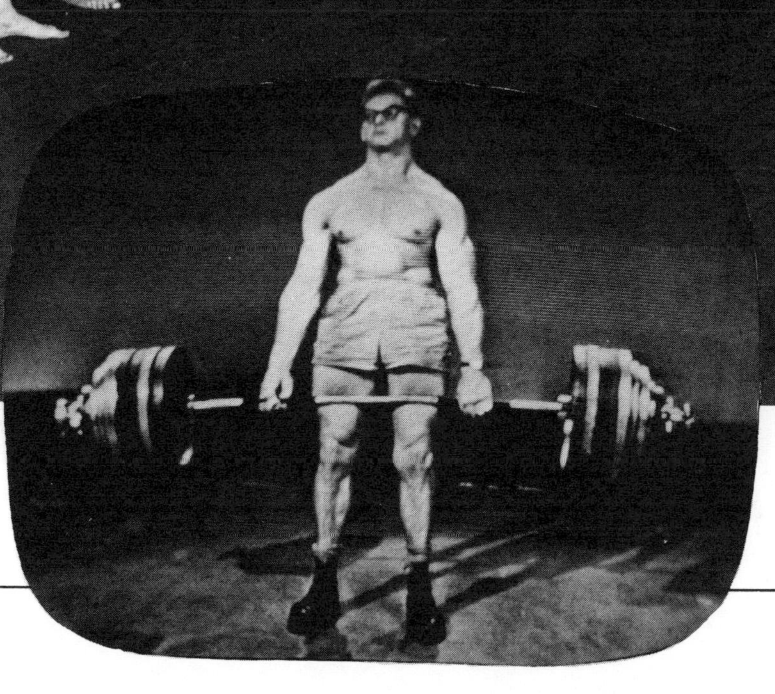

ABOVE RIGHT: GOLD FOR LOUIS MARTIN AT BUDAPEST. **ABOVE:** THE LINE-UP FOR MR UNIVERSE 1960. **RIGHT:** A BRITISH RECORD – 678¾ lbs.

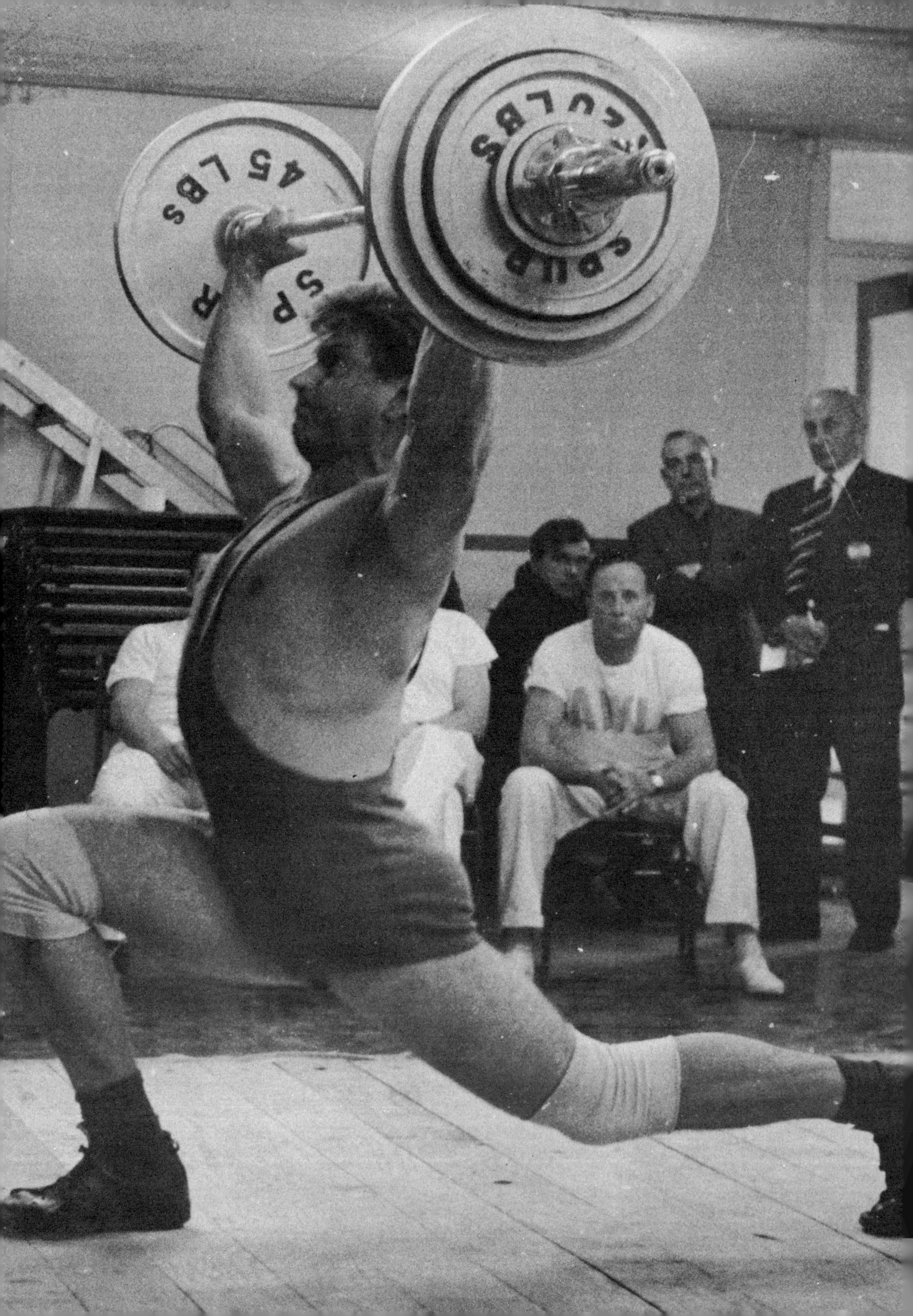
45 LBS

Chapter 2

GETTING A LIFT UP IN LIFE

In 1962 I came to the peak of my fitness and won the British Olympic Weightlifting Championship and so qualified for international competition for the first time. It was Empire and Commonwealth Games year and the Games were to be held in Perth, Australia. This was the big carrot that was dangled under every athlete's nose, weightlifters included. I always remember, when I was alone at last in the changing room after that competition, feeling as if I was on a cloud of joy. 'I'm the best weightlifter in the country,' I kept on thinking to myself. People kept on knocking at the door and coming in and saying 'Well done, Dave' and things like that, but I could hardly speak to them, I was in my own private world of ecstasy. The next thing I knew was that, back in Bristol, I received a letter from the British Weightlifting Association congratulating me on winning the title and informing me that I had been selected to join the team to go to the World Championships to be held in Budapest. The sting came in the tail '. . . Unfortunately, the resources of the Weightlifting Association are such that they can only afford to send three lifters, and regretfully we must ask you to meet your own travelling expenses . . .'

It was a great honour to be asked. I went to Regional Pool Promotions, where I had worked for a while, and asked for their help. They held a whipround, and everybody contributed so generously that they sent me to Budapest. But it was a disaster from the word go.

We arrived in Hungary after a terrible train journey all the way across Europe, to find ourselves placed in a huge teachers' hostel in Budapest. Wally Holland was the team manager (who later became secretary of the Weightlifting Federation). Al Murray was the coach. The team consisted of Louis Martin, the great mid-heavyweight, who had been World Champion in 1959 and was strongly tipped to regain the championship this year; there were two other coloured lifters – Carl Goring, the lightweight champion, and Sylvanus Blackman the other, lifting at light-heavyweight; and Mike Pearman, another well-known light-heavyweight was along as I was, selected but paying his own way.

The bill of fare at this hostel was vienna schnitzel for breakfast, lunch and dinner, so if you didn't like vienna schnitzel, which I didn't, there was not much else to eat. I went off my food straight away, which is of no use to a weightlifter. In addition, we were told strictly not to touch the water – or the fruit, which could be bought plentifully in the markets – because of the danger of dysentery.

It was a wonderful experience for me, a virtual newcomer to the game, to be competing with all these great lifters, the Americans, the Russians, who were just legends to me. But ghastly things were happening to the new boy. In the first place, the team manager Wally Holland, was going around putting out silly, exaggerated stories about my prowess, for no-one had heard of me. He was saying things like: 'When Vlasov (the Russian champion) finishes, this man starts.' Vlasov was like a walking lifting machine, the most perfect weightlifter I've ever seen, and there was no way I could live with him in competition. Far too much was expected of me from the advanced publicity.

We were allocated a gymnasium for training and

OPPOSITE: ON THE WAY TO BECOMING BRITISH CHAMPION.

alternative times – ten o'clock in the morning or seven in the evening. I wanted to train in the evening, which was my normal style, but the officials didn't want their social evenings spoilt, so they opted for the morning, against my wishes. I was, to re-emphasise it, the new boy, and so didn't have much say in things. But I felt that they didn't worry about me. Their whole effort was spent on Louis Martin, because he was the guy in with the real chance, and I felt left out. This feeling was reinforced the next morning when training dutifully, I pulled my trapezius muscle and ended up with a very stiff neck, which helped my lifting no end! Al Murray the coach, said to me, kindly enough, 'Well laddie, I don't think there's much use in your trying to train with the rest of the team. You'd better make your own

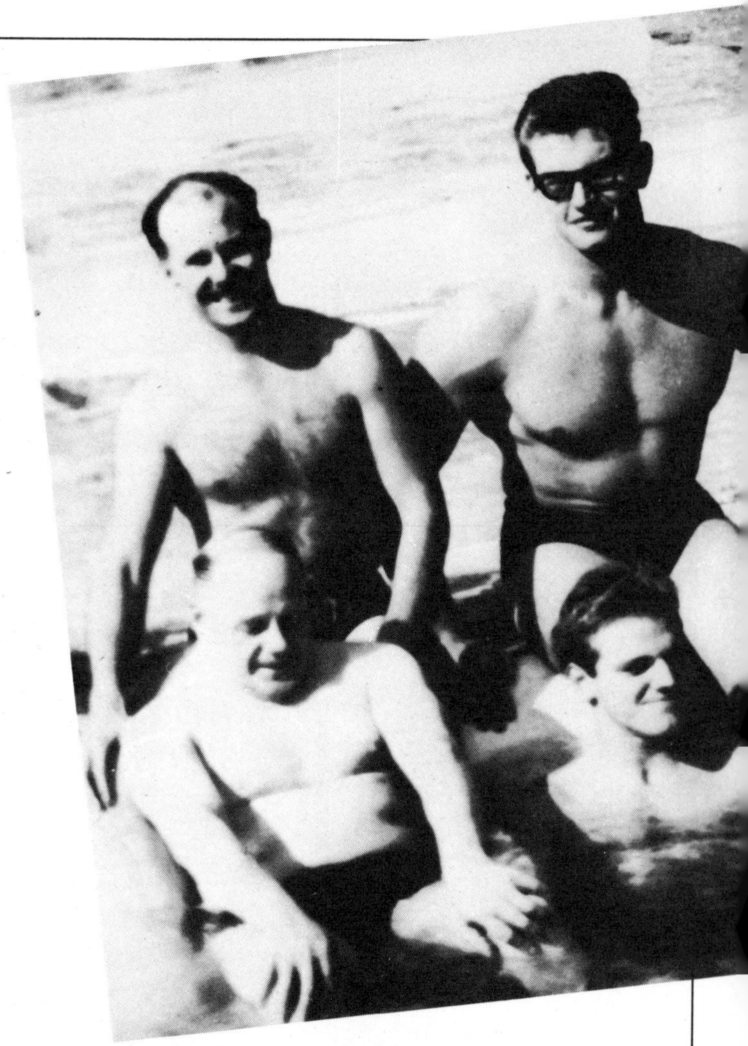

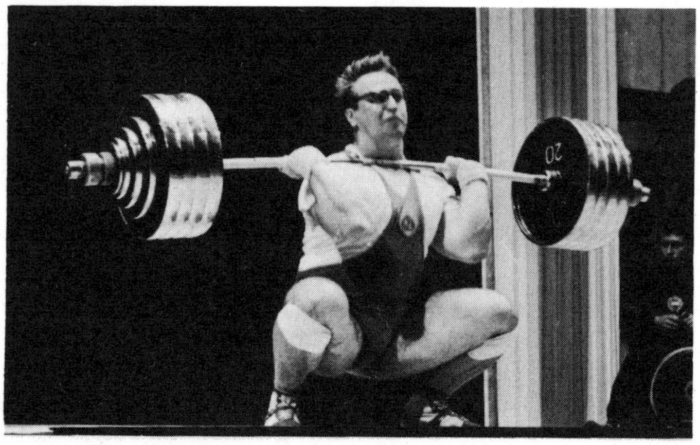
THE GREAT YURI VLASOV.

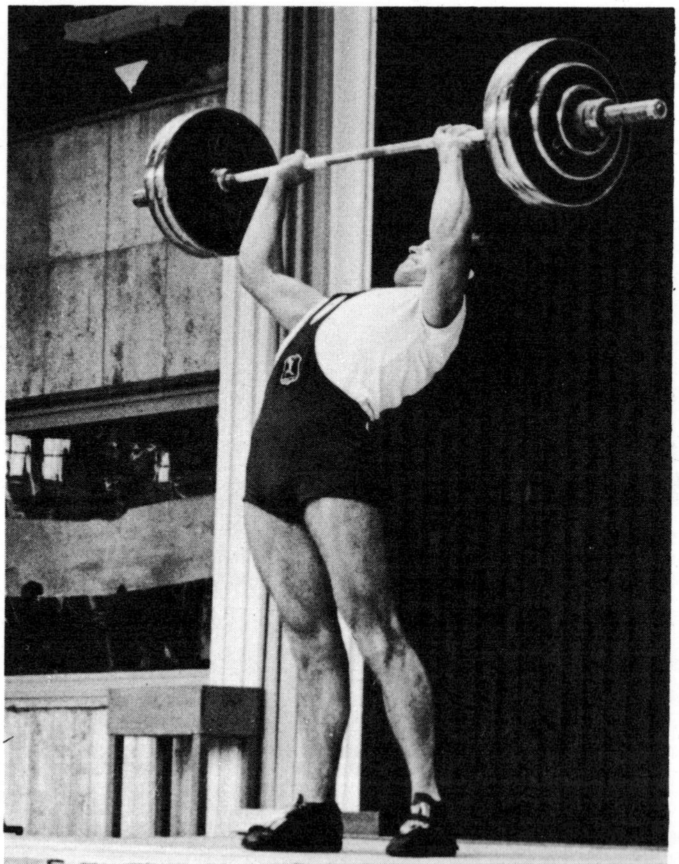
ME AT 17st 13lbs.

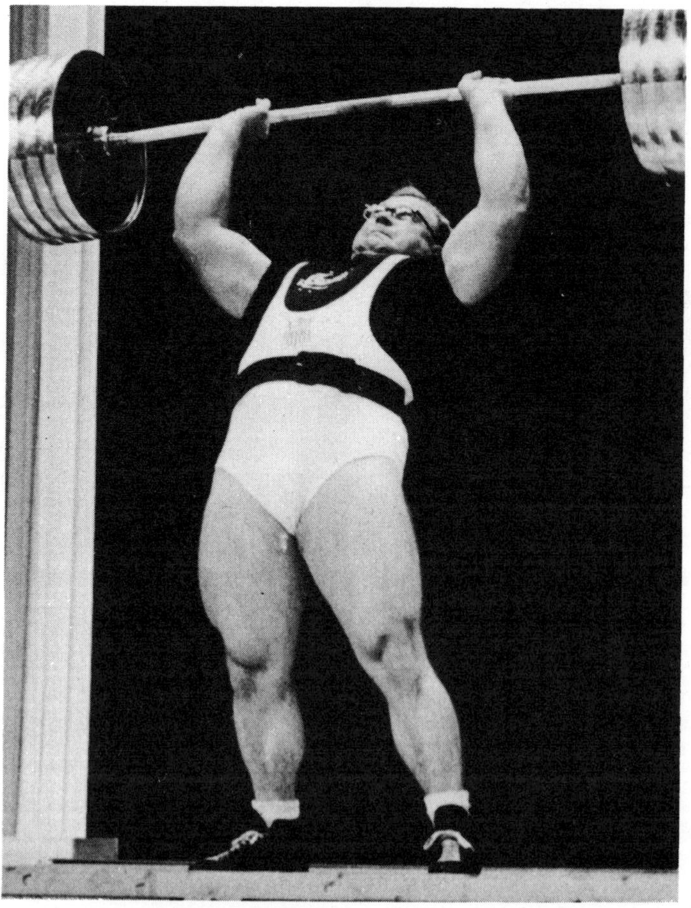
SCHEMANSKY AT – ? ? ?

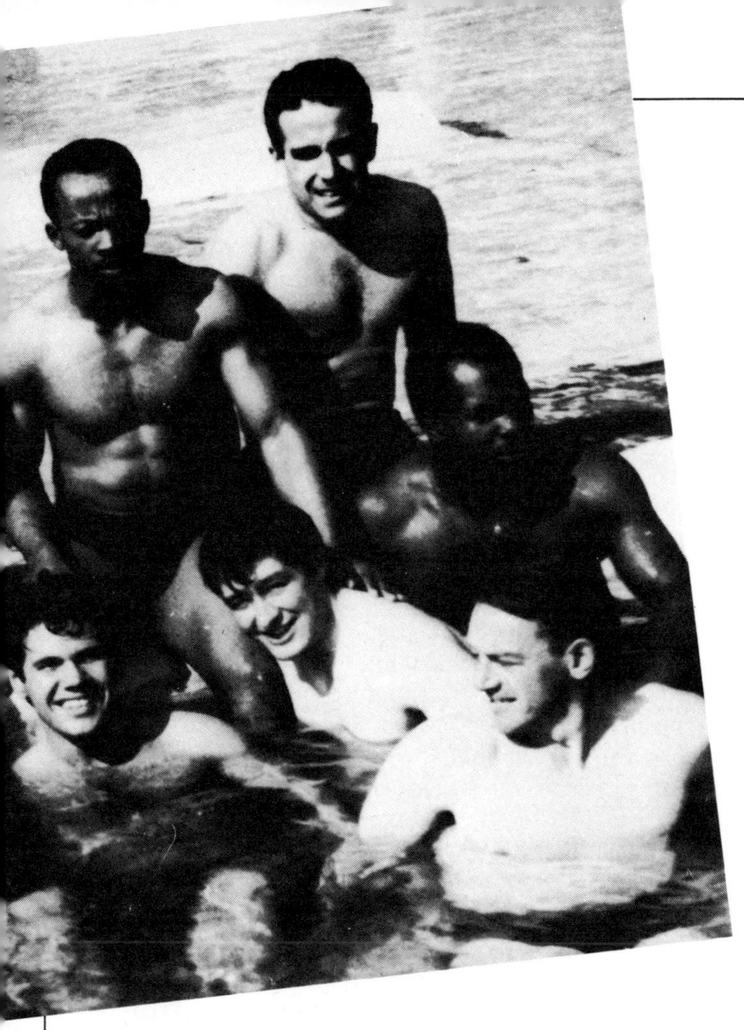

BRITISH TEAM AND FRIENDS IN BUDAPEST.

arrangements.'

The team is under the control of the manager and coach, who are essential to the success of each individual. Each man has three goes at each lift, and his weights are decided by him and the manager together to put as much pressure on the opposition as possible and to exploit his best lifts. There's always a great deal of politicking at a championship, with each manager trying to find out what the opposition is doing. I admit I was a bit of a handful, but I believe that on that particular trip too much attention was paid to the established lifters and I, a beginner at this level, was left to fend for myself.

I felt really annoyed, not only was it my first international competition, but I'd been made to pay my own way and here I was, shoved off on my own. It was all part of their preoccupation with Louis, who subsequently became a very good friend, incidentally.

But things were made even worse when I went off and by chance bumped into a Rhodesian, Tony Assaro, who was all by himself as well, and was lifting for South Africa. We decided to train together, and we were helped by the Austrian national coach. I'm no racialist, far from it, but the other members of the team, three of them black, decided that this was just what I was, and ostracised me for the rest of the time in Budapest. They even stopped letting me know when and where they were going out.

I was there when Louis won back his World Championship. It was a fantastic piece of lifting, and I felt ecstatically happy for him. And yet, remembering how I'd felt when I'd won the British title, I knew that I did not wish to spoil the moment for him – I didn't want to impose, somehow. So I didn't go up to him immediately afterwards, and didn't go back to the dressing room, like the rest of the team. Later I was bitterly accused of bad sportsmanship, lack of generosity, selfishness – they threw the book at me. In hindsight, I can see that perhaps I should have gone straight up to him, but there it was, I followed my deepest feelings, and made a mess of things.

So here I was, properly in the dog-box. My training was going badly, and to add to my misery, I ate some fruit and got dysentery, just as they had said I would. Believe me, you can't lift weights, if you've got dysentery.

About a week before my division, the heavyweight lifting took place, I was trying to buy some stamps in a little shop in Budapest, and the woman behind the counter was being no help at all. They often don't care for strangers in Budapest. Suddenly a gentle voice said from behind me, 'Can I be of help?' She was from heaven, a little old lady. She bought my stamps for me and on the pavement outside, she found out all about me, how miserable I was, what I was doing, how I couldn't eat the food and so on. It turned out that she was British, and had food parcels sent to her from home. She invited me to her flat, and there was Typhoo Tea and steaks, the lot. She gave me a grand meal, and invited me to eat there for the rest of my stay.

This was marvellous, I was eating regularly, and getting the sort of food I was accustomed to, and my training began to improve. Then, three days before I was due to lift, the old lady said to me, 'I've got another surprise for you tonight. I want to introduce you to my daughter.'

Her daughter arrived that evening, with two cousins. Her name was Agnes, and she was a stunner! I don't know if it was because I hadn't seen a good-looking girl for a while, but she bowled me over. The old lady took us all out for a fabulous meal at Budapest's luxury hotel, the Geilliart. Agnes was training to be a physiotherapist, but she couldn't speak any English whatsoever. Her older cousin, who had a few English words, asked me to come with him to the toilet, and when we were out of earshot of others, he let me know in no uncertain terms that Agnes had, shall we say, hot pants for me. 'Agnes she jig-a-jig, you know,' he said, again and again, making the appropriate signs.

Well, I wasn't too sure about that, I was in Budapest to lift weights. After dinner, we went back to the flat, but I didn't go in, and Agnes and I had a very passionate session outside before I staggered back to the hostel in the early hours. That was the Thursday evening. On Saturday I was due to lift in my competition. I hadn't seen anything of the rest of the team, so they left me a note saying that I'd be picked up at five o'clock on the Saturday to be taken to the arena; and their faces were pictures when I turned up with this marvellous blonde girl on my arm! The team didn't take very long to put one and one together and make five.

That evening I made a complete fool of myself. I promise you, it was nothing to do with Agnes. Perhaps I wish it had been! In the British Weightlifting Championships I pressed 315 lbs; that night I did 281, which was a disgrace. On the snatch I did 231, and fell flat on my face the first two times, just managing to get it up the third time. And on the clean and jerk I took my starting poundage, which was 330 lbs, and could hardly get it up to my chest. As I bent to jerk it up, I could feel the dysentery biting. It was as if I was going to unload my whole stomach onto the floor. I didn't even try to lift the weight. I just put the bar back down on the floor as gently as I could manage and walked off, having failed to make a total, which is a terrible crime in any weightlifting competition, let alone a world championship.

I went back to the dressing room in despair, and Al Murray came to see me and gave me hell. I had nothing to say; I was feeling so guilty at having let down those friends of mine back in Bristol, who'd dived into their pockets and handbags to send me to Budapest. My shame knew no end and this was added to on the return journey, when I was pointedly ignored by the whole team. Al Murray and the manager also said they were putting in an adverse report about my conduct, or misconduct, but I couldn't have cared less. The one bright spot was on arrival at Dover. We all leapt for an English newspaper, only to see the headlines on the sports page that I had been chosen to represent England at the Commonwealth Games in a couple of months' time, in Perth. I didn't deserve it, but they'd given me a second chance. The officials were livid!

There was a much better atmosphere on my second international trip. When we arrived in Perth we found the whole team housed in a bungalow in the new Olympic Village. The manager and coach bagged one bedroom, and there were three beds in the second and two in the third. Our team consisted of four negroes and myself, and promptly one of the coloured lads took one of the two beds into the other room making four in there. I protested, but they said, 'We thought you'd like to be on your own.' Mindful of my Budapest experience, I said, 'Not on your life,' and as no-one would move in with me I moved the last bed in with the other four. Five in one room, and we had the time of our lives!

This was a totally different experience. We all trained to the utmost, the weather was marvellous, and the England team cleaned up – three golds and a silver. All except me – again.

This time the reasons were different. I've never felt fitter and more ready for a competition. As I've described, the two hands clean and press had to be performed with the legs stiff on the press. A new technique had been developed the previous year by a man who had won a world championship, which was strictly illegal, whereby he was able to 'whip' the knees straight at the same moment as he pressed upwards. This bow-like effect enabled him to lift considerably heavier weights than before, and he won his world championship. As I say, it was strictly illegal, but it was not until the films were analysed in slow motion that the judges discovered what he was doing. By this time it was too late. So everyone began watching this new technique. But what's suitable for a normal-sized man can look clumsy in someone as big as I am – everything's exaggerated – and in any case the judges in Perth hadn't really been in touch with modern developments.

I should just explain that there are many different ways by which a lift is judged 'foul': if the knees are bent in the 'press'; if there's too much hip kick; if the back is bent back too much; if the weight stops on the way up; if it twists on the way up; if there's not complete control at all times; in the snatch: if the weight 'unlocks' at arm's length; if it doesn't go from floor to the full extent of the arms in one movement; in the clean and jerk: if the weight goes to arm's length, unlocks and then is pressed out again; if the weight's not under control.

Anyway, I selected 295 for my first press – the highest starting weight I'd ever tried. I was feeling very good, and genuinely in line for the bronze medal. I bent to the weight and up it went, smooth as a whistle. No hesitation at all, no strain. I put it gently to the ground, and strolled off, only to hear the crowd booing. I looked back. There were three red lights – a foul lift! I went to Al Murray, but he was just as much in the dark as I was. I went back for the second lift, and this time it went up just as easily. More booing. This time there were two reds and a white – still a failure. On the third lift – my last chance, Al Murray told me to get it to my chest and then press up absolutely rigid, not a whip, not a motion. I was so angry that I didn't even feel the weight. I stood stock still, knees totally locked, and pressed 295 lbs to the full extend of my arms. To my utter astonishment, I got three reds again. Later, we found out that they thought I'd twisted my arms on the press, but I still can't understand it. And that was the end of my second international tournament – another disaster.

But this time I got a good report for behaviour, and I loved Perth. I'll go back there one day. Perth's the city which switched on all its lights every time the first American astronauts were orbiting the earth. It acted as a sort of beacon to them and that's why it's been called the City of Light ever since. It's the City of Light for me too.

We came back from Perth to the terrible winter of 1963, when Britain was snowed up for weeks on end, and no football could be played. The papers had no sport to write about, and therefore when we had a lifting match against West Germany at Tottenham in London, they all went absolutely spare, and I had some of the greatest publicity I've ever received. I beat a chap called Huppfer – and at last I had a win in an international competition.

Until this time, all my training had been done in the back garden, in all winds and weathers. Sometimes I had to chip the weights out of the ice to start. I couldn't train indoors – a hundred pound weight doesn't do much good to the floor if you drop it. But about this time a livewire called Denis Welch had formed the Empire Weightlifting Club in Bristol in the basement of an abandoned church, and Mecca had donated their first Olympic barbell. They asked me to train there for, as British Champion, I gave the club a bit of kudos.

At the same time I was offered some coaching help by a German, Wolfgang Peter, who was working in Newport for a few months. Wolfgang was a super guy, and coach to the German national team, and I made more progress in the few months he trained me than at any

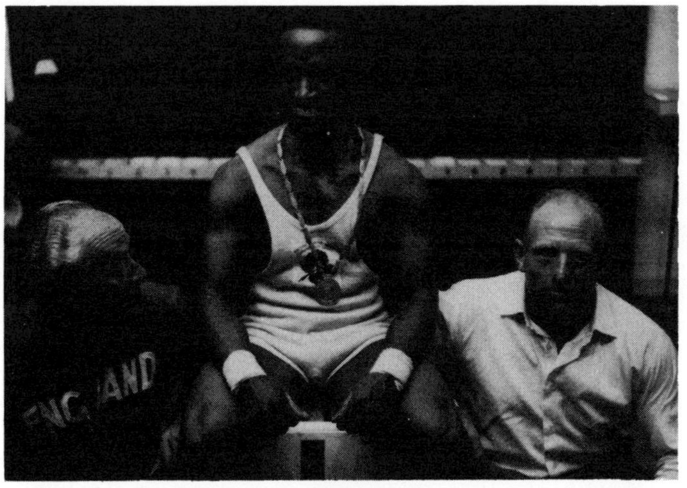

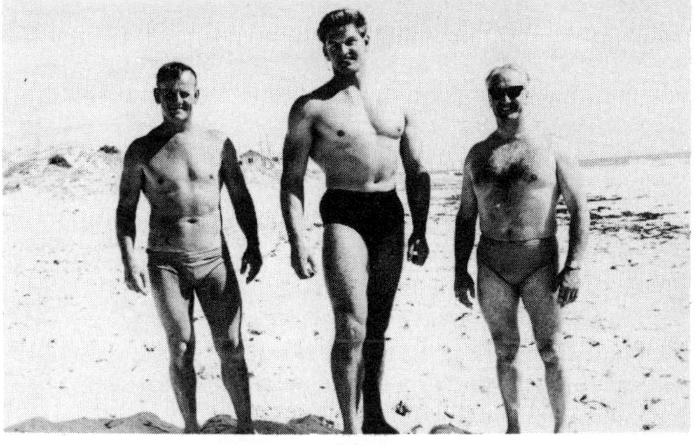

TOP: GEORGE NEWTON, EMPIRE LIGHTWEIGHT CHAMPION.

ABOVE: ON THE BEACH AT PERTH WITH AL MURRAY.

other period. I always said I became the British Champion too quickly. To become a good weightlifter you really have to know your technique, and I was very green at the time. It took me virtually two years to learn to do one of the Olympic lifts correctly; and even when I went in for top competitions I never knew whether I was going to land up on my arse or I was going to do a perfect lift.

My biggest problem was that I started off weightlifting as a very big strong man. When I was at the lake, I used to think nothing of picking up 360 lbs, heaving it up to my shoulders, bumping it over onto the back of my neck, doing, say six squats, bumping it back over to my chest and putting it back on the floor. And yet, after two years of the best technical coaching, I couldn't lift 360 lbs above my head without ending up nearly doing the splits. I'd gained in technique but I'd lost power. I wasn't putting the two together and getting the best out of both, and this is what Wolfgang was helping me to do. I finished at the beginning of 1964 by doing a total, for the three lifts, of 936½ lbs, which was an English native record.

I moved to a job in Croydon, selling sports goods for an American firm, and as part of the job I helped organise the 1963 Mr Universe competition in Croydon. My firm brought over as a celebrity attraction a former winner of the American version of the Mr Universe, George Eiferman, who must be just about the nicest guy I've ever come across. He couldn't be more grateful even for the smallest service you could do him. He was a bit past his best, but he was celebrated for having the biggest chest muscles (pectorales) in the world. To be crude, they looked like big tits. He did a speciality strength act in which he'd pick up a girl and hold her over his head with one hand, go down and do a number of squats while playing the trumpet with the other hand. Or he'd sit the girl across his shoulders and he'd do one legged squats and play the trumpet with both hands. He wasn't the world's greatest trumpeter, but he was a great performer.

He stayed over for a bit after the Mr Universe job, and his company organised a trip around Scotland for the pair of us. They've always liked strong men in Scotland. This was the week before I was due to get married, and we toured Glasgow, Dundee and Aberdeen, ending up in Dundee on the Wednesday. We had a fantastic reception everywhere we went. George did his trumpet-blowing, and I ended up by lifting against two men. I managed to hoist about 360 pounds above my head, and the other two lifters together on one bar, managed 380 pounds – it was a great feat of co-ordination

When any visiting strong man goes to Scotland, you have to test your strength on their 'manhood stones'. In the olden days, many country estates had these round stones at the gates, and a visitor had to prove his manhood by lifting them onto the pillars before he was allowed to enter. We went to Inver which has a great, egg-shaped granite boulder lying on the village green. If you can pick this up (it weighs 268 lbs) and carry it across to the pub on the other side of the green, the landlord will give you a free pint. We did all that and ended up, true to tradition, at a place called Patrach, to lift what are called the Dinnie Steens (stones).

GEORGE EIFERMAN.

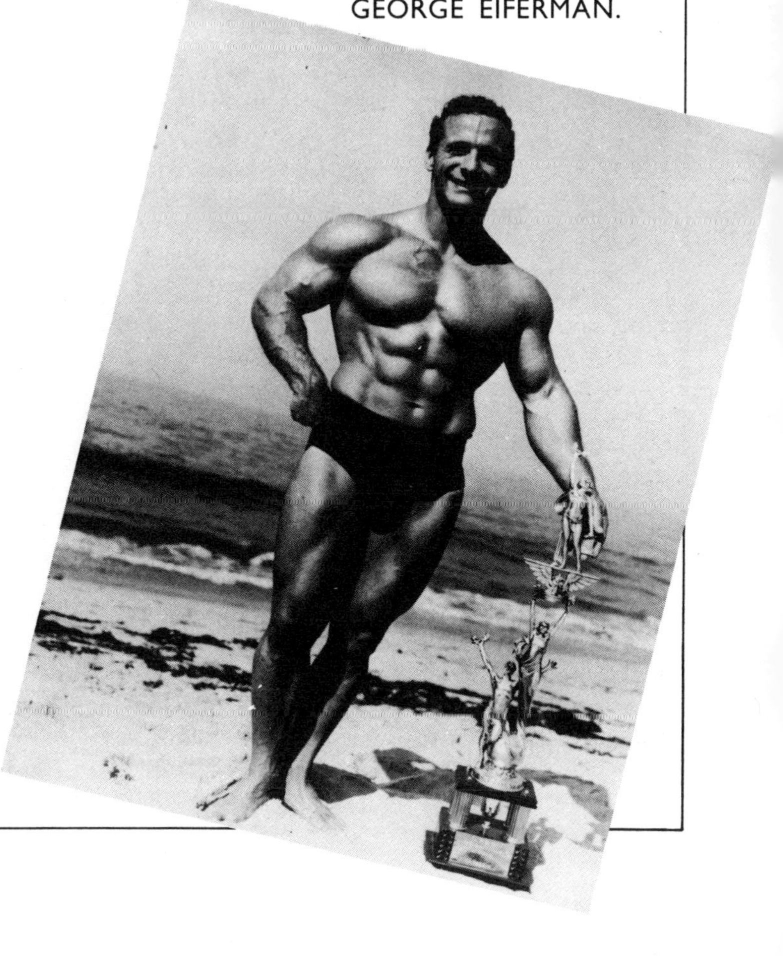

In the last century, Donald Dinnie, who was a famous Highland athlete, was reputed to have been helping his father, a bricklayer, to point the brickwork on the bridge. The horses started to stray, so the father shouted to Donald, 'Bring the steens,' which are the stones they used to tether the horses to. So Donald picked up the two stones and walked across the bridge with them, a distance of 18 yards.

When they weighed the stones afterwards, they found that one weighed 340 lbs, the other 440 lbs – more than seven hundredweight. They both have rings on top, to which the horses were tied, and which help in getting hold of them. Well, until I went there, no-one had lifted the stones since Donald's day, though many had tried. Of course without telling us, they'd got TV cameras and the Press there. The stones looked pretty formidable.

The chap who took us down advised me not to try to pick them up in the usual manner, with one on each side of me. He reckoned this could have taken all the skin off the sides of my legs. His advice was sound, so I tried in a wide straddle, with one stone at the back and the other in front of me. I picked up the first stone, the lighter one, a few times, to get the feel of it, and then I tried the heavier one. I asked if I could use wrist straps, which help your grip and transfer some of the weight from your fingers, and they said this was alright. So I arranged myself in the straddle position, and picked the two up. No problem at all, the first time since the great Donald. That was easy; the real problem was to move.

With this straddle position I found I could only shuffle a couple of inches at a time, and there was no way that I was going to make 18 yards. So I put the stones down, and they crowded around and said, 'Well, you didn't do what Donald did.'

I answered, 'Yes, well, do you want my honest opinion?'

'Yes, please, Mr Prowse.'

'I think he was a bloody liar.'

They were a bit indignant at my calling their national hero a liar, and I explained that I thought this was one of the stories that had built up over the years. The probability was that Donald carried them over one at a time, and the story, like Topsy, just growed. For even with all his other (accurately recorded) feats, I knew that Donald Dinnie couldn't deadlift anywhere near as much as I could.

I don't think that they appreciated it, and poor old Donald was probably turning over in his grave, but that's still what I think. Incidentally, like the four-minute mile, once one man had done it, many other strong men since have lifted the Dinnie Steens, but none has walked with them along Donald's 18 yards.

Then I rushed back to London, drove to Bristol and was married on the Saturday. We made a disastrous tour of Cornwall for a honeymoon – disastrous because I didn't have any money and it rained without stopping the whole time. I always said I married my wife for her money, because she had £40 in the bank at the time, and I had nothing. Anyway, our cash ran out and I had to get back to Bristol to borrow money from my father-in-law to get us back to our new flat in London. At least I'd rented that furnished, so we had somewhere to go to.

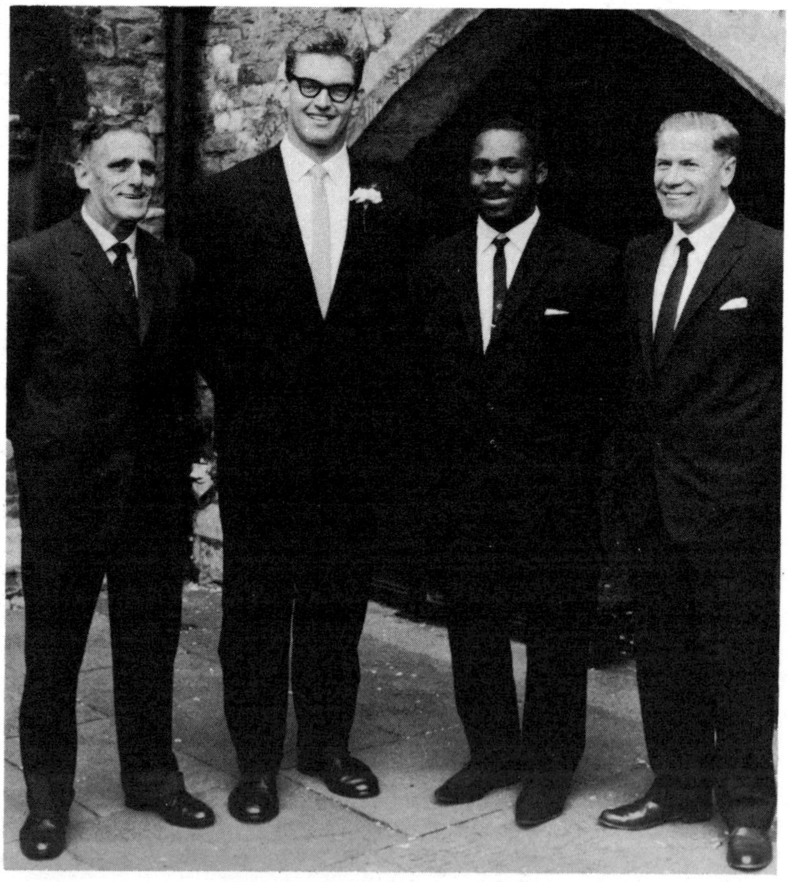

DON LEE, LOUIS MARTIN
AND BILL MILLER AT MY WEDDING.

Chapter 3

'BRITAIN'S STRONGEST MAN'

Nineteen sixty-four was the big year for every athlete, including the weightlifters, for it was the year of the Tokyo Olympics. As British Heavyweight Champion I felt well in line for an Olympic place. At the beginning of the weightlifting season the British Weightlifting Association told us all that selection for the team would depend, not only on our performance at the Olympic trials, but on our consistent performances throughout the year. That's not necessarily the best way to choose, for you try to build any athletic performance up towards a peak, but I thought that if that's the way they want it, then I'll compete in any and everything I possibly can.

After a number of club events, the first international was in May against Sweden, and I won that with the highest total ever put up by an English heavyweight in the three Olympic lifts – 936½ lbs (press, snatch and jerk). In June I won the English Championship; in July I won the British Championship and won an international against Wales; in August I won return matches with Denmark and Sweden. I was the only person on the entire British team to go through the season undefeated, and when the Olympic team was announced they decided not to send a heavyweight. It was a bad blow. The only thing I could think of was that the heavyweight standards in this country were far below international levels, but this was so at all weights, with the exception of Louis Martin at mid-heavy. In fact he disappointed expectations by getting the silver medal. Nobody else did anything.

At the same time, I'd been having plenty of troubles with the Weightlifting Association over my amateur status. I was hauled up before them on a number of occasions for minor infringements and quizzed. Even when I'd appeared on local TV in Bristol to talk about weightlifting (I thought I was doing well to publicise the sport) some busybody reported me and I had to appear before the Association to explain myself and was ordered to pay my £25 fee (all but £2 'expenses') to the Association. I was sick and tired of the petty officialdom of the Association. I enjoyed lifting, I enjoyed the competitions, but I didn't enjoy kowtowing to the officials who knew next to nothing about the sport, and were only there for the glory. They even tried to prevent my employment as sales manager for the Weider Organisation (the sports firm which I worked for in Croydon) on the grounds of professionalism. So not being chosen for the Olympics was the last straw. I turned 'pro'.

There was nothing dramatic in this. I just informed the Association that I was no longer available for selection for their events, and set myself up (I still held the heavyweight lifting title) as 'the strongest man in Britain', and started to do exhibitions and physical culture shows for money. At the same time I was asked to appear in a professional play, but I'll come to that later (in Chapter Four).

Then Dave Webster, who was at that time assistant secretary to the Scottish Council of Physical Recreation, an old acquaintance in the weightlifting business, suggested I should try my hand at the Highland Games – tossing the caber and so forth – at which, he said, I could pick up quite a bit of cash as well as advance my reputation.

There's a lot more to the Highland Games than wearing a kilt and tossing telegraph poles about. You compete on seven different events. You put the shot, which is done with a granite boulder rather than the conventional metal shot; you put a 16-pounder and a 22-pounder. You then throw the Highland hammer – a shafted hammer rather than the wire-handled hammer usually used in international competitions; again, there are two hammers, 16 lbs and 22 lbs to be thrown. You then 'throw the weight for distance' – you have a 28 lb block weight like the one the coalman uses, and you twist round in a discus-like spin and throw it as far as you can. Then there's throwing the weight for height, in which you toss a half-hundredweight block (56 lbs) over a bar, like a pole-vault bar. You stand with your back to the bar and swing the weight up from between your legs and over the bar above your head. It's the equivalent of tossing a small boy over a double-decker bus. We used to put the weight over about 14 feet. And lastly there's tossing the caber, which is basically a tree trunk like a telegraph pole and weighs anything from 90 lbs to 150 lbs. It tapers, and you lift it by the thin end, with the heavy end waving about in the air. You toss for straightness, not distance, and the optimum is for the caber to land straight in front of you at 12 o'clock. A good toss is anywhere between 9 o'clock and 3 o'clock.

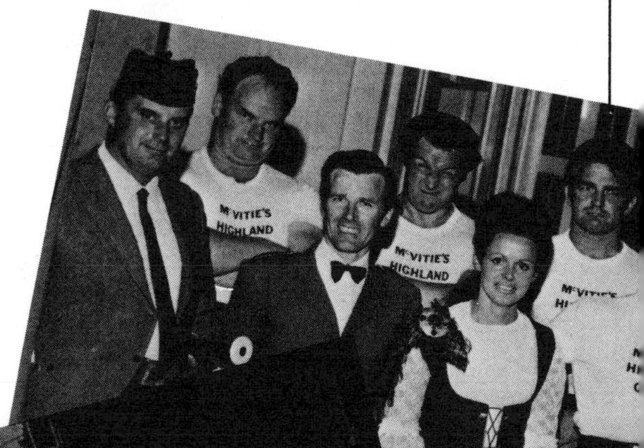

ABOVE RIGHT: McVITIE'S TEAM IN SAN FRANCISCO.

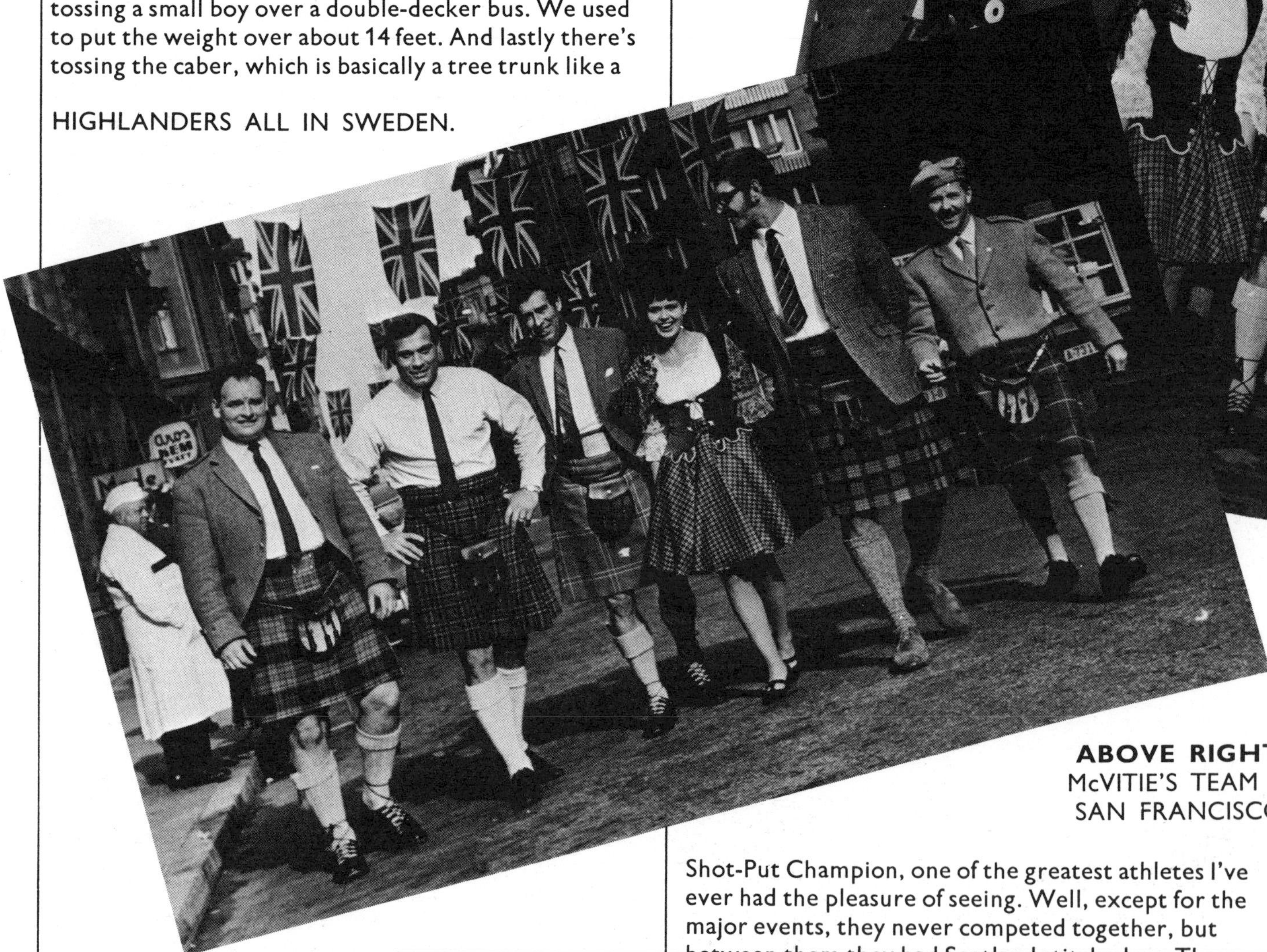

HIGHLANDERS ALL IN SWEDEN.

I went to Glasgow and got measured for a kilt and then Dave took me to Duck Bay Marina on Loch Lomond; and there, under the tuition of one of Scotland's finest Highland athletes, Jay Scott, I learnt to toss the caber, throw the hammer, and put the shot.

But I weighed up the position and it became very obvious that the whole of the Highland Games scene was carved-up between two great athletes. One was Bill Anderson, from Aberdeen, a nineteen-stone rugged, powerful man, and Arthur Rowe, former European Shot-Put Champion, one of the greatest athletes I've ever had the pleasure of seeing. Well, except for the major events, they never competed together, but between them they had Scotland stitched up. There wasn't much hope of my splitting these two, so I decided to set my target on the world caber-tossing championships. The second year I tried I got third place – Arthur was first, Bill was second.

It was quite a problem training in the south for caber tossing. No-one wanted their nice soccer pitches cut up by a dirty great pole. So I found derelict building sites to practise on. I'd go out at night and chop down a tree to throw around. Eventually I decided to get myself some proper cabers and landed up at Banstead telephone exchange.

'Oh yes,' they said, when I asked them if they had any old telegraph poles. 'Plenty out at the back. Help yourself.'

'How much?' I asked.

'Oh, I don't know. Three and sixpence each.' That's about 17 pence in new money . . . but it cost me eight pounds to hire a furniture van to lug them away.

After my third place, Dave Webster invited me to join a Highland Games troupe which he formed and hired to United Biscuits (McVitie's) for promotional

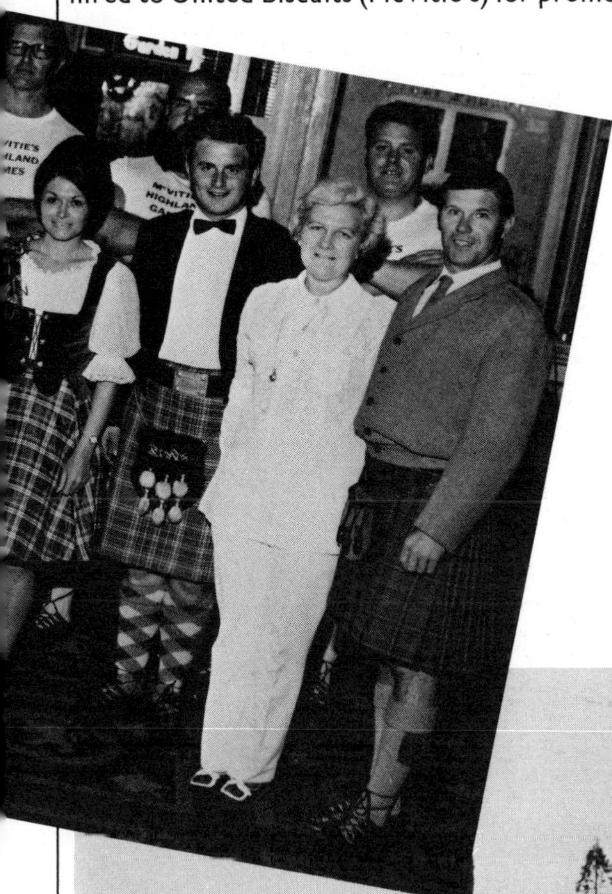

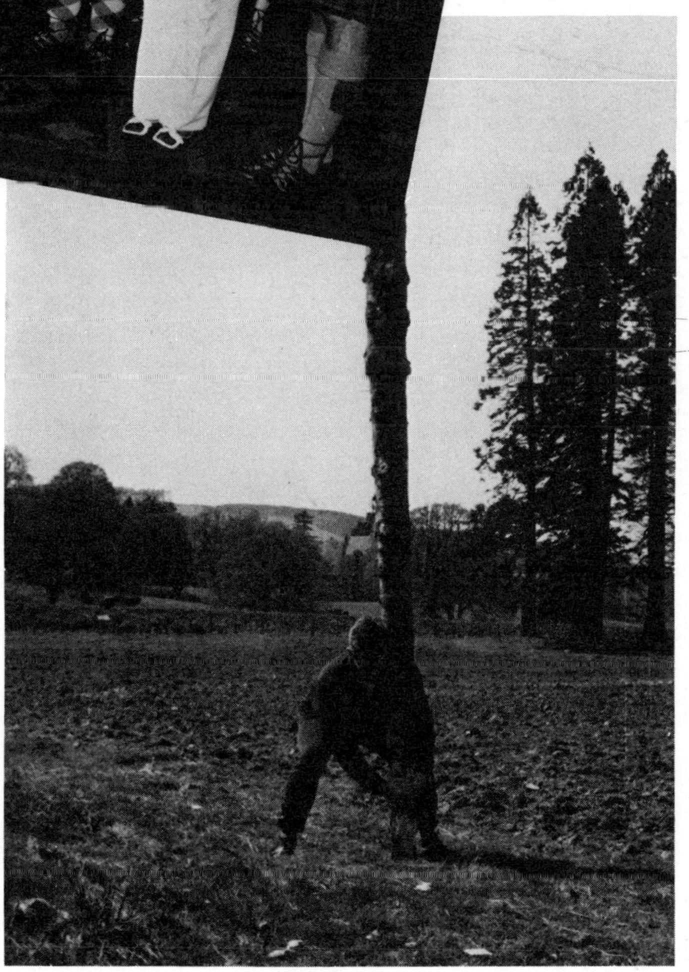

BELOW: MY FIRST CABER.

tours. There were Highland wrestlers, weightlifters, dancers, pipers, the whole works, and for three years we went to British Export Weeks all over the world. We did fortnights in Sweden, Tokyo and San Francisco, and had a marvellous time. Unfortunately for us, after that the British Export Weeks were discontinued.

It was in 1964 that I first went to the National Sports Centre at Crystal Palace. I performed at the opening exhibition at the National Sports Centre before the Duke of Edinburgh. I was most impressed with the facilities there, and afterwards I went back to see Emlyn Jones, the director, and asked him for permission to train at the Centre. I was then going for the Olympic team.

To my astonishment he refused. It was against the rules, he said, for any individual to use the Centre's facilities. They were intended only for the use of clubs and associations. So, reluctantly, I formed a weight-training club through the auspices of the Central Council for Physical Recreation (CCPR) and ran it there for five years or so. So far as prestige was concerned, it did me a power of good, for I used to describe myself as Director of Weight-Training, National Sports Centre, although I never received a penny out of it. I ran it until I decided to open my own gymnasium in 1969.

Meanwhile, I'd also ventured into journalism – and burnt my fingers badly. I'd left the Weider Organisation and become a sales agent on my own, selling Weider equipment and a number of other lines, vitamin pills, health equipment and swimming suits. I had also started endorsing the Bullworker (see Chapter Eight for a description of this), which became the biggest selling single piece of physical exercise equipment in the world. I acted as a consultant for the organisation selling the Bullworker, and an obvious next step was to form an association or club for all the proud possessors of physical training equipment. It made sense, and business sense too, to maintain their interest and help them develop their physiques. So I formed the Bullworker Club of Great Britain, with some three to four thousand members.

Just at this moment, the firm which had the Bullworker franchise, Honour House Products, went broke owing me thousands of pounds. Frankly they weren't very businesslike, but it left me out on a limb. So I decided to strike out on my own anyway. It was a period when the literature of health and physical culture in this country was at a low ebb. The Weider Organisation's magazine *Muscle Power* was fading fast; they did another one called *Mr America* which became a sexually-orientated publication. *Health and Strength* came out when it felt like it and there was a publication which catered for weightlifters called the *Strength Athlete* which was a tiny thing.

I felt that the time was ripe for a magazine which brought all the various interests together, making it as topical as possible. It was called *Power*. I wrote it, edited it, and took pictures for it, and within a few months I had a circulation of some four thousand. It went out by post free to all my Bullworker Club members and it contained my own advertisements for my own products – vitamin pills, weights, clothing and equipment. That was

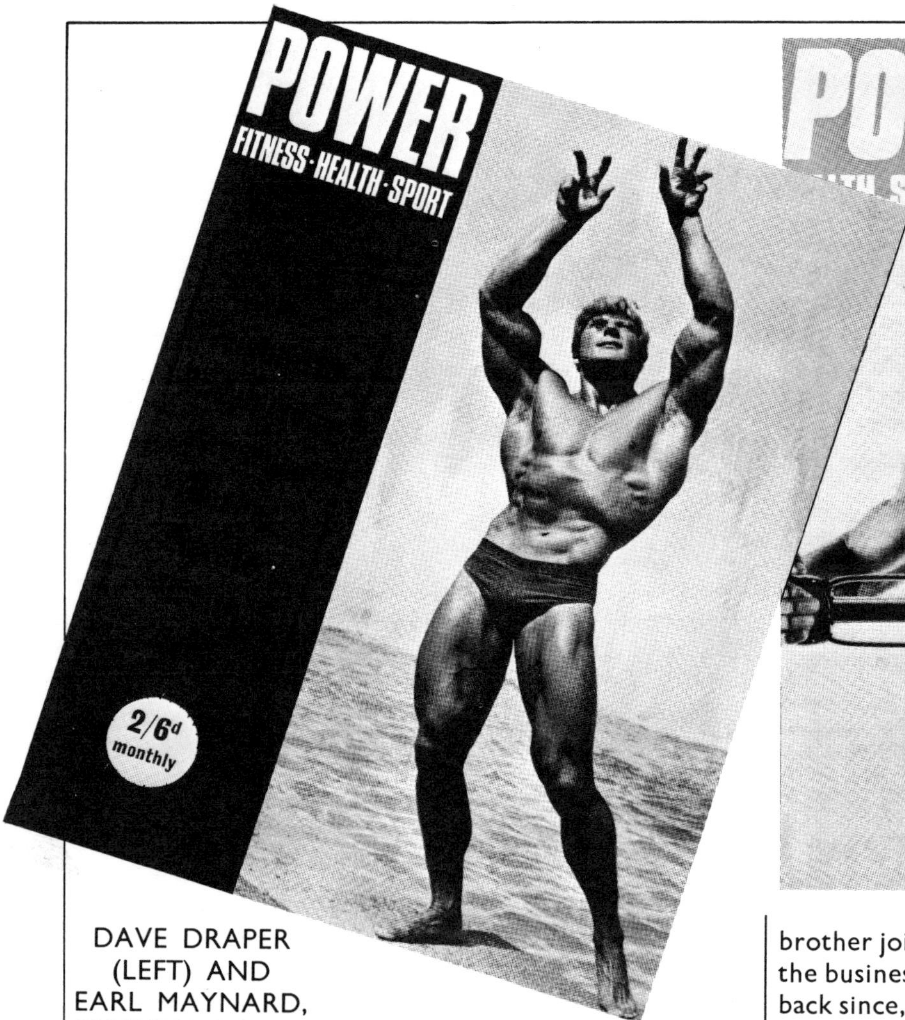

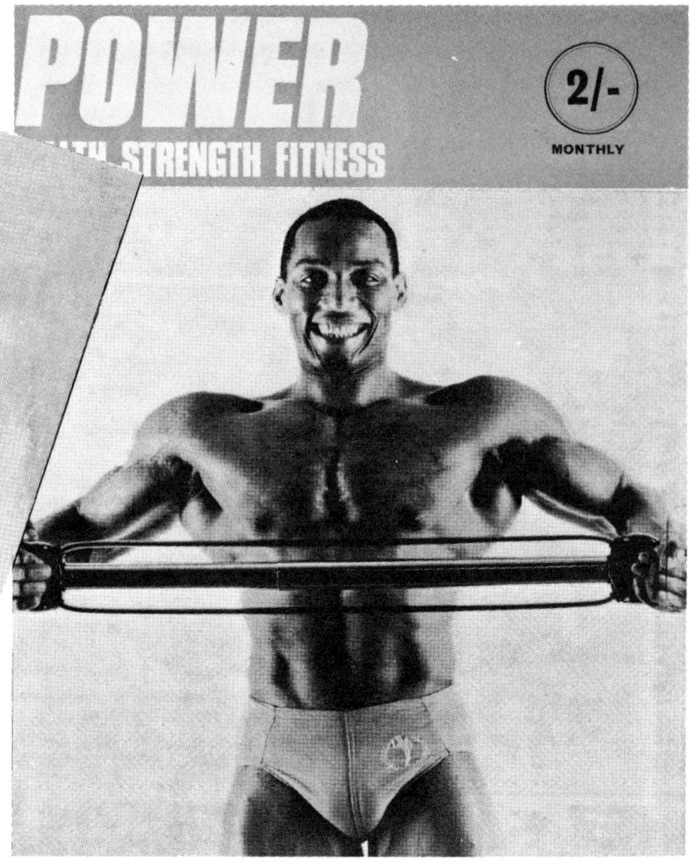

DAVE DRAPER (LEFT) AND EARL MAYNARD, 'POWER' COVER MEN.

how I made my money – selling the products. In next to no time I was making a profit of around £200 a month after all costs.

I did this for about eight months, and then I made my big mistake. I enlarged the magazine, increased the print run and marketed it through normal retail outlets. I thought things were going well but after four months, I found myself around £15,000 in debt. Bailiffs arrived to take away the office furniture and I was at my wits' end to know where to turn when some friendly creditor did me the best favour he could have done – he put me into liquidation.

I must admit to feeling really low – really defeated – when I trailed into the Official Receiver's office in Inveresk House in London for the examination of my accounts. Still, it all worked out in the end and I managed to salvage about 600 rusty weights from the equipment side of the business. We worked on these; wire-brushed, cleaned, polished and painted them. They were the foundation of my equipment when I opened my new exercise gymnasium a few months later, in December 1969.

At first, because I was undercapitalised (again), I didn't have the cash for promotional activities and things moved very slowly. I had to be away from the gymnasium, which we called the Dave Prowse Exercise Advice Centre, for three days a week. Although customers came in gradually, after two years I was on the verge of packing it in. But at that moment my brother joined me as business manager, and suddenly the business began supporting itself. We haven't looked back since, although my brother is now in Saudi Arabia and we have a new business manager. We called it the Advice Centre because, although there's a fully-equipped gymnasium there, it's more than that. Individuals, clubs, local authorities and so on can come to me there for advice on exercise training and equipment and I've fitted out gymnasia and exercise centres in many parts of the country. It's a sort of consumer exercise consultancy.

In the meantime, apart from my film and TV work, I've been engaged in two other exercise consultancies. The first, which has been going now for eight years, is with Harrods, the great London store. I had sold equipment to Harrods for some time, and when I returned from a trip to the United States in 1969, I brought along with me a new computerised horoscope to show to Harrods. This was something new for me, and I was very enthusiastic. They passed me round from department to department and eventually I was talking to the management.

They didn't seem to be very interested in computerised horoscopes. Every time I talked about horoscopes they talked about exercise equipment. Eventually they asked me to write down all my ideas about how to equip, staff and run a keep-fit shop. (They allowed me to put the computerised horoscopes in on a trial basis for a fortnight. We sold one – at eight guineas.) I came back with four foolscap pages of typing on a keep-fit operation for Harrods. They adopted my ideas and I joined them as a consultant, at first on commission, and later on salary. It's been a most fruitful operation, and is now part of Harrods' great Olympic Way, probably the biggest commercial sports complex in the world. I've met many people there from all walks of life, but perhaps the most surprising was John Wayne. The big man was poking about among the sports equipment, and I asked him if we could help.

'Sure,' he said. He really is a big man – tall as me and built like a battleship all the way down. 'I'm looking for some rope – or a rope ladder.'

It turned out that he was in England working on a film and he had been placed in a modern hotel suite many floors up and with no obvious fire escape near his suite. He was looking for alternative means of escape; he confessed he was scared to hell of fire. I directed film's toughest guy to a camping shop down the road.

My second consultancy was more recent – to Grosvenor House, the well-known luxury hotel. A gymnasium and swimming pool had been operative there for years, managed by a highly respected expert, Edward Hine. He'd been there for 15 to 20 years and had taught the royal children to swim. Mr Hine, who was 68, had a heart attack and died.

Grosvenor House, or rather Messrs Trust House Forte, approached me to take over. I joined them as a consultant and drew up full plans for modernisation, re-equipping and so on.

I was at Grosvenor House for two years, supervising their gymnasium, and met some extremely interesting people there. Among them was Mr Heath, who at first came only for the swimming. But he joined in with the exercise programmes after a while. He surprised me with his fitness. He was very strong, and could pedal away on the exercise bike long after most people would have collapsed. But he was very stiff, hardly mobile at all, and had no idea of how to touch his toes. He used to wear a light blue track suit (what else?) and I came to like him very much indeed as a person. In fact, I must say I've never met a man whose public image I disliked, but whom I liked more, in private.

I was also introduced there to the Crown Prince of Saudi Arabia, Prince Khalid Bin Sultan Bin Abdul Aziz, who came in to see me for remedial exercises (he was overweight). We got on like a house on fire, and eventually he asked me to return with him to Saudi Arabia, to build and equip two gymnasia to the highest standards, and to stay with him as his personal consultant. It was a tempting offer, but I had a great deal going for me in Britain, so I reluctantly turned him down. Instead, I supervised the whole operation for him, going out four times last year; and my brother Bob left the gymnasium and now works full-time for Khalid in Saudi Arabia. It's a very happy arrangement, and Prince Khalid is a fine and generous employer and friend.

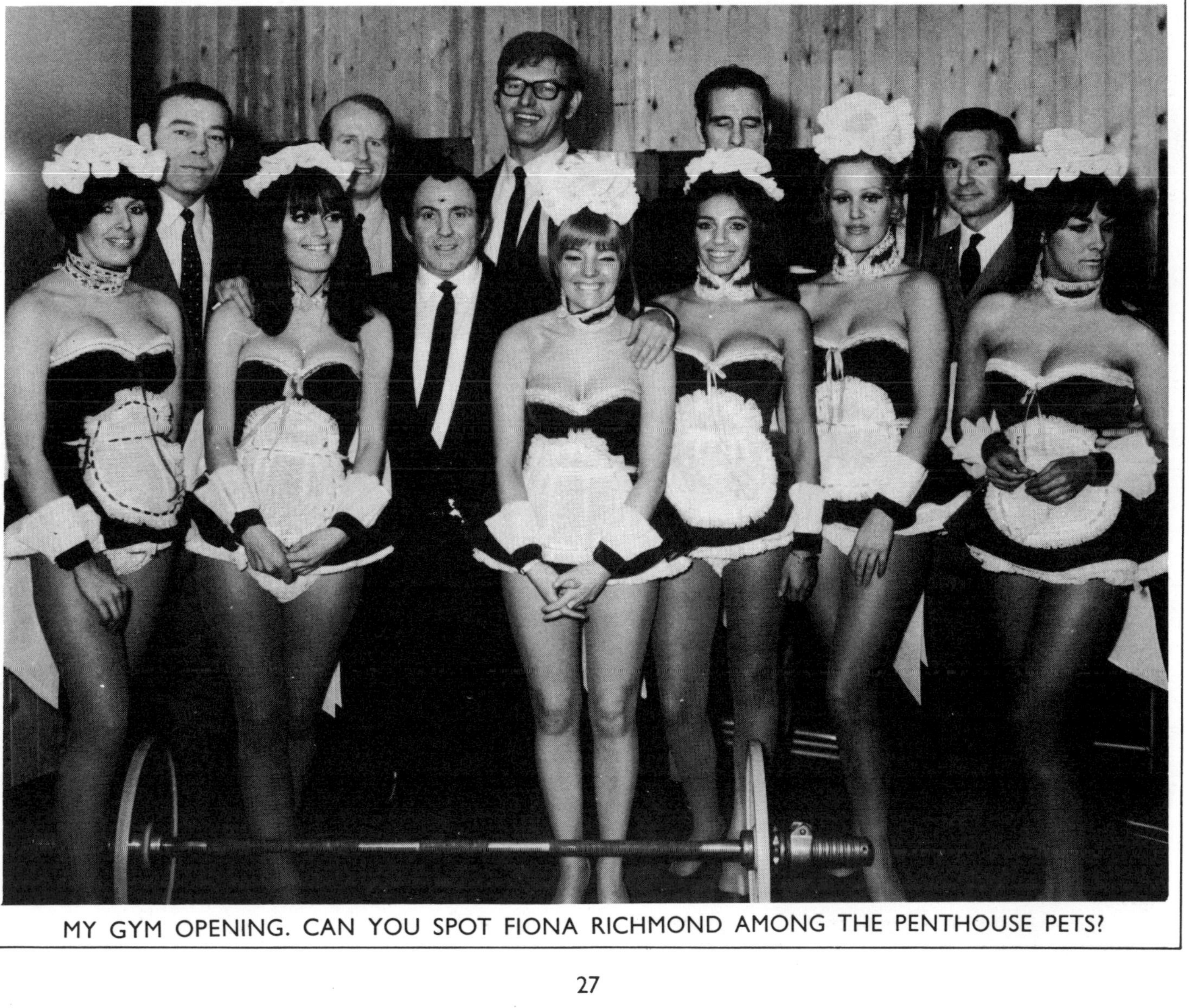

MY GYM OPENING. CAN YOU SPOT FIONA RICHMOND AMONG THE PENTHOUSE PETS?

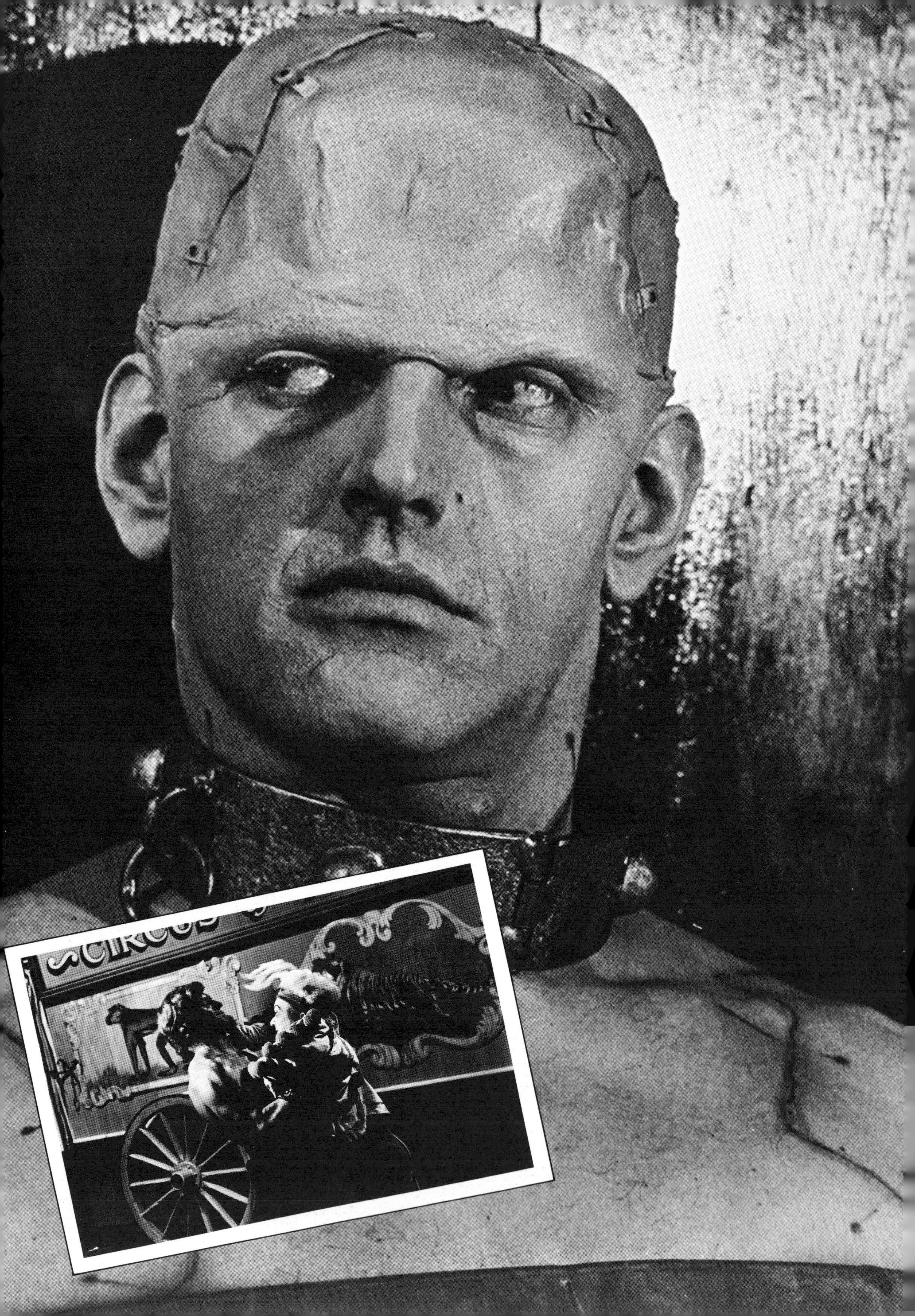
CIRCUS

Chapter 4

'CAN YOU DO IT TWICE A NIGHT?'

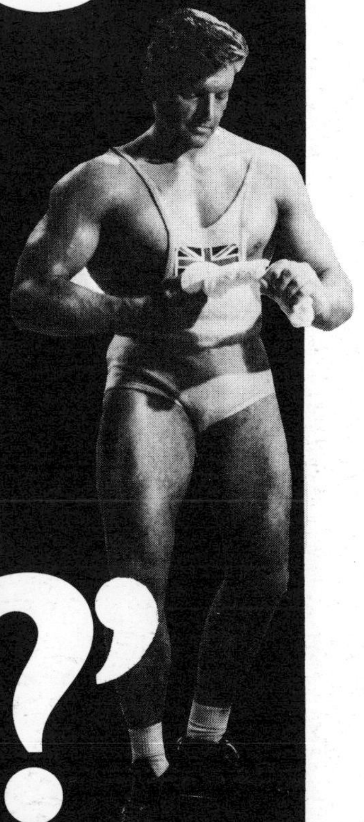

My show business career began in 1964 when I was a salesman, calling on various firms. One of my clients was the Tough Guys Agency, who supplied musclemen, stunt men, and stand-ins for films and TV work. One day they rang me up and asked me if I'd like to go along to the Mermaid Theatre where Bernard (now Sir Bernard) Miles was producing a Terence Feeley play with Kenneth Griffith, Caroline Mortimer and Liz Fraser. It was called *Don't Let Summer Come*. The finale called for Death, in the form of a very strong man, to pick up Kenneth Griffith and waft him off the stage. Bernard Miles had been auditioning actors for the part, but nobody could pick up Kenneth Griffith. When I got to the Mermaid they were rehearsing on stage, and Mr Miles thanked me for coming, but said they didn't think they were going to go ahead with it, because Kenneth Griffith had been dropped six or seven times, and was getting fed up.

I said, 'Tell me what you want done, and I'll tell you if it can be done.'

'All we want is him picked up and carried off stage,' he said.

I walked across to where Kenneth Griffith was lying on a bed wrapped in red velvet, picked him up (he weighed about nine stone) strolled across to Bernard Miles with the actor held out at arm's length and said, 'There you are. What d'you want me to do with him?'

'Can you do that twice a night?' said Mr Miles.

'As many times as you like,' I said. So I got the part, and with it an Equity ticket.

So for the next few weeks I turned up at the Mermaid Theatre at around eight o'clock and eleven o'clock, donned a black shroud, and carried Kenneth Griffith off stage twice nightly.

I was still 'Britain's strongest man' at this time, and I did a TV ad for Hotpoint, trying to wring water from a towel they had spun dry. More TV ads followed. I played the heavies in *The Saint* and *Department S* – small parts – and then I was called to an audition at the BBC for a part in a *Before the Fringe* production, starring Hermione Gingold. At the BBC Theatre were dozens of big blokes in dress suits, all with hungry gleams in their eyes, like me. Miss Gingold came in and sat down, and for some reason which I can't explain, I moved over and sat in the seat behind her. Perhaps it was just to be near a star.

After a few minutes, she turned round and asked me if I had a copy of the day's paper. I hadn't but offered to find her one, and after a bit of a search found her a *Times*.

OPPOSITE: STILLS FROM *THE HORROR OF FRANKENSTEIN* (TOP) AND *VAMPIRE CIRCUS*.

About ten minutes later we were all called up on stage for the audition. Hermione came out, didn't look at the other chaps, but pointed straight at me. 'I'll have that one,' she said. All I had to do was to carry her hat on and walk off; but it was my first BBC part.

After that I had small parts in all sorts of programmes, mostly comedy, working with the Goodies, the two Ronnies, and other well-known comedians.

Then I got a call to go to Shepperton Studios for a part in a sketch with Peter Sellers in the prestige film of the year, *Casino Royale*. The part was 'Super-Poo' a huge Teddy Bear who was supposed to haunt Sellers in his dreams. I looked around, and there were five or six other big men again, so I got hold of the second assistant on the film, who was responsible for casting, and told him that I thought I was working on the film, and didn't expect to audition. It was very cheeky, as I hadn't been near a film set before, but he just said 'Oh really?' and sent all the others home. The 'second assistant' was Dominic Fulford who has since become an outstanding director in his own right.

All that week I turned up for work, at £30 a day. It wasn't until the Friday that we started filming the sketch. I climbed into my costume, Peter did his stuff, and then they said that was that for the day and come back next Monday to complete the sketch. Well, apparently Peter's contract had expired and he was too expensive to hire on a daily basis, so he pushed off to Europe and the sketch was abandoned. A few days later I had another call from the studio asking if I was the man they'd measured for Frankenstein's monster's mask. It wasn't me, but they offered me the part anyway, so I did appear in *Casino Royale* after all.

My next big job was six weeks' location shooting in Portugal, near Estoril, on Irving Allen's *Hammerhead*. That film made a number of firsts. It was Vince Edwards' first film under contract to Irving Allen; it launched Judy Geeson; and it was Diana Dors' comeback film. Peter Vaughan played Hammerhead, an international pornographer, and I was the guy who did all his dirty work for him. Vince Edwards injured himself three-quarters of the way through, and most of his shots were taken sitting down. It was all great fun, but the film wasn't too successful.

In 1970 I played Frankenstein's monster in Jimmy Sangster's send-up of the famous horror film *The Horror of Frankenstein*. Peter Cushing wasn't available, so Ralph Bates got his chance to play Frankenstein. Nowadays Hammer Films make a complete plaster cast of your body, so that they can chop it up and bits of you appear in the vats when necessary and they can take a rubber mould at any time so you can slip it on; but when I worked for Jimmy Sangster I used to spend $2\frac{1}{2}$ hours in the make-up chair every day.

That film wasn't too well received either. One horror film society voted it one of the ten worst of all time. It was a bit too jokey. I think that Jimmy Sangster just decided to have a bit of fun with it.

I also appeared in *Vampire Circus*, for Hammer Films. It was one of the best horror films I've ever seen, but that too ran into difficulties. It was directed by Robert Young – his first, and he was very good. But when you're working for Hammer Films you have to deliver within schedule and within budget. If you're left with three or four days shooting at the end of the contract they just don't get done, and you have to cut the film accordingly, no matter how important they might have been. That's what happened to Robert, and the film could have been very much better.

My last horror film was *Frankenstein and the Monster from Hell*, also for Hammer Films, directed this time by Terence Fisher, the doyen of horror film directors. It introduced me to Peter Cushing for the first time. Both men were marvellous to work with. In one scene, I was on the rampage in the laboratory, and Peter, who's no chicken, saw me breaking everything up, took a flying leap onto the bench, grabbed a bottle of chloroform, smashed it into his coat, and then bounded onto my back, wrapping the chloroformed jacket round my face. I staggered around, with Peter Cushing fastened to my back, like an aeroplane spin in wrestling, until the choloroform took its effect and I collapsed to the floor unconscious. The whole set, the director, the film crew, everybody stood up and applauded. It was a great experience.

Before that I'd worked with Stanley Kubrick on *A Clockwork Orange*; and it was in this film that I made my major step forward. It didn't begin propitiously. I had a call to go to Stanley Kubrick's house at Elstree to talk about the film. It takes me an hour and a half to drive through London from home to Elstree, and when I got there I was kept waiting for half an hour before someone told me, 'Mr Kubrick can't see you now.' So I drove back to Croydon. The following Wednesday the scene was repeated. I was told Mr Kubrick had been delayed. This got up my nose a bit, and I told the intermediary that the only possible time I was available was at ten o'clock at night the following Friday. I was being as awkward as I could.

Sure enough, at ten o'clock next Friday night there was Stanley waiting for me. I read for the part of Julian, the bodyguard to Patrick McGee in the film, and I think Kubrick liked me because I wasn't an actor. He could mould me to the part as he wanted. I seemed to be the only person on set that he could talk to on normal matters outside the film – the news, what was on TV last night and so on. Everyone else seemed to live in dread of his temper. He certainly was a demanding director.

I got an inkling of what he was like as a director when I had to go to Harlow Hospital, where they were doing a scene with a psychiatrist; I arrived at the hospital at eleven o'clock and they were on 'take 30'. They eventually finished the scene on 'take 78' at three in the afternoon. And they used something like 'take six'.

The first scene I had to do myself was to answer a door. I had to run up three flights of stairs, open the door, catch the character (Alex) as he fell through it, pick him up and carry him down the three flights of stairs and hold him while he carried on a conversation with the writer (McGee). Still holding him, I had to run up three flights of stairs and dump him in a bath. We did this all day, time and again, without stopping. At the end of the day I couldn't move my arm, so strained were my

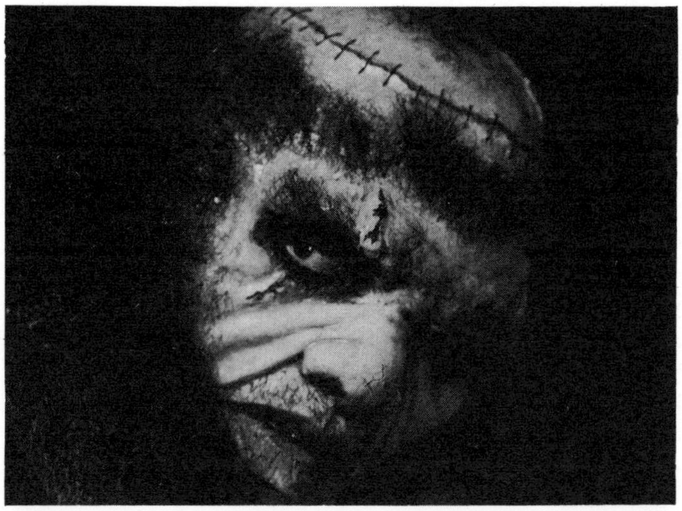

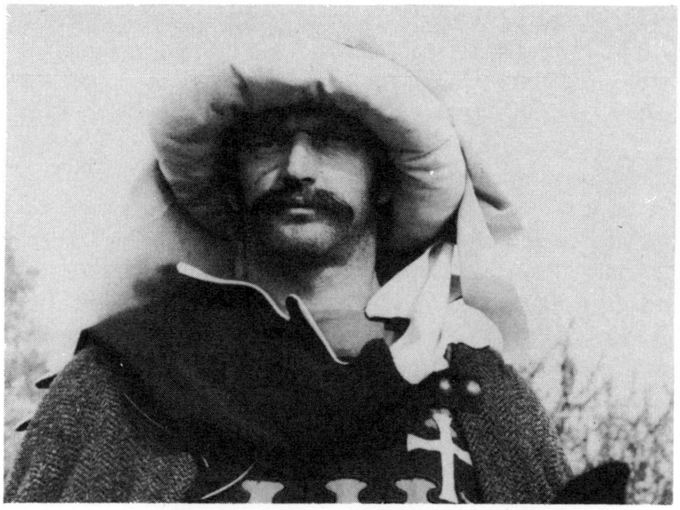

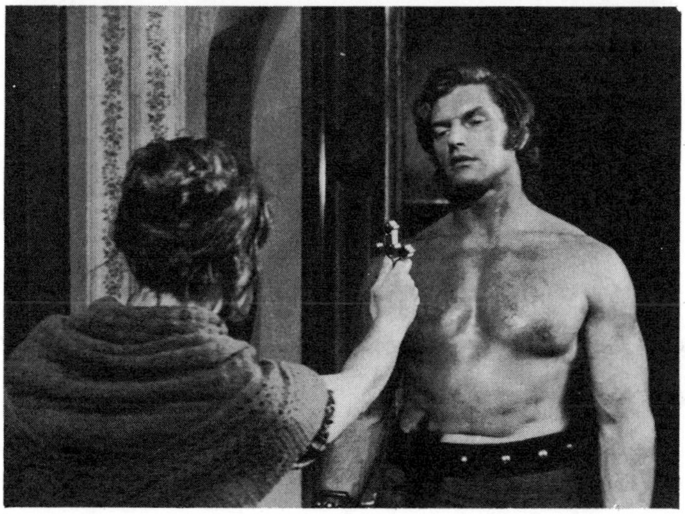

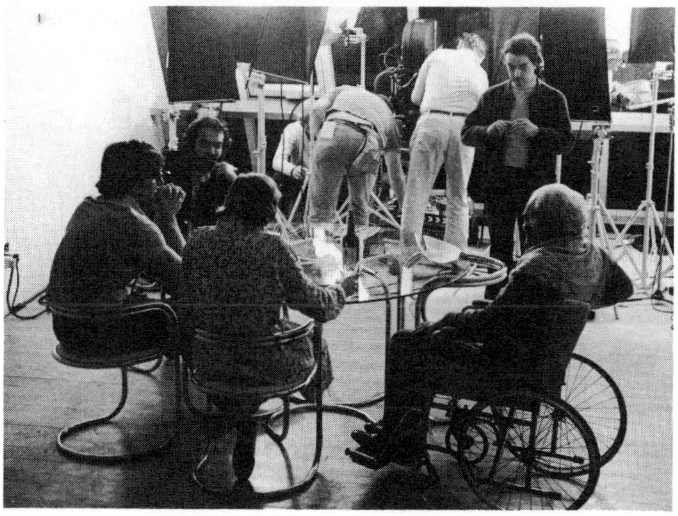

TOP LEFT: *FRANKENSTEIN AND THE MONSTER FROM HELL,*
TOP RIGHT: *UP THE CHASTITY BELT,*
ABOVE LEFT: *VAMPIRE CIRCUS,*
ABOVE RIGHT: STANLEY KUBRICK'S *A CLOCKWORK ORANGE.*

muscles.

A couple of days later Stanley told me: 'This is where you carry the writer in his wheelchair down the stairs.' Patrick McGee weighs a firm 13 stone and the wheelchair was heavy too. I had to carry them both down the three flights of stairs and put them down as if it was no trouble at all.

I said, 'Stanley, you must be joking.'

'What's the matter? You're a strong man, aren't you?'

'Yes, I am. But you don't know what you're asking. And your name's not One-Take Kubrick.'

There was dead silence. I think everyone expected me to get the sack. There was a pause and a broad grin came over his face.

'Don't worry, we'll shoot it as quickly as we can.'

We did. In six takes. And I didn't drop him. But each time Stanley would complain that there was a funny noise coming over the microphone. There was. It was my breath, forcing its way out through clenched teeth as I tried to appear nonchalantly unconcerned at the effort.

Clockwork Orange did me a great deal of good. It got me known in the United States, and it gained me acceptance not merely as a strong man, but as a bit of an actor too. After all, if you worked for Stanley Kubrick, people said, you're good enough to work for us. From then on, jobs improved dramatically, in number and quality.

I went to Barbados working for Russ Mayer for five weeks and then worked in *Up Pompeii* with Frankie Howard. That went quite well, and I was asked to be available for the next *Up* film – *Up the Chastity Belt.* They asked me on the phone if I could ride. I'd never been on a horse in my life – you never say no to anything – and I agreed airily that I could. A couple of weeks later they rang again to fix an appointment to talk about the 'jousting scenes'. This really did put the wind up me, and I went straight along to some local stables and learnt to ride. I went out every day for a fortnight, and at the end of that time I was thoroughly enjoying it and quite competent – even jumping. When I went to the conference I learned to my astonishment that I had a stunt man and stand-in – that I wasn't going to joust at all. All I had to do was to look good on the horse afterwards. I was Baron Grunwald de Grunt, and finished up without any trousers on, racing up the jousting field.

Christmas 1975 marked a major turning point in my career. My agent telephoned to ask me to go to see a man called George Lucas at 20th Century Fox in London. I didn't have a clue who George Lucas was, and my agent didn't know the name of the film involved, so it didn't seem much at the time.

I went to some rather imposing offices in Soho Square and was made very welcome by a charming American girl called Bunny Allsopp, who was Mr Lucas's secretary, and after waiting for about five minutes in came this slip of a boy – beard, dark glasses, looking just as if he'd just come down from college. This was the great George Lucas. He offered me one of two parts. – 'Take your choice,' he said. The first was a character called Chewbacca, a hairy Teddy Bear of a character who goes through the film on the side of the goodies. The thought of being wrapped up in a great smelly costume was too much, so I asked George what the other part was.

'He's Darth Vader, the big evil villain of the film,' said George.

'You needn't say any more, George,' I said. 'That's the part for me.'

'Why are you so sure?' he asked me.

'In my opinion, people will always remember the villain,' I said. 'They can never remember the names of the goodies.'

I went under contract in February 1976; and almost at the same time I had a call from the BBC, who were casting for the Open University Drama Course, offering me the part of the Executioner in Jean Genet's *The Balcony*. This was real drama, normally way outside my scope, and a great opportunity. In addition, Norma and I were still broke to the world and this BBC contract was something we did not expect at all. Normally you get paid a salary by the Beeb, and then you get repeat fees as the thing goes on; this time, because it was part of the Open University course, they wanted to repeat the programme say six or eight times, they offered me a treble lump sum to buy me out of repeats; so for a fortnight's rehearsals and a couple of days shooting there was this thumping big cheque.

Straight from that we started filming *Star Wars*; and I was on that all the way through the summer, at Elstree Studios. The others did in fact go to Tunisia for all the desert sequences, but I wasn't involved in them. All my action was on the Death Star.

At the beginning of the year, too, I'd been asked to pose for pictures by Ogilvy Benson and Mather, one of the country's top advertising agencies, for some road safety pictures for the Green Cross Code campaign for children aged four to eleven. The campaign had already been launched, using sports stars, but they'd found that the kids related to the star, rather than the code and so the campaign wasn't working as well as they'd hoped. So someone hit on the idea that they'd have a 'Bionic Man' as the Green Cross Code Man.

We did the test pictures on a freezing cold morning in the wilds of Clapham, and the pictures were submitted to the Central Office of Information. The COI went to the Department of Transport, who liked them, and so it came back down through the COI and Ogilvy Benson's (some three months later). We were now in the middle of filming *Star Wars*, and they asked me if I was available to 'go for an audition'. This seemed a bit odd, as I'd already posed for the pictures which were approved, but they said I'd have to win the part in open competition to prove to the Department everything was above board.

At first, it was decided that the commercials would go out on television twice a year. But after the first time they were shown there was a snag. Many mothers wrote in to say that their four- and five-year-olds were still running out into the middle of the road without warning, and when remonstrated with, they answered, 'Oh, the Green Cross Code Man will be there to save me.'

Of course, this was quite reasonable really, because we'd introduced the effect of my appearing and disappearing on the roads like magic, and my protection was implicit in the words with which we finished the film: 'Every time you cross the road, Always use the Green Cross Code.' So we made a second set of commercials which finished, 'Always use the Green Cross Code, Because I won't be there when YOU cross the road.' Not so hot on metre, perhaps, but effective.

In the second year of the commercials, the makers hit on the idea of sending the Green Cross Man out into the country to make personal appearances in schools to meet the children there and to drum up publicity locally for the campaign. In a word, to give the national campaign local impact. Since then, this has become a twice-a-year chore, and a most enjoyable one too. For five weeks or so during the period when they are showing the commercial on TV, I tour various areas of the British Isles. I usually 'do' three towns a week, covering two schools a day for three days. So far I've done five tours, visiting about 15 towns per tour, and I've visited over 70 towns in England, Scotland, Wales and Northern Ireland, talking to the children at more than 170 schools, meeting between 300 and 500 children each time . . . work out the total numbers for yourself.

I've always loved it. I didn't know anything about talking to kids en masse – but really it's an extension of talking to my own kids. When I began I'd learned the Green Cross Code by heart – I'd repeated it often enough – but once I started to lecture I went into road safety much more deeply. I've certainly become much more aware of road safety myself – when I'm driving, and when I'm on foot. And of course, I'm much more aware of how to talk to children, how to approach them, get their confidence and so on. It's like having a huge family – and one that's always recognising me in the street wherever I go.

I usually talk to the children about the Code for half an hour or so, and then spend 15 to 20 minutes on what I call 'fun', when I answer their questions, dish out badges, lift them up to show them how strong I am, take them out into the playground to demonstrate how to cross the road, and so on. I've appeared on local TV and radio shows all over the country, and given scores of press interviews. It's become much more than a job – more of a vocation for me. Conversely, of course, it's been very lucky for me. Normally any TV advertising campaign lasts a few weeks and then is forgotten. This has continued now for three years.

I was lecturing in Belfast when a bomb went off nearby. I was standing there looking huge in my green and white uniform, and an eight-year-old kid looked up at me and must have seen the apprehension in my face, for he said: 'Don't worry, mister, tis only a bomb. . . .'

Since the Green Cross Code campaign started, the accident rate in the four to eleven years age group has *dropped* by 24 per cent throughout the country, which is another reason why it's turned into a vocation for me. Long may it last.

I went back and completed shooting on *Star Wars* which was taken over to the United States for the special effects to be added; and immediately I became the special guest star for Gerry Anderson in *Space 1999*. The episode was called 'The Beta Cloud' and I played the monster who invaded the space ship *The Eagle* to steal its life support systems. I had a great time, I was electrocuted, poison gassed, shot, burned, beaten up – the lot. But I was immune, and finished by having a smashing time, breaking up the control room of the spaceship. 'This is your show, Dave,' they said. 'Just don't throw anything at the camera.' And they all retired behind barriers while I wrecked the set . . .

I went straight from there into Terry Gilliam's film *Jaberwocky*, a medieval film about a monster terrorising a village. First I got a call asking me to play the part of the 'Good Knight'. I said sure, and would they send me a

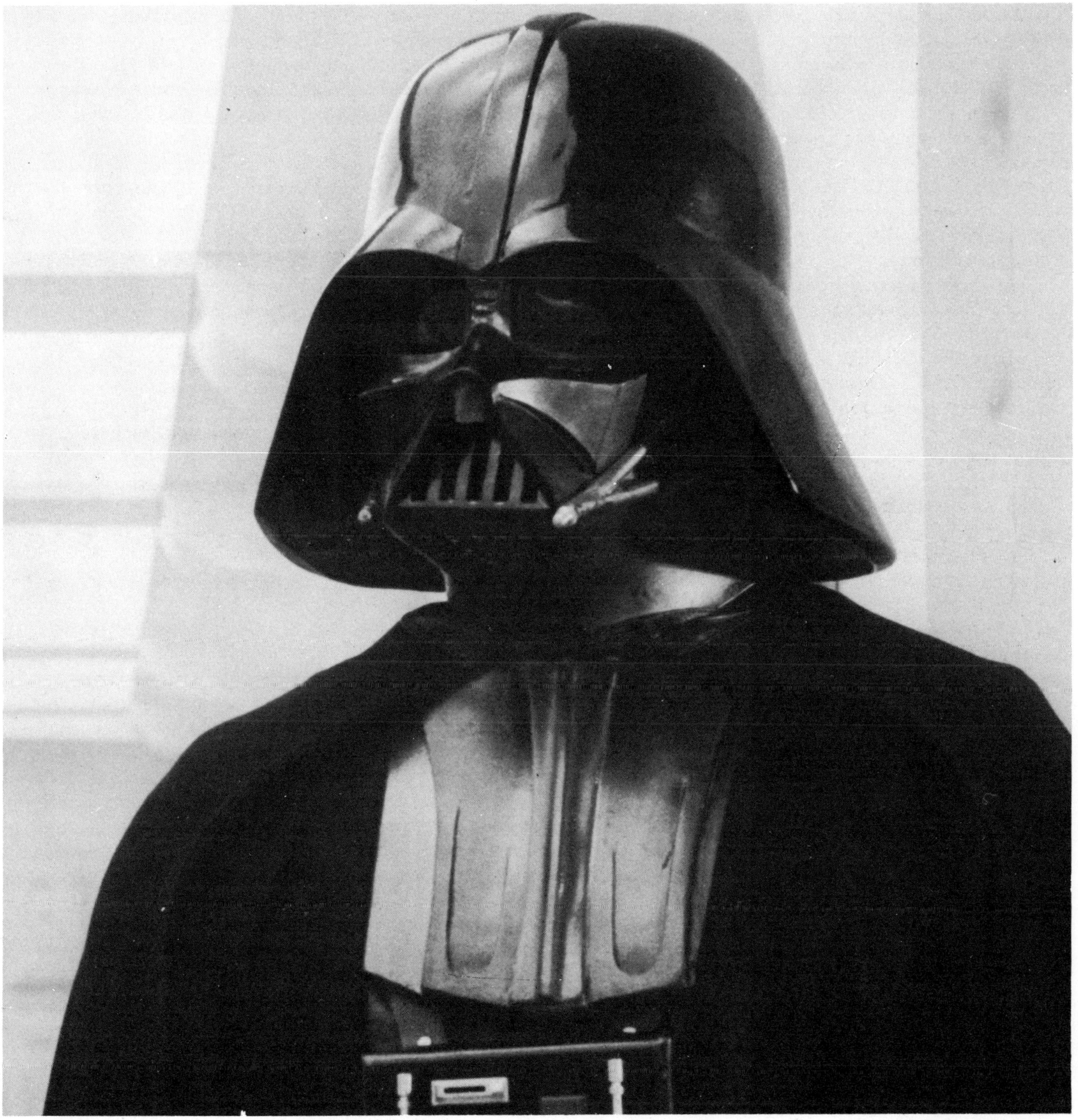

AS DARTH VADER IN *STAR WARS*.

script. 'Oh, you don't want a script,' they said, 'there's no talking.' So I asked what the Good Knight did, and they said that he had a fight with and gets killed by the Black Knight. 'Oh,' they said. 'D'you think you could play the part of the Black Knight as well?'

'Sure,' I answered, 'But what does *he* do?'

'He has to fight the Monster,' they said. 'You couldn't play the monster too, could you?'

Eventually a tall skinny dancer went into the Monster's costume and I finished up as the two Knights. It was great fun. We had some problems in filming it, down at Pembroke Castle. I had to do a fall off a horse in full metal armour weighing 50 or 60 lbs. They had to guide the horse into the right spot, where all these boxes and mattresses were to break my fall. My job was to slash away with my battle axe, slash too far and topple off the horse. I kept falling off this damned horse all day, and I was bruised and battered and cross. I was also having trouble with my stirrups – what with their size and the armour on top I had to jam my feet into them, so getting out of them was a major operation, let alone falling off. The horse wasn't too co-operative either.

Right towards the end of the day, on take umpteen, I leaned out, smashing the air with my battle axe, and – crash, over I went. But this time I didn't get my feet out of the stirrups, and the horse decided to bolt. So now here I am, bouncing along the floor in my armour at full speed, my feet stuck in the stirrups, absolutely helpless. We were filming at the base of a quarry which was filled with water, and if I'd gone in, I must have been a goner. But before anything awful could happen, the horse's girth snapped, and the whole saddle came toppling off on top of me.

Everyone came racing along, stood me upright, felt me over for breaks, and said, 'Super. Great. Just what we wanted. Marvellous shots. Are you all right?' In roughly that order.

When it was all cut and edited, of course that was the take that was used – it was by far the most spectacular. But – if you look very closely at that fall, which of course takes place in medieval times – you'll see the camera follow me, crash bang wallop, past a background of a Hertz Rent-a-Van filling the screen.

In the meantime, the Green Cross Code campaigns have been filling my time – and my life. It has been both a privilege and an honour to be connected with something that is not only useful to children, but enyoyable to do. Once the first impact of the Green Cross Code had been proved to be a success, someone in the Ministry hit on the idea of taking the Green Cross Code Man out to meet the children. So in the past two years I've made four big tours, of England, Scotland, Wales and Northern Ireland. I've visited 70 cities, and seen two schools in each city, talking to about 300 children at each school. That's an awful lot of children. In that time, in the four to eleven age group with which I'm concerned, the accident rate has dropped by 17 per cent; even last year when accidents as a whole showed an increase, in this four to eleven group there was still a five per cent decrease. What more could you want? On top of the visits, of course, I've done scores of press

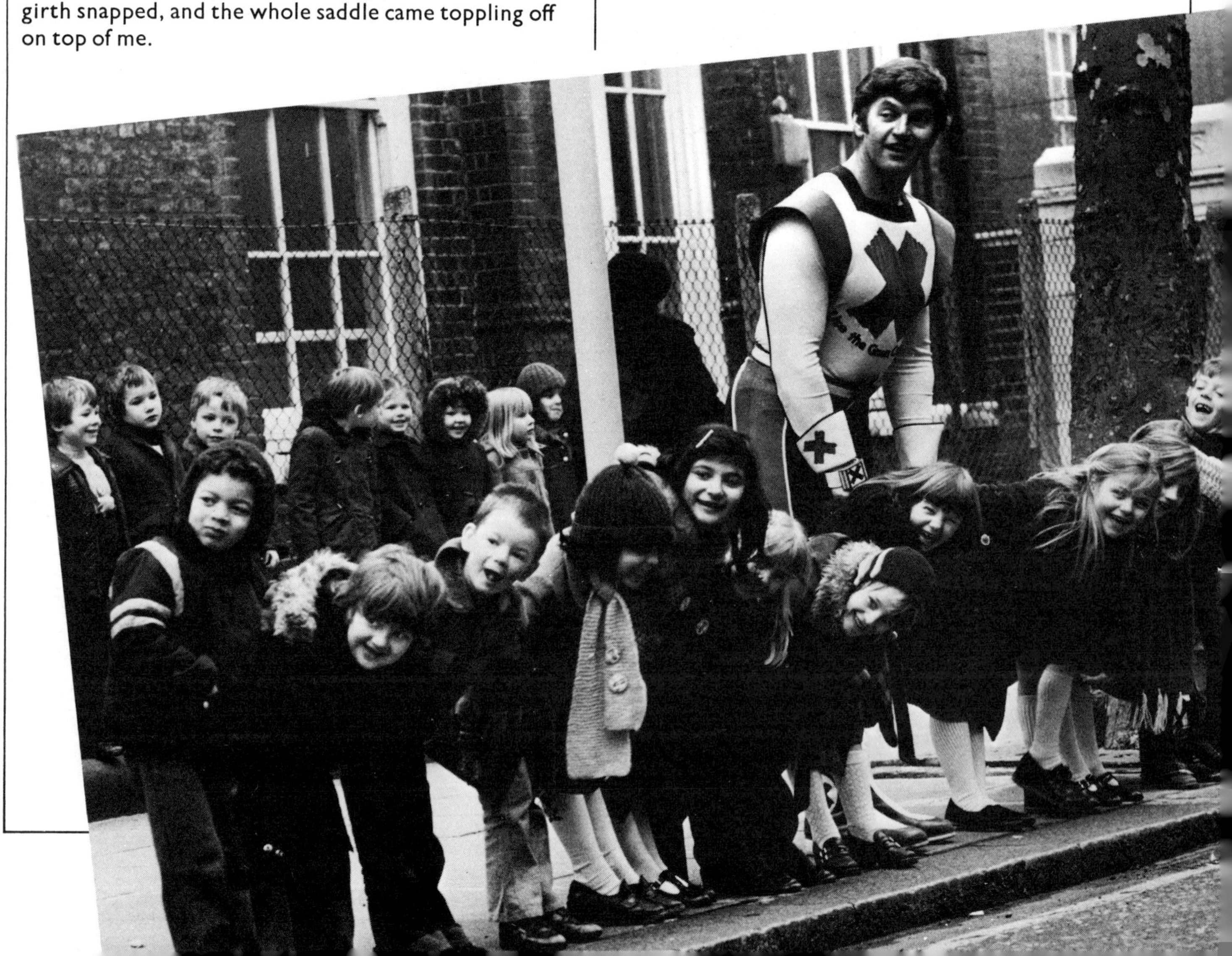

interviews, dozens of local radio and television shows, all of which has been free publicity for the campaign. It's almost become a vocation in itself.

When I went into *Star Wars*, neither I, nor any of the rest of the cast, believed it was going to be half as big as it turned out to be. It was just another part. In fact, I was a bit perturbed about going in for it as I didn't know whether I wanted to play another masked part. I'd been a succession of monsters and knew I didn't want to play Chewbacca; but it wasn't until I was well into the film that I realised that Darth Vader was masked. By then it didn't matter; I was sufficiently wrapped up in the whole thing by then.

I learnt all the lines, and throughout the whole shooting of the film I spoke them. I never really knew if my Bristol accent, which wasn't too bad, was acceptable or not; I went to George Lucas, and he didn't know, or rather I don't think he'd thought about it. In fact, much of the picture developed as it went along. I don't even know whether at the time they thought of Darth Vader as a type of robot or whether in fact he was human underneath the black robes and the mask. Even the main plot developed. They found they'd got plenty of action at the start of the film, and at the finish, but they hadn't got enough in the middle, so they had a script conference, called Alex Guiness in and asked him if he'd mind being killed off in the middle of it . . . it was that sort of set up.

I didn't know what was happening at all until after the film came out, when I had a letter from Russ Meyer in Los Angeles saying that *Star Wars* was out and that

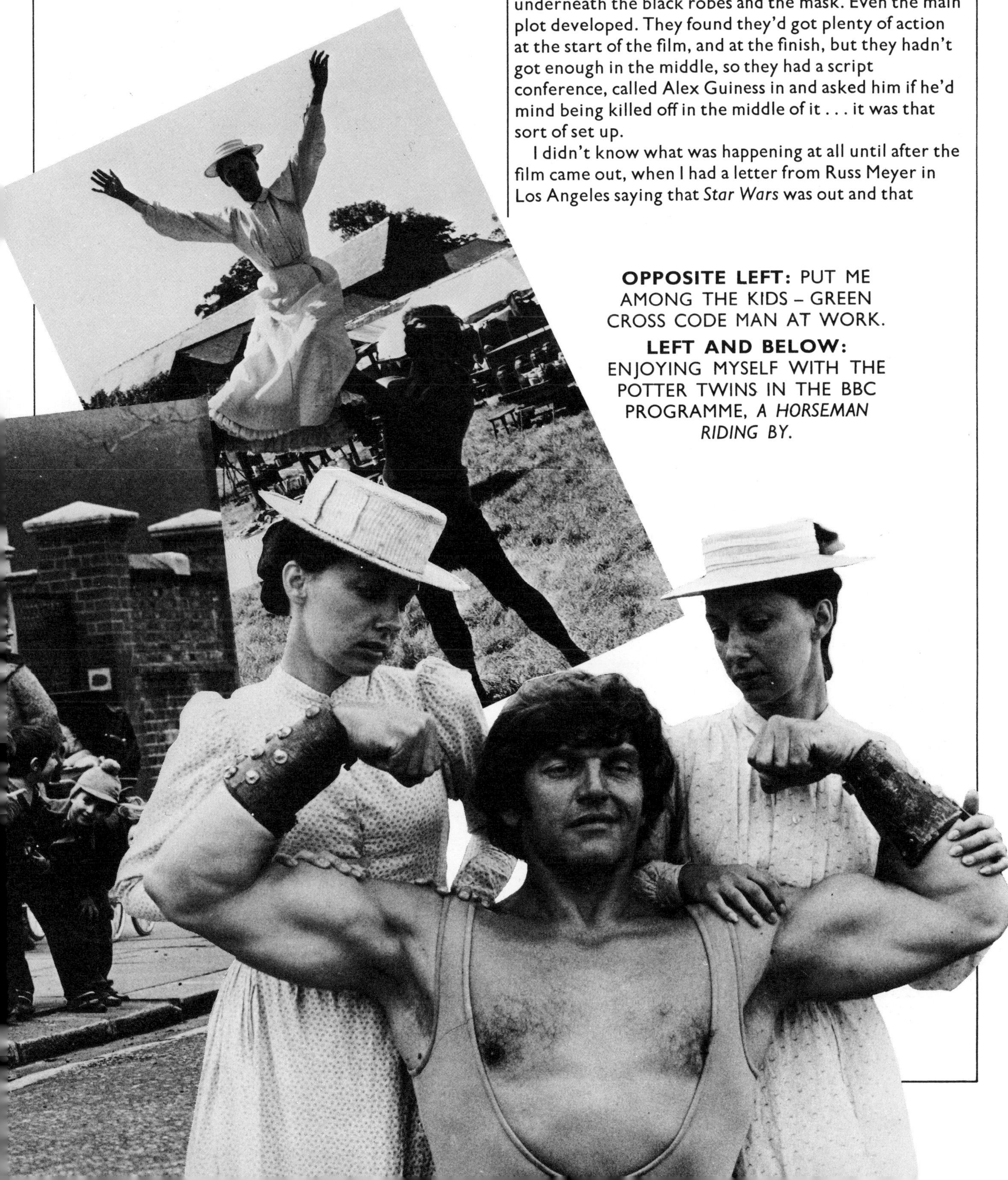

OPPOSITE LEFT: PUT ME AMONG THE KIDS – GREEN CROSS CODE MAN AT WORK.
LEFT AND BELOW: ENJOYING MYSELF WITH THE POTTER TWINS IN THE BBC PROGRAMME, *A HORSEMAN RIDING BY.*

James Earl Jones had dubbed my voice. I was disappointed, and indeed I'm told that James Earl Jones didn't want anybody to know he'd done the dubbing. But in fact, strangely, because of the success of the film, it's become a back-handed compliment to both of us and we've both had much more publicity through the dubbing than we'd have got otherwise. In my case, they tried to disguise the fact that it was Dave Prowse inside the costume, so everyone started clamouring to find out who it was.

One benefit of playing masked is that, of course you're not stereotyped. I can play any number of Darth Vader parts without being recognised, which allows me to step off into any other roles I like. But I still feel I've missed a great deal in not having been through the mill – drama school, repertory, pantomime and so on. I feel a great sense of envy when I hear the genuine old pros talking about the Hippodrome here, the Palladium there, and so on. And yet I feel that I'm in near the start of a whole new resurgence in films and television plays. So one day I'll be an old-timer in my own right.

It's a bit early to say in this book what difference *Star Wars* and its success has made to my life. Financially, so far, not much difference, as I was paid a fee for the film and I spent that long ago . . . but there will be more *Star Wars* films to come and if they have the same success, we shall see. Certainly now I'm better known everywhere I go, and I'm getting better film and TV parts. I'm now getting more genuine acting roles – at the moment I'm rehearsing *As You Like It* for the BBC – with dialogue of my own too. And even my relatives occasionally write for my autograph.

As to the future, I can see it lying more in films and television than in business. It's what I really enjoy doing and I hope I'm doing it better each time. My body has brought me success; it's taken me from being a dance-hall bouncer to being an internationally-known personality. I've always sought success, and I'll continue doing so – whether as Darth Vader, the Green Cross Code Man, or plain Dave Prowse.

While I was working on *Jaberwocky*, I tried – unsuccessfully – for the film part of Superman. But they couldn't have an Englishman playing an American folk-hero. One day I had a call from the director, Dick Donner: 'We've found our Superman,' he said. 'We want you to look after him, hand, foot and finger, and see what you can do with him in six weeks.'

I did it. I got him vitamin pills and supplements, special drinks and diets, and in six weeks I got him up from 13 stone 7 pounds up to 15 stone 2 pounds, and all of it good hard muscle on his chest and shoulders. They particularly wanted a big V-shape, tiny waist and big shoulders, and this we achieved. He maintained the weight all the way through the picture and everyone was very excited about what we had done, particularly the manufacturers of Nutrament. He used to drink the stuff by the caseful.

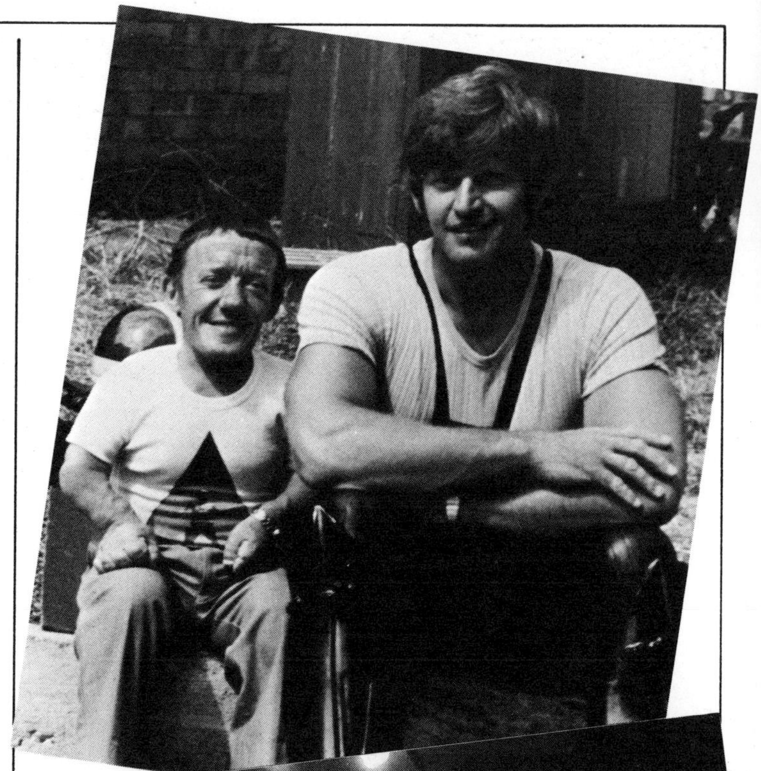

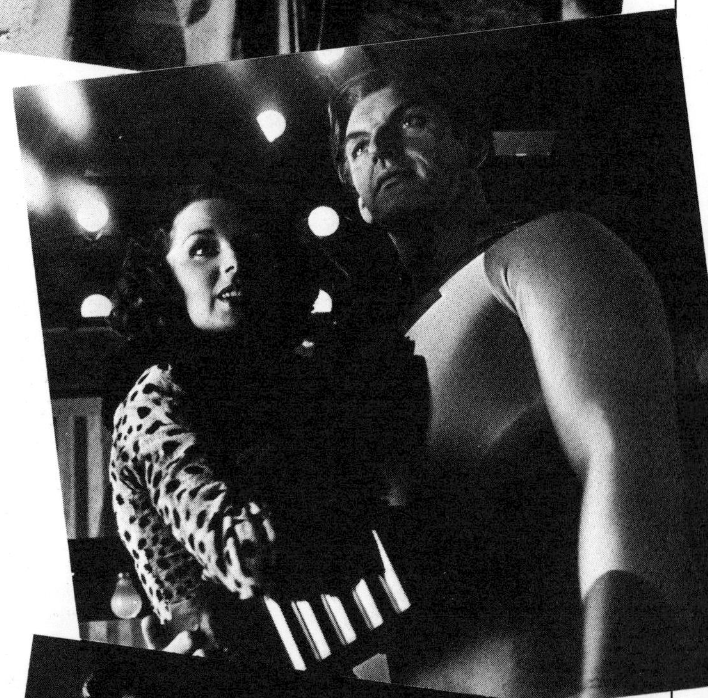

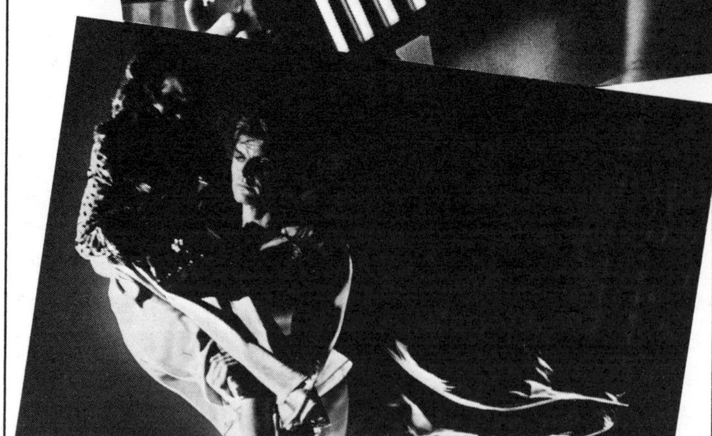

TOP: RELAXING WITH KENNY BAKER R2D2 OFF THE SET OF *STAR WARS*. **MIDDLE AND BOTTOM:** PLAYING SUPERMAN FOR MAX FACTOR.

Chapter 5

LET ME GET YOU FIT FIRST

When I began exercising in 1951 it was to build up my body after being in and out of hospital for the past four years. For a year I'd lain in hospital with suspected tuberculosis of the knee, and for three years I'd been encased in a leg-iron. At the age of 13 I was a well-set-up five feet nine inches tall; at 17 I was a skinny 6ft 5ins, weighing eleven stone. Since then I've been involved in exercise training for a variety of reasons, ranging from straight body-building to weightlifting to training directly for the sports in which I've been interested.

Through the years in my work in exercise gymnasia, I've come to realise that, like most people, at first I had got it all wrong. Almost invariably, people exercise for cosmetic reasons, and this is what I did originally. Although ostensibly I wanted to get fit again, to run and jump and play rugby football, at the back of it all I know there was the thought that I might become Mr Universe, or certainly a muscleman. The fact that the exercises I was going to do would improve my heart and respiration and general fitness was purely incidental. I didn't give it a moment's thought. What I was interested in was the showiness of my physique, the ability to demonstrate to the world my muscles and my power. It wasn't until I entered the Mr Universe competition itself that I came to realise how sterile my ambition then was.

No matter who you are, what shape or sex or size or age, the most important muscle in your body is your heart. If that's working correctly, everything else about you will improve. You'll think more clearly, your stamina, your sex-life, the whole quality of your life will be altered radically for the better. Closely allied with the heart, of course, are the lungs. So the next object of exercise training is to improve your respiration. Then, in order come strength and suppleness and lastly, mere physique.

So, the objectives in this book are:

1. Cardio-vascular fitness; which means your ability to recover from physical exertion;
2. Strength;
3. Suppleness and mobility;
4. Figure improvement.

Before we get down to the exercises themselves, there are a number of important points to remember if you haven't done exercise training before. The programmes are progressive; that is they become more difficult as you work through the book, so don't try to go too fast by plunging into the middle. You'll soon find out how much you can do in any one area of training. Secondly, they can be safely undertaken by anyone in normal health between the ages of seven and seventy, but if you have any doubts whatever about your fitness, particularly about your heart and your blood pressure, check up with your doctor before you begin, and tell him what you intend to do.

Warming up

Always warm up before beginning exercise training. You'll find the first two exercises in Programme No 1 are warming-up routines to limber up the waistline and lower back. Most muscle damage is caused by stretching when the body is cold. For the same reason, wrap up warmly. Many health studios like girls to exercise in leotards and tights with plenty of mirrors around – the object being that you will see the ghastly state you're in and be inspired to work to correct your appearance. I set about it the other way. Wear leotards and tights, fine, but with a track suit or sweater and slacks on top, well buttoned up at the wrists, ankles and neck. The body functions best when it's warmed up, like a car engine. Apart from anything else, plenty of warm clothing helps you to perspire, which is most important for toning up the body.

Diet

Eat what you like, within reason. The average person these days worries far too much about his (or more particularly her) diet and not nearly enough about general basic fitness. Of course, if you're definitely overweight, watch your fluid intake and stick to low-calorie, high-protein diet; if you want to gain weight and build yourself up, maintain a high-calorie, high-protein diet. In Chapter Eighteen, I explain the relationship between exercise and training and how you can combine the two to attain your personal objective. We hear a great deal about slimming, but it's true that almost as many people want to gain weight as to lose it.

Training in company

Try to get someone else to train with you. There's nothing like a little competition and a common objective to keep you going. We've found that particularly among our family, exercise training is not only fun but it helps our togetherness. One person can help the other, too, supporting during some of the exercises, pointing out faults, and so on. For example, doing 20 press-ups doesn't help me much these days; I'm long past that stage. But doing ten with my wife Norma on my back is getting me somewhere!

Train regularly

Try to make a regular time for your training, if you can. Obviously the optimum is to train daily, but three or four times a week may be quite sufficient for most people. And don't abandon hope if you can't do an exercise the number of times specified in the programme. What I am giving is the 'set' to work towards. In most cases you'll find that after a week or two, you'll be able to go through the whole programme easily. At that stage, begin trying to repeat the 'sets'. For example, if I specify 20 press-ups and you find you can do that easily, take a breather and then try for another 20. Generally speaking, the optimum number of 'sets' in any one exercise is three.

Girls and muscles

Many women and girls worry that undertaking a programme of exercise training can lead to their developing 'muscleman' outlines or figures like those East German girl swimmers at the Olympic Games. The anxiety can manifest itself after a few weeks' training when the muscles seem tauter, the body harder, and the outline more defined. Let me put your mind at rest. Much as I admire the achievements of those remarkable swimmers, the last thing I would want my daughter to do would be to grow up with a hugely developed back and shoulder muscles; and there's no chance of my recommending anything like that.

In the first place, a woman's body will only develop like that if subjected to thousands of hours of training designed to develop specific areas of the body. These enormous latissimus dorsi (back) muscles came about after years of training, with weights as well as in the pool, for six to eight hours a day, plus a very high daily diet of protein. Even a man's body will only develop in this way after years of training and dieting. The relatively tiny amount that most people will do through this book – say, in all, an hour and a half a week – is designed for your fitness, not to create a breed of supermen and women. That 'firming-up' you'll experience in the first few weeks is merely the (desired) loss of fatty tissue, allied to the toning and strengthening of the muscles, the essential preliminary to improving your health.

Some myths about weight training

And while I'm about it, there are one or two other 'old wives' tales' I'd like to scotch in relation to fitness training. It's often thought that weightlifting has to be done with the feet close together, and that if you lift with your legs apart you're wide open to a rupture. The truth is that ruptures or accidents occur in lifting when the lifter overbalances and is trying to re-establish his base. For example, if you try to pick up a sack of potatoes with your feet together and half way up the sack pulls you off your narrow base your natural reaction is to stick your feet out to try to re-base yourself. It's then the accident occurs. Stand up straight with your feet together and ask a friend to try to push you over and you'll see what I mean. He'll manage it easily. Now stand with your feet apart and ask him to try again. With a nice solid foot position you can resist all his efforts.

Many girls think that weight training will give them big muscles. The mere mention of weight training conjures up visions of large arm and shoulder muscles. Ask a girl to use a rowing machine and she'll imagine she'll end up looking like the Boat Race crews. *Weights are used merely to make exercises more difficult. The introduction of weights to the exercise programme makes exercising more difficult and less time-consuming.*

Can you get 'muscle-bound'?

Finally, the most widespread fear. Will I get muscle-bound? Well, there's (almost) no such condition. Many people think that men with large muscles are restricted in their movements and can't perform normal bodily functions like combing their hair or crossing their legs. The fact is that most well-developed athletes are more supple and mobile than the average man-in-the-street, because they work all their muscles over the complete range of movement. Muscle, being soft tissue, does not restrict your movements. The term 'muscle-bound' can only apply when one muscle which has its own action is developed to the detriment of its opposing muscle which has its opposing action.

Perhaps I can explain this: every muscle in your body

moves the joints in certain ways; i.e. the biceps muscle raises the forearm with the fulcrum at the elbow joint so that the wrist comes up to shoulder level. (It also tends to supenate – twist – the forearm but I won't go into that here.) The biceps' opposite number is the triceps which is a three-headed muscle at the back of the upper arm. Its sole function is to straighten the upper arm when bent. To get into a muscle-bound condition one would have to over-develop the biceps muscle by spending hour upon hour upon it and paying no attention to the triceps. Then you'd eventually arrive at a condition whereby the biceps muscle would be stronger than the triceps, which would be too weak to keep the arm straight. Don't worry, there's no chance of that if you follow my programme.

How hard should you exercise?

Don't worry if you puff and pant and your heart thumps away like a steamhammer after some of the exercises. That's exactly the object. You are imposing deliberately on your body a certain work-load, designed to raise your pulse-rate and to increase your oxygen intake. If you have to work hard, it means that the exercise is improving your physical fitness, unlike many others, which although they're geared towards strengthening certain muscles, don't distress you much at all. Remember, don't try to do too much too soon and, if you've heart or blood pressure problems, see your doctor before you start.

Breathing correctly

One last point. Correct breathing is essential to all exercising. As a general rule, breathe in deeply at the start of each exercise and breathe out once you're over the hard bit. Remember that the body runs best on a full tank of oxygen. This applies to all exercising, but in some cases you'll find that I specify exactly when to breathe. Have fun, and get fit.

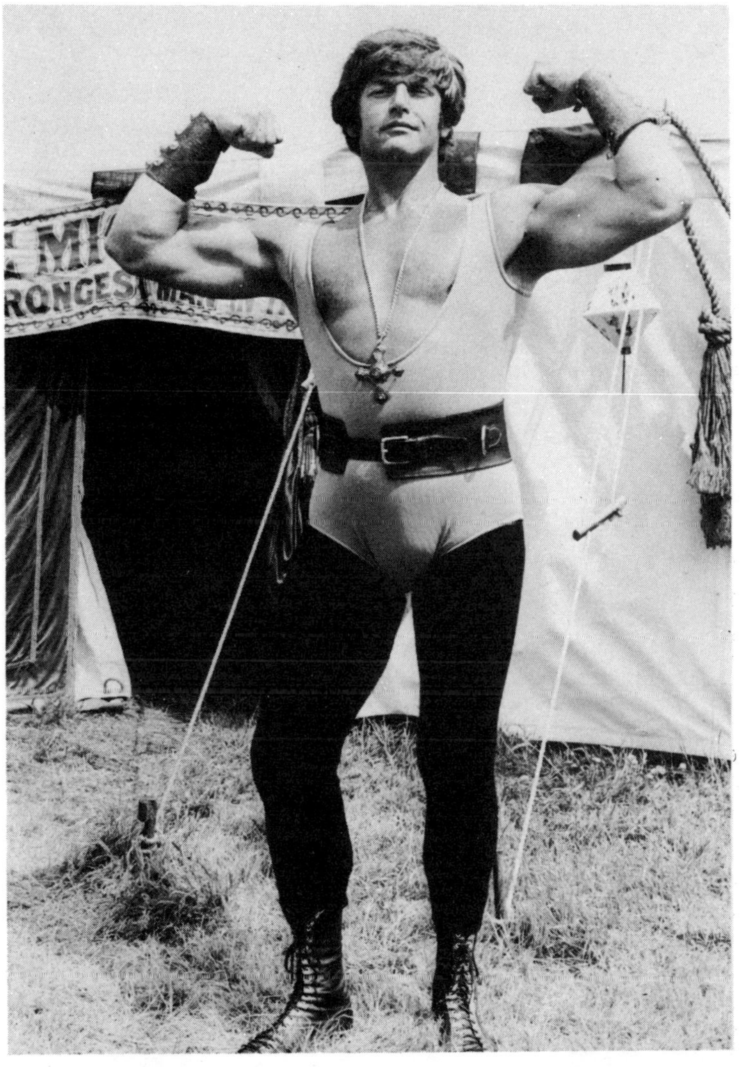

ON LOCATION IN DEVON FOR THE BBC PRODUCTION OF *A HORSEMAN RIDING BY*.

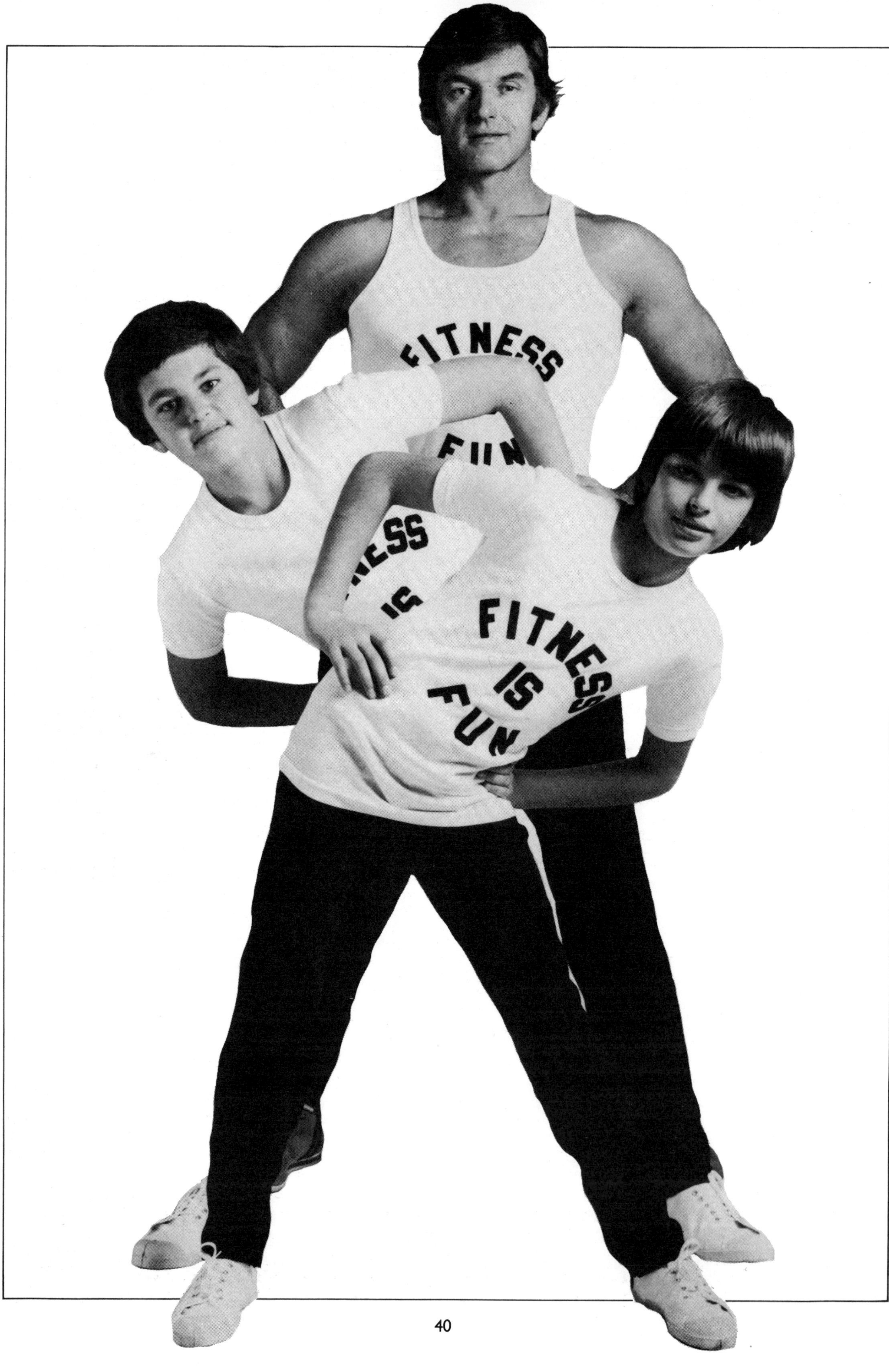
FITNESS
IS
FUN

Chapter 6

MAKE IT A FAMILY AFFAIR

Picture if you can a weightlifter or a body-builder. My bet is you'll have one of two images. In the first, your muscleman is tucked away in dim corners of an unlikely gymnasium, sweat pouring down his face and body as he grunts, groans, and twists himself into impossible attitudes in pursuit of his ideal. He's a loner, a dedicated masochist in the cause of the body beautiful, and he suffers self-imposed tortures way beyond the endurance of the ordinary fellow. If he's not that, he's a thick, beaming knucklehead of a chap, surrounded by adoring females, with hyper-bulging muscles and no conversation.

Naturally the truth is somewhere between the two. Body-builders are people, like anyone else, with better-than-average physiques (or a desire to improve). Weight training can be a lonely business, but, as I found out when I got married, it can also be fun.

At the start of my marriage, when Norma and I were struggling to make ends meet, I was also struggling to become a champion weightlifter. I couldn't afford expensive equipment, nor pay for training courses. But something had to be done, so together we turned Norma into my trainer. First, I took her to all the weightlifting competitions I could, and told her everything I knew. She quickly learned to spot when an exercise was not being completed properly; when a weight was being lifted incorrectly, when the posture was wrong. And then, at home, she began to train me. As I went through the routines, night after night, she would criticise, correct and advise me where I was going wrong; and in those two or three years I reached the peak of my strength and fitness.

This 'togetherness' continued when we had a family. We found exercising together was not only good for us as a family, but it helped keep everyone of us really fit.

Norma has exercised religiously after having had each of the children and I swear that she has a better figure now than when I married her. I train to keep in shape all the time but work harder when I have a film or TV part coming up. I never push the kids but they always want to join in and as a result they feel and look better. I even use the kids as weights, using them to make the exercises more difficult for myself. It all adds to the enjoyment of exercising and when we say, 'Fitness is Fun', we really mean it.

Try it for yourselves.

Anyone can join in.

Family Exercise Programme No I

1. Side bends

Stand upright, feet astride, hands comfortably on hips.

Keeping the hips still, bend your body as far as possible to the right, bending your right knee slightly as you do so.

Return briefly to the upright position and then bend your body to the left still keeping the hips as still as you can. Bend the left knee slightly.
Repeat 20 times.

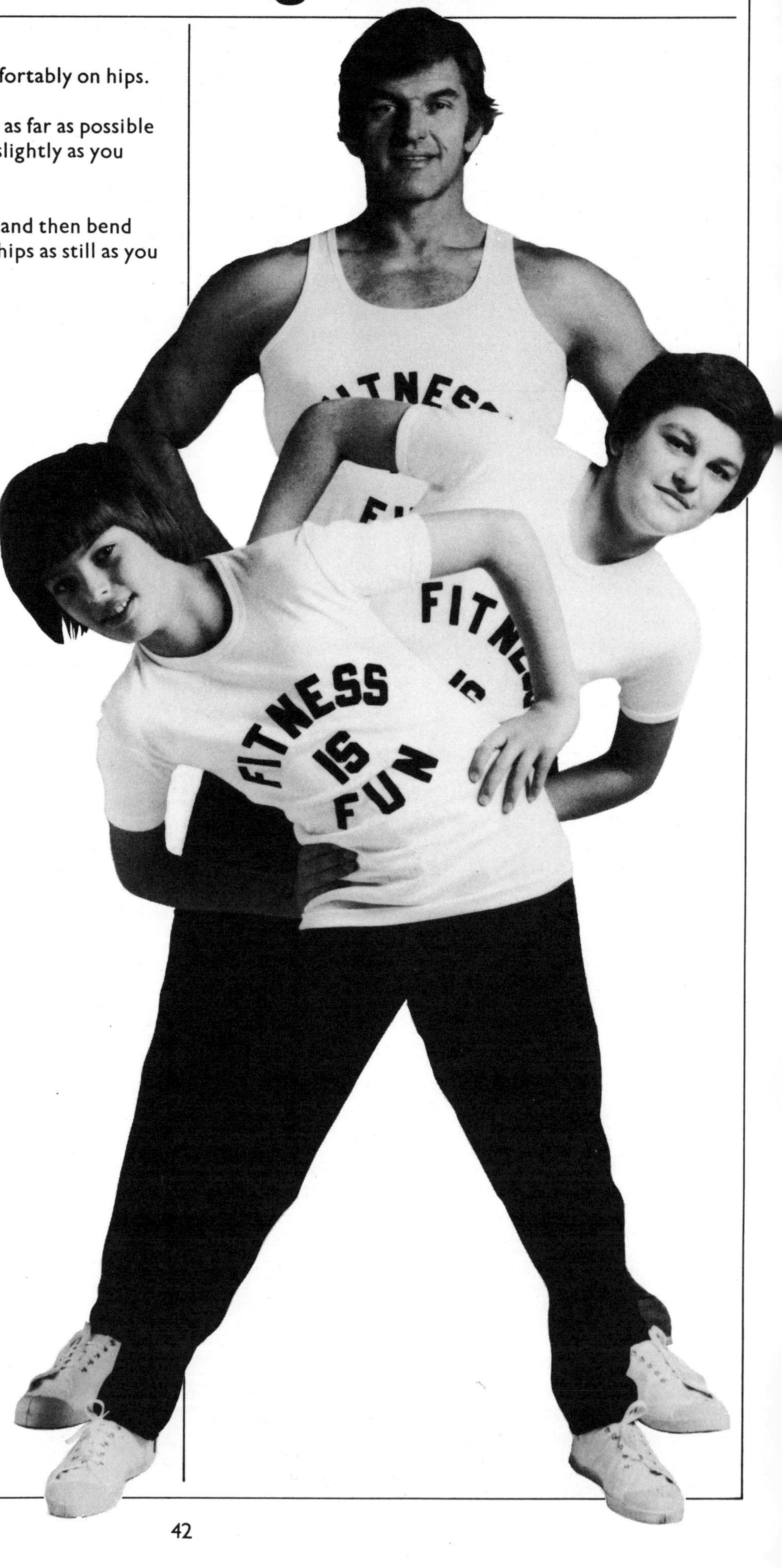

2. Free good mornings

Stand upright, feet astride, hands comfortably on hips.

Bend forward as far as you can go, keeping the hips still.

Come to the upright position, as you do so push your hips forward with your hands and arch your back. Repeat 20 times.

NB The object eventually is to make your shoulders touch your knees.

As a variation, hold your hands in front of you and touch the floor on the down bend. As you grow more supple, you reach further in front of you.

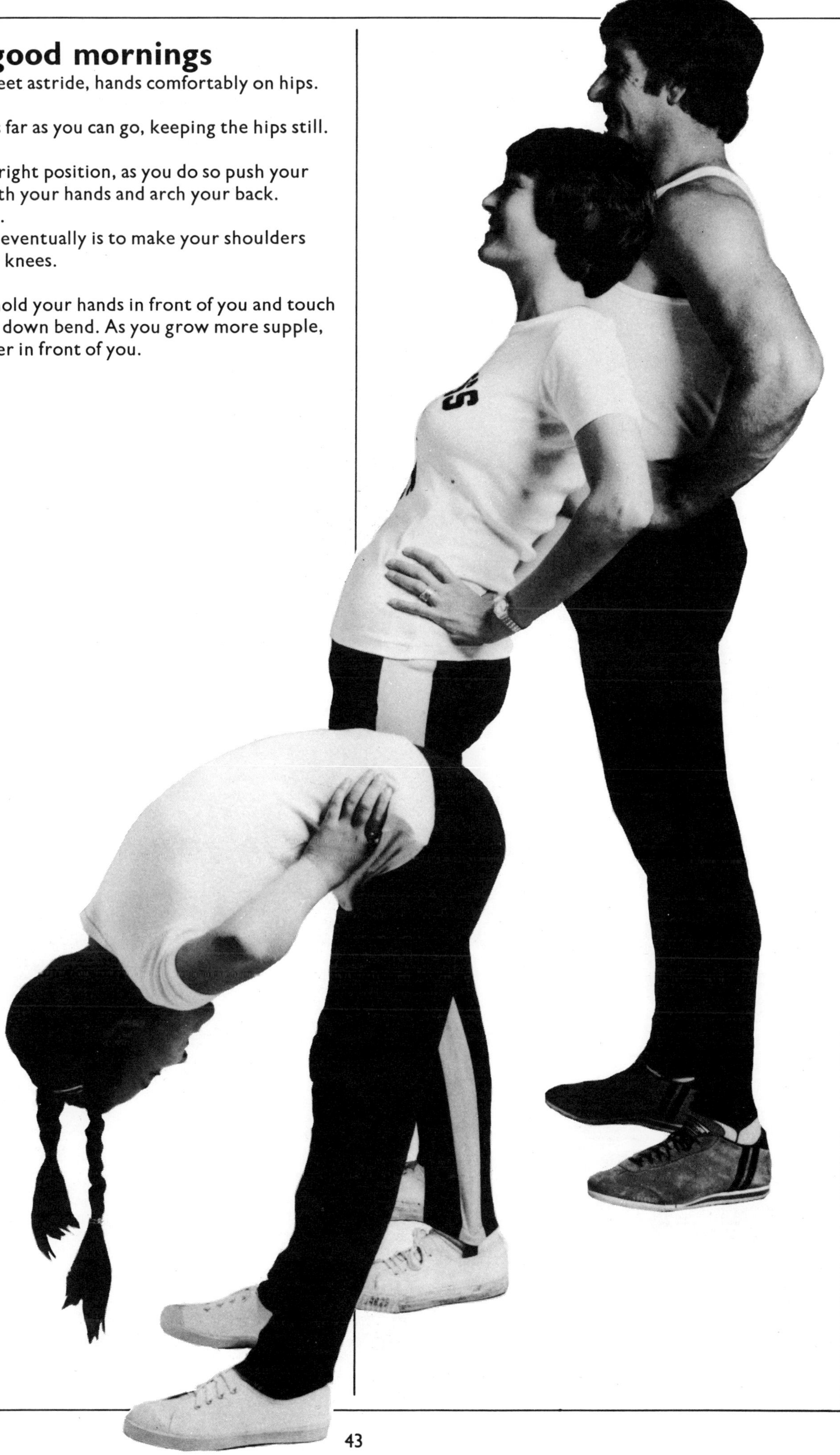

3. Seat stretch

Sit on floor with legs stretched out straight, as widely spaced as you can get them. Elbows on thighs, arms relaxed.

Rock forwards as far as you can, keeping your arms still. Repeat 20 times.

IN THE PICTURE OF RACHEL AND ME WE SHOW A VARIATION WHERE YOU ROCK FORWARD WITH YOUR ARMS OUTSTRETCHED TRYING TO REACH AS FAR FORWARD AS POSSIBLE.

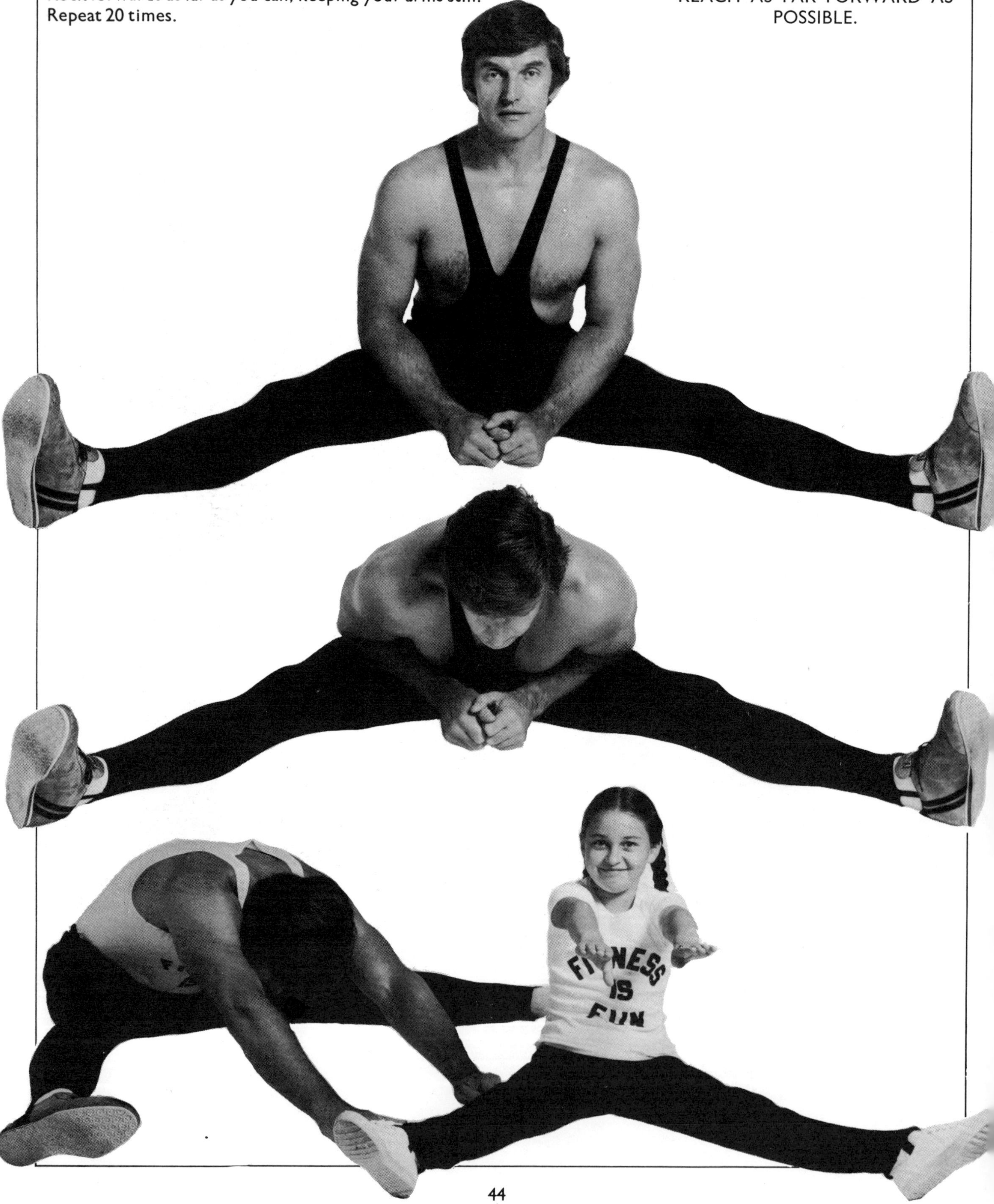

4. Seat turn

Sit on floor with legs stretched widely. Face down left leg, place right hand on left knee and stretch left hand towards left toe.

Rock forwards and back until your nose touches your knee.
Repeat 10 times.

Reverse position to face right leg. Place left hand on right knee and stretch right hand towards right toe.

Rock forwards until your nose touches your knee.
Repeat 10 times.

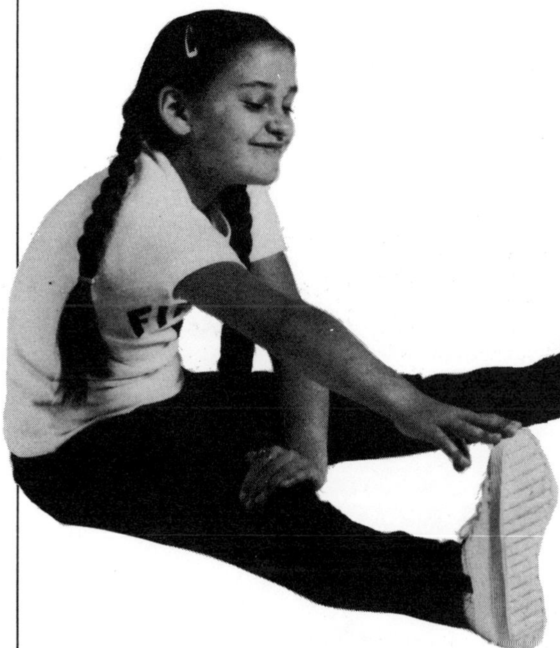

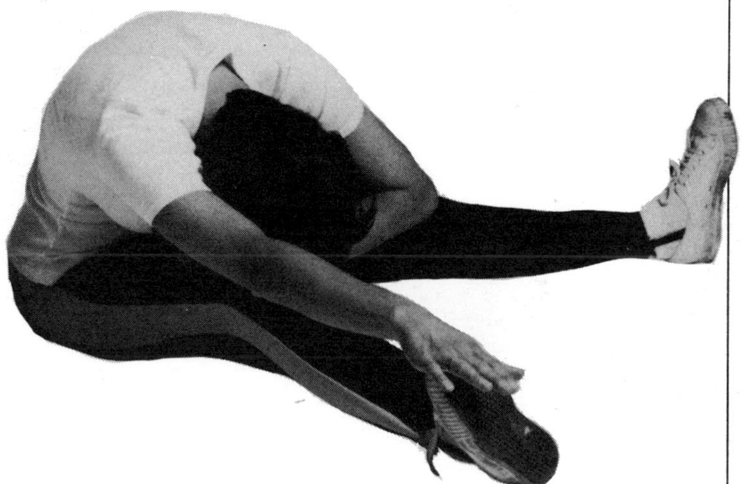

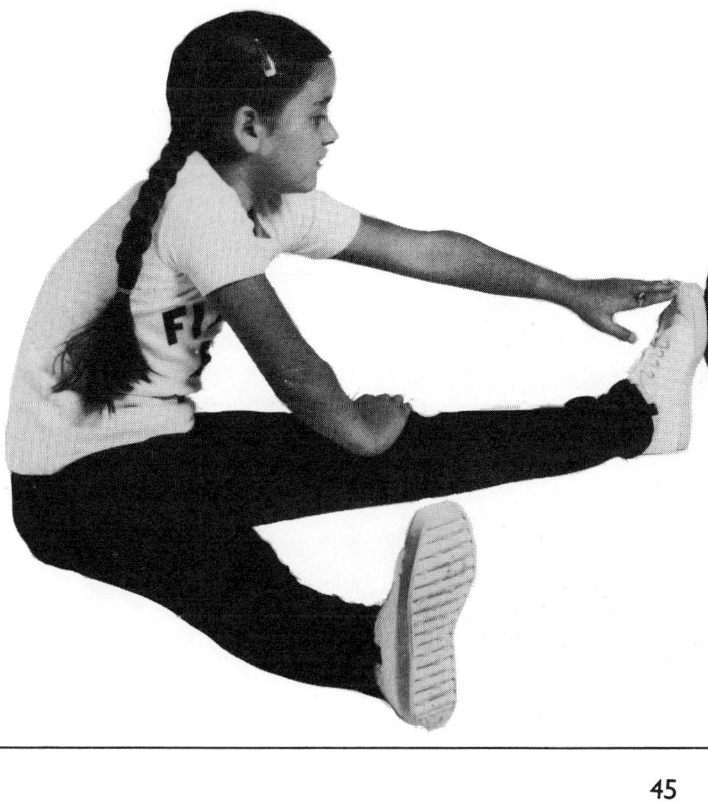

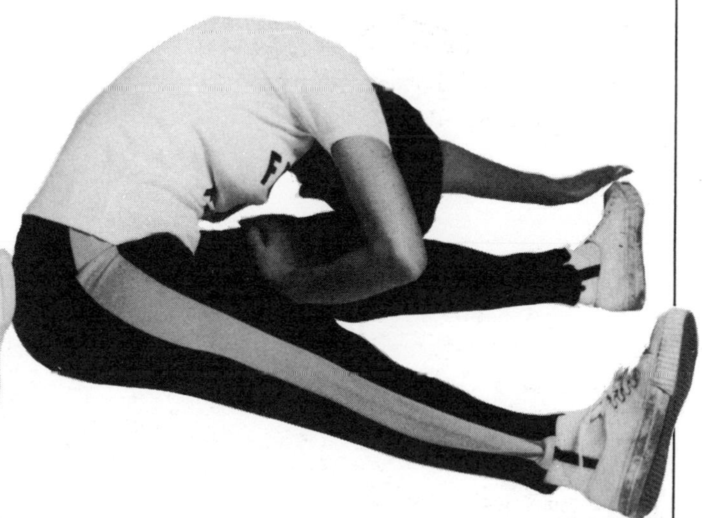

5. Leg raises

Lie flat on floor on back. Clasp your hands together under your buttocks.

Raise your legs, keeping them straight and pointing toes, to about 60 degrees.
Repeat 20 times.

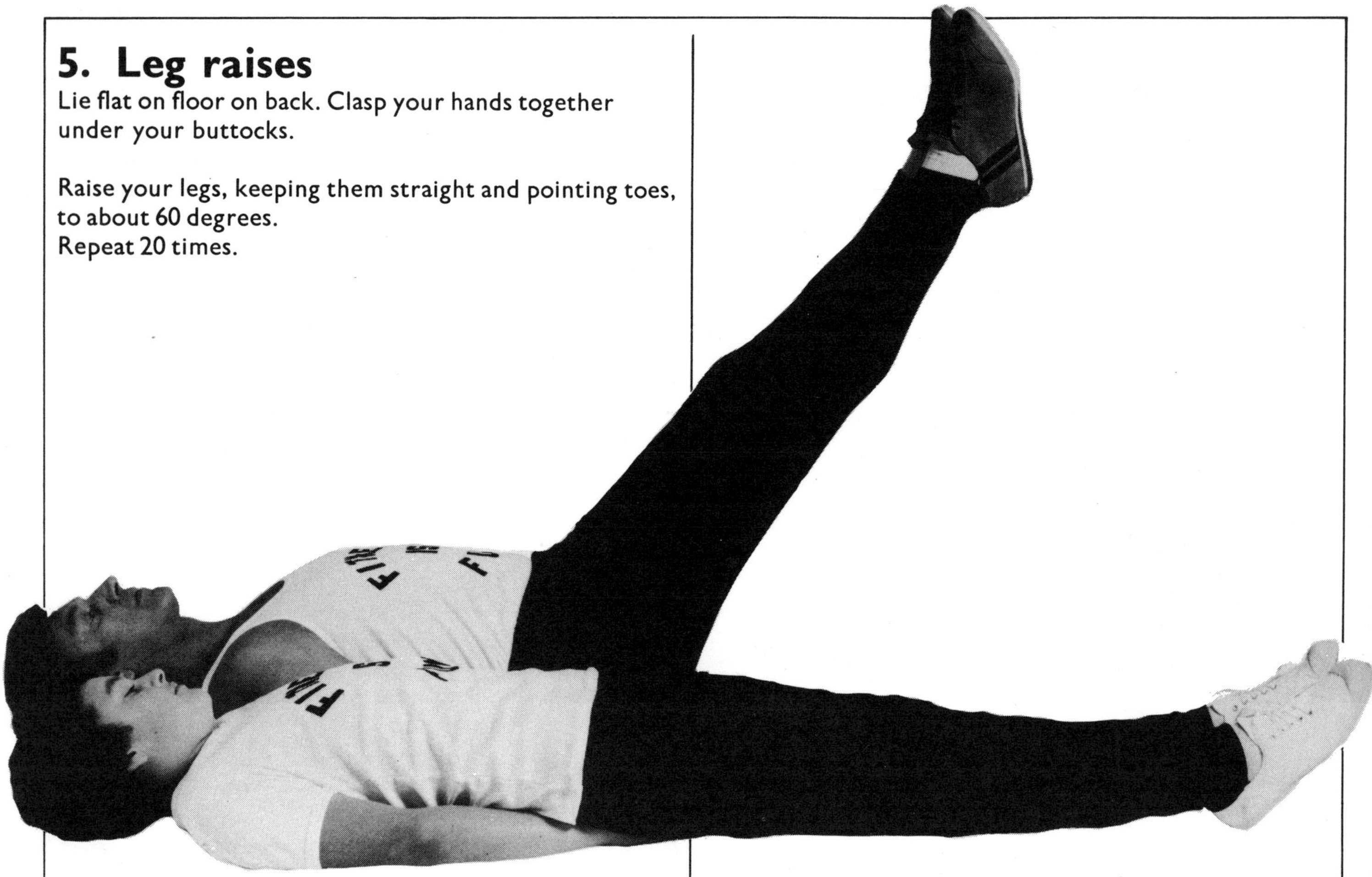

6. Half sit-ups

Lie flat on floor, legs straight, hands on thighs.

Using stomach muscles alone, come up to a half-sit position of 45 degrees. Bend knees slightly.
Return slowly to floor, without stopping, return to 45 degrees position.
Repeat 10 times, working up to 20.
NB At no time in this exercise are the stomach muscles relaxed.

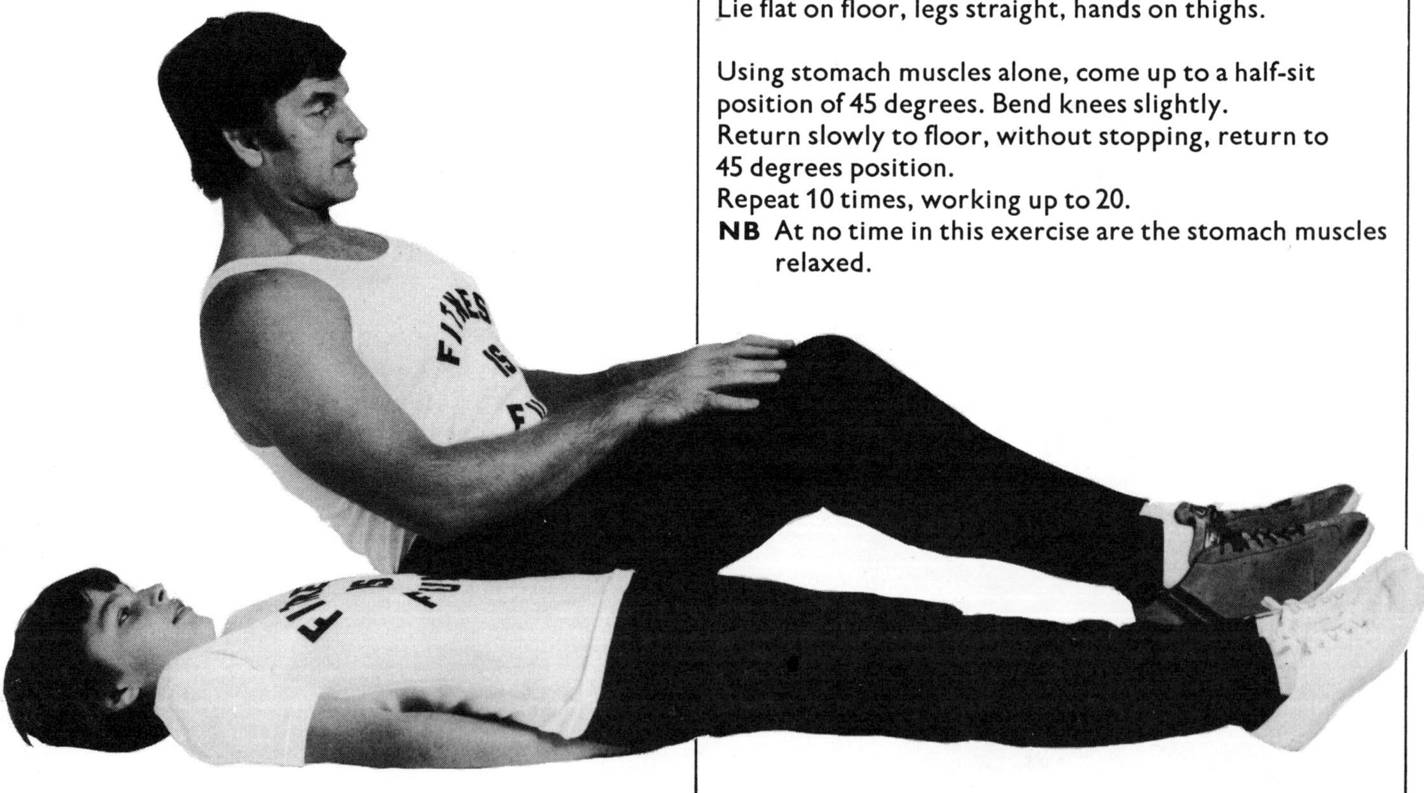

7. Waist-aways

Lie on back on floor, hands clasped under your bottom.

Bend knees and bring them up together under your chin.

Thrust legs out together to about 45 degrees.

Lower slowly to start position.
Repeat 20 times.
NB Whole exercise is done slowly.

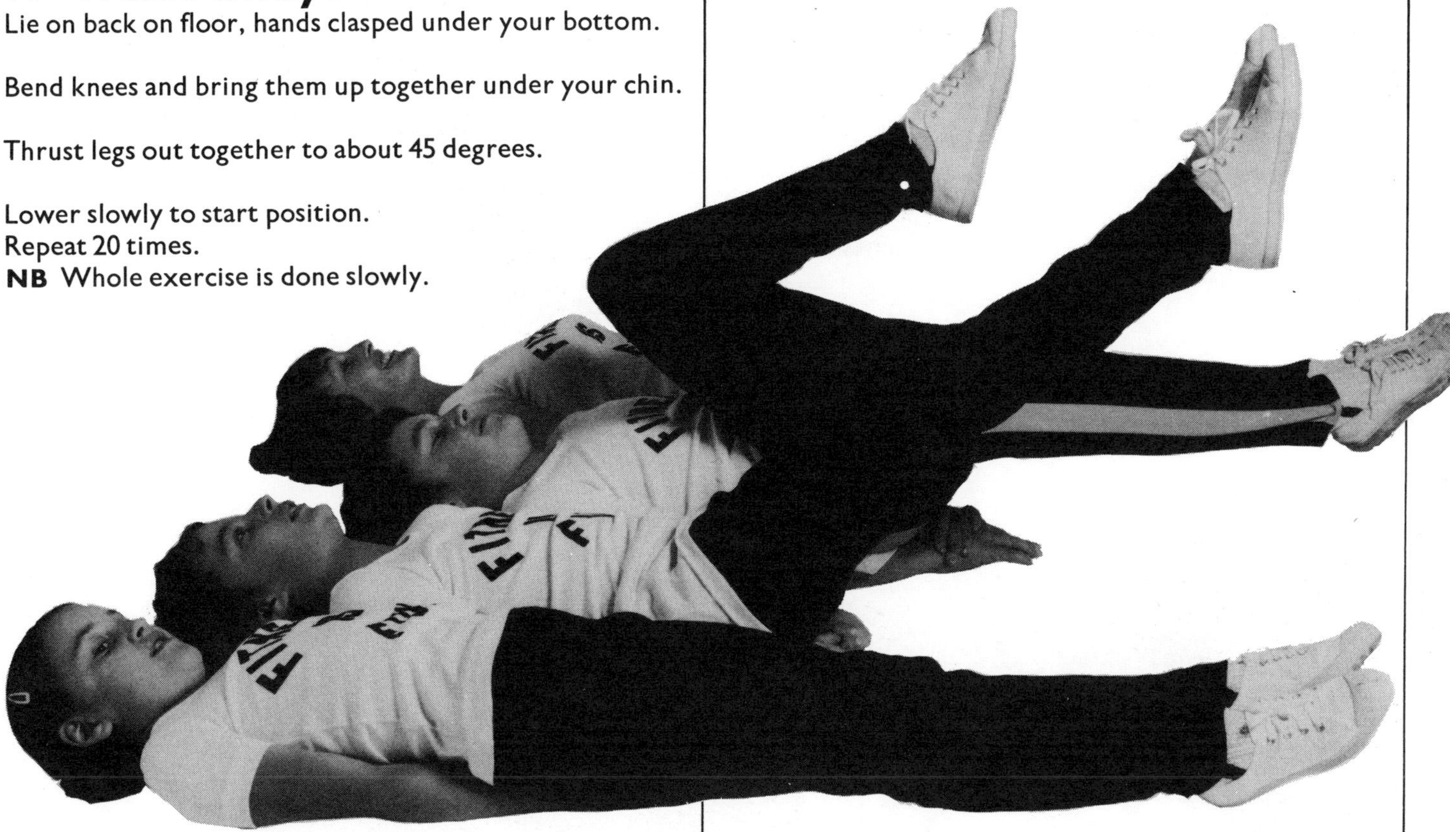

8. Scissors

Lie on back on floor, legs straight, hands clasped together under your bottom.

Raise legs 18 inches off floor and then criss-cross one under the other in scissors movement, keeping legs straight.
Repeat 50 times.

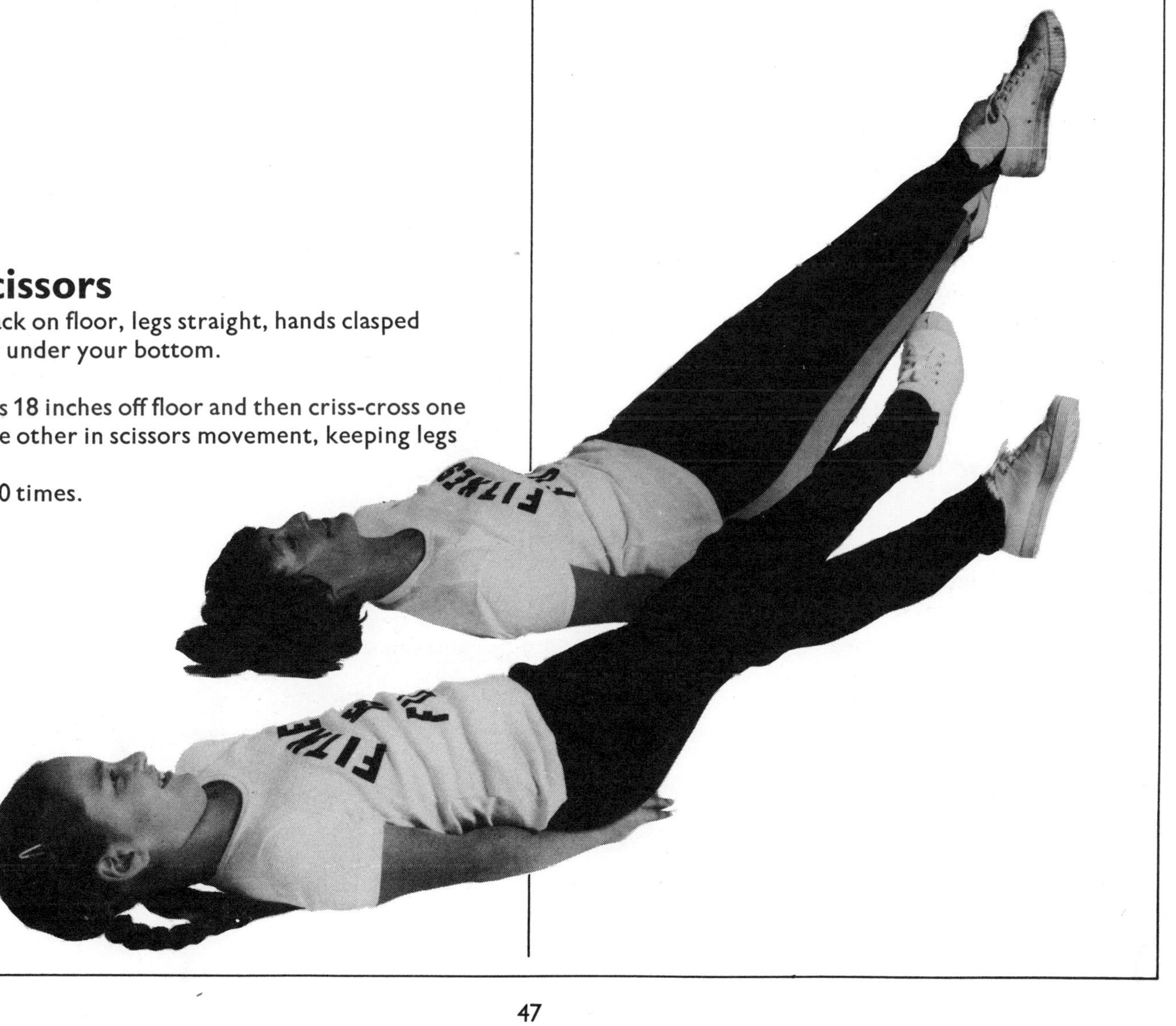

9. Side leg raises

Lie on right side, head in right hand leaning on right elbow. Place left hand on floor in front of you.

Raise left leg slowly, high as you can.
Return to original position.
NB Make sure you do not shift from your side, otherwise the exercise loses its purpose.
Repeat 20 times; turn over and repeat 20 times on left side.

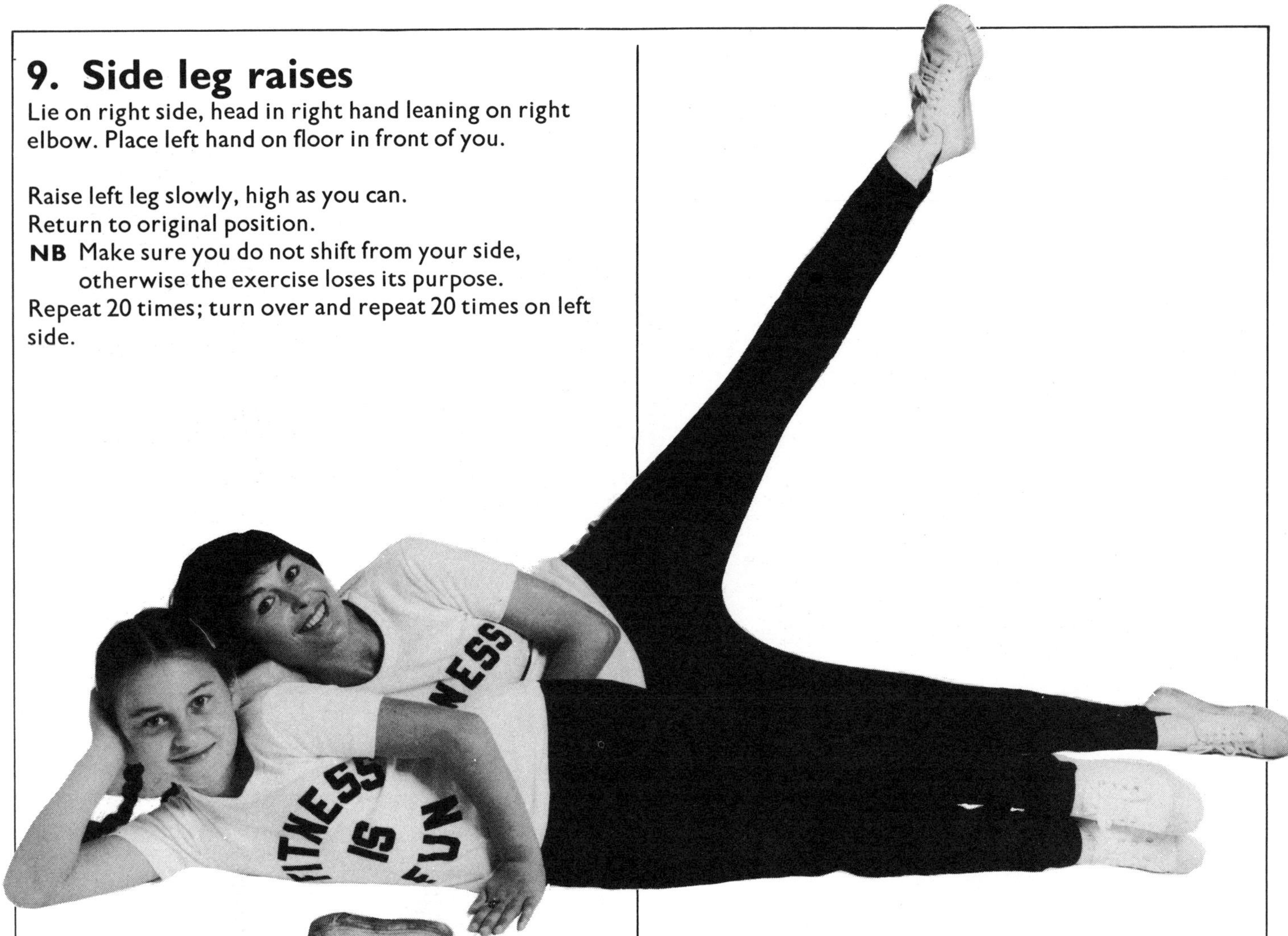

10. Hip kicks

Take up position on all fours.

Bring right knee up under chin.

Kick right leg backwards and upwards.
Hold position then lower leg slowly back under your chin.
Repeat 20 times with each leg.
NB Exercises 9 and 10 are particularly suitable for women, who are advised to leave out Exercises 13 and 14 in this programme. If they wish, men may leave out 9 and 10 and include 13 and 14. But the choice is optional.

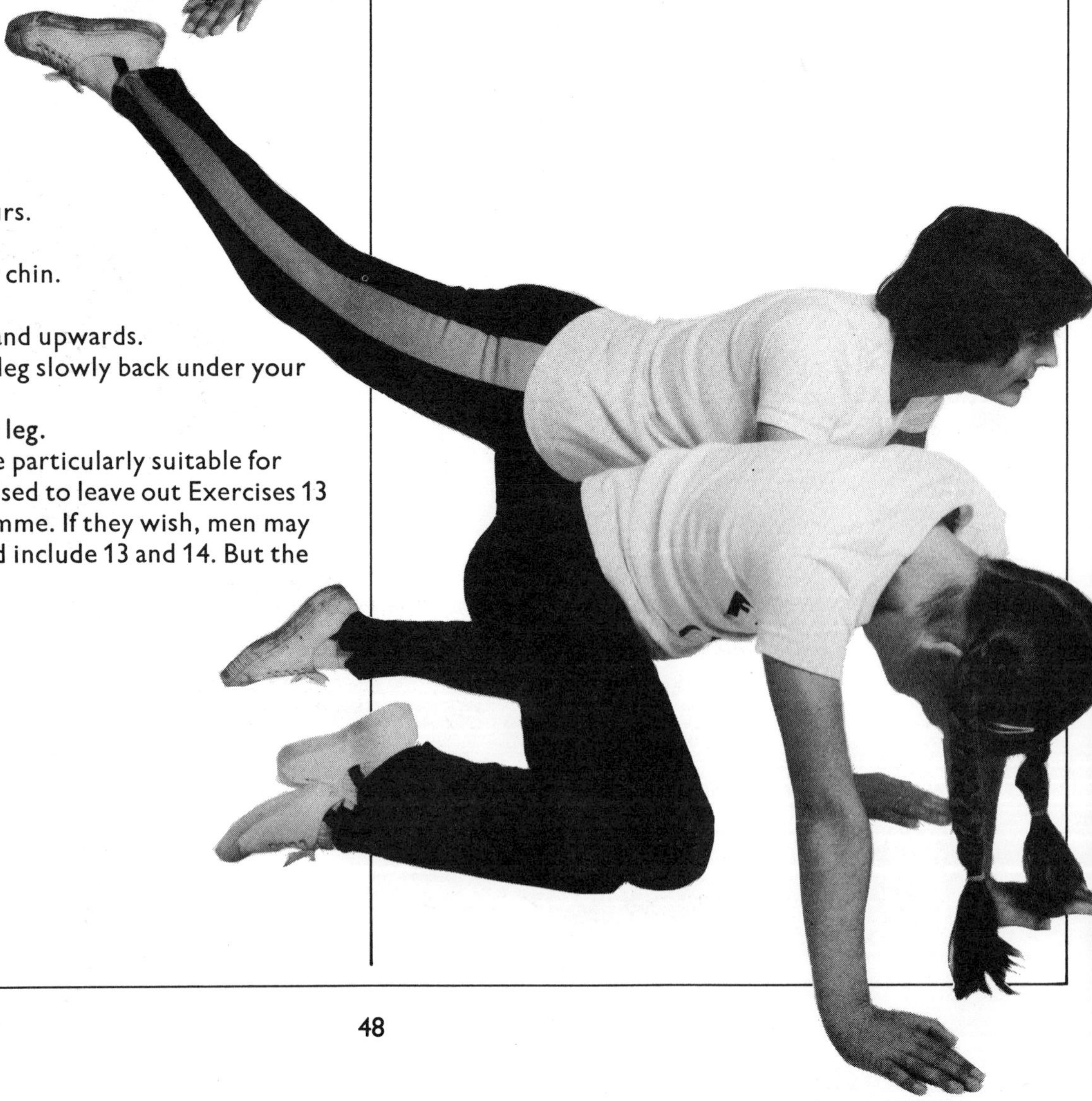

11. Press-ups

Lie face downward on floor, with hands at shoulder position.

Keeping body stiff, push arms straight.

Bend arms slowly and lower body to floor.
Repeat 20 times.

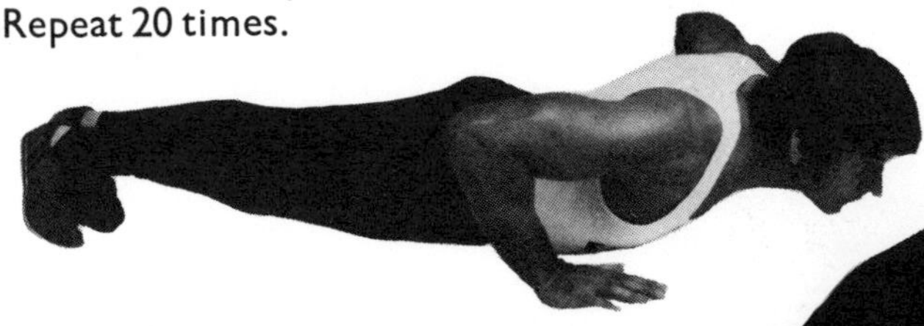

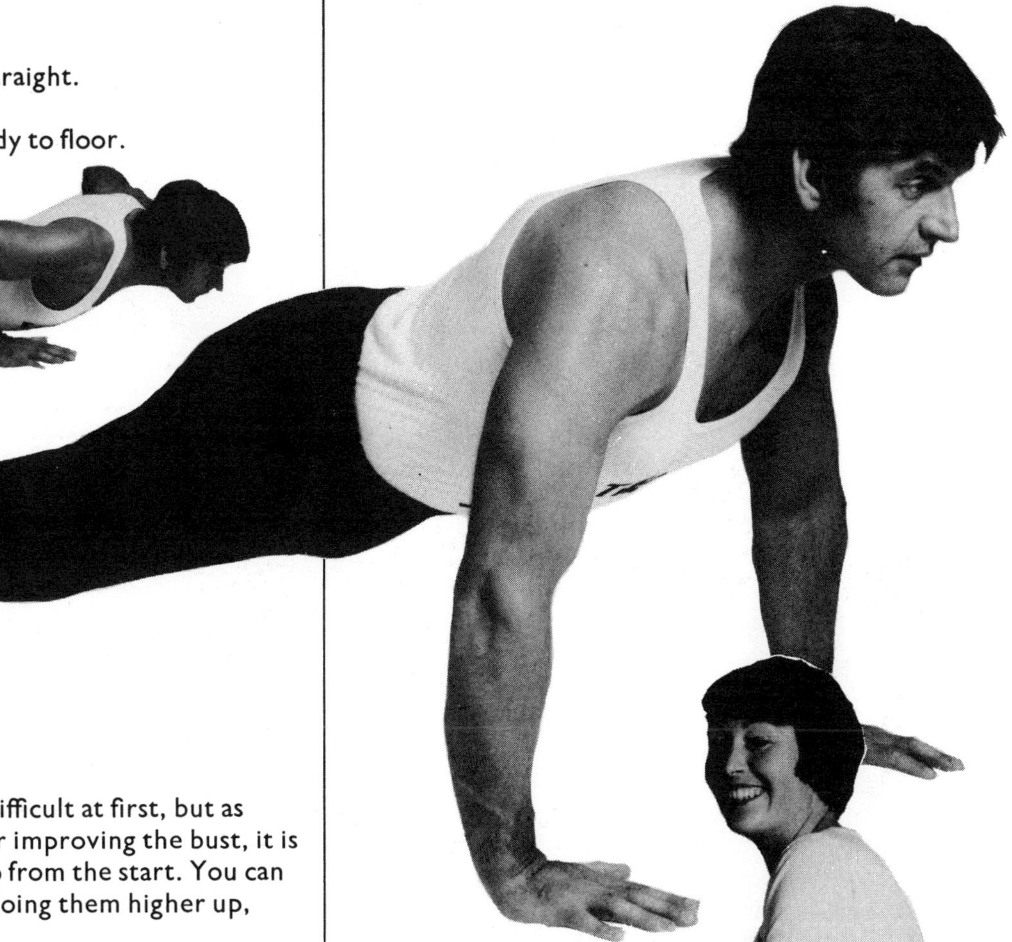

NB Many girls find press-ups difficult at first, but as this is a superb exercise for improving the bust, it is one they should try and do from the start. You can make press-ups easier by doing them higher up, using a table, like this

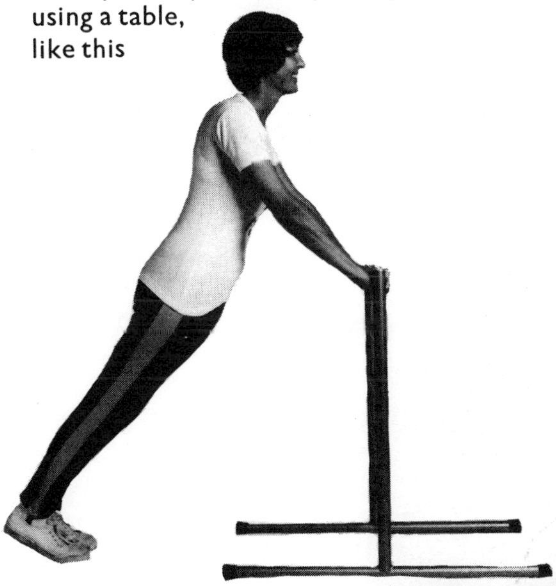

Or, if you find three 'sets' of 20 press-ups a doddle, you can step up the pressure; like this.

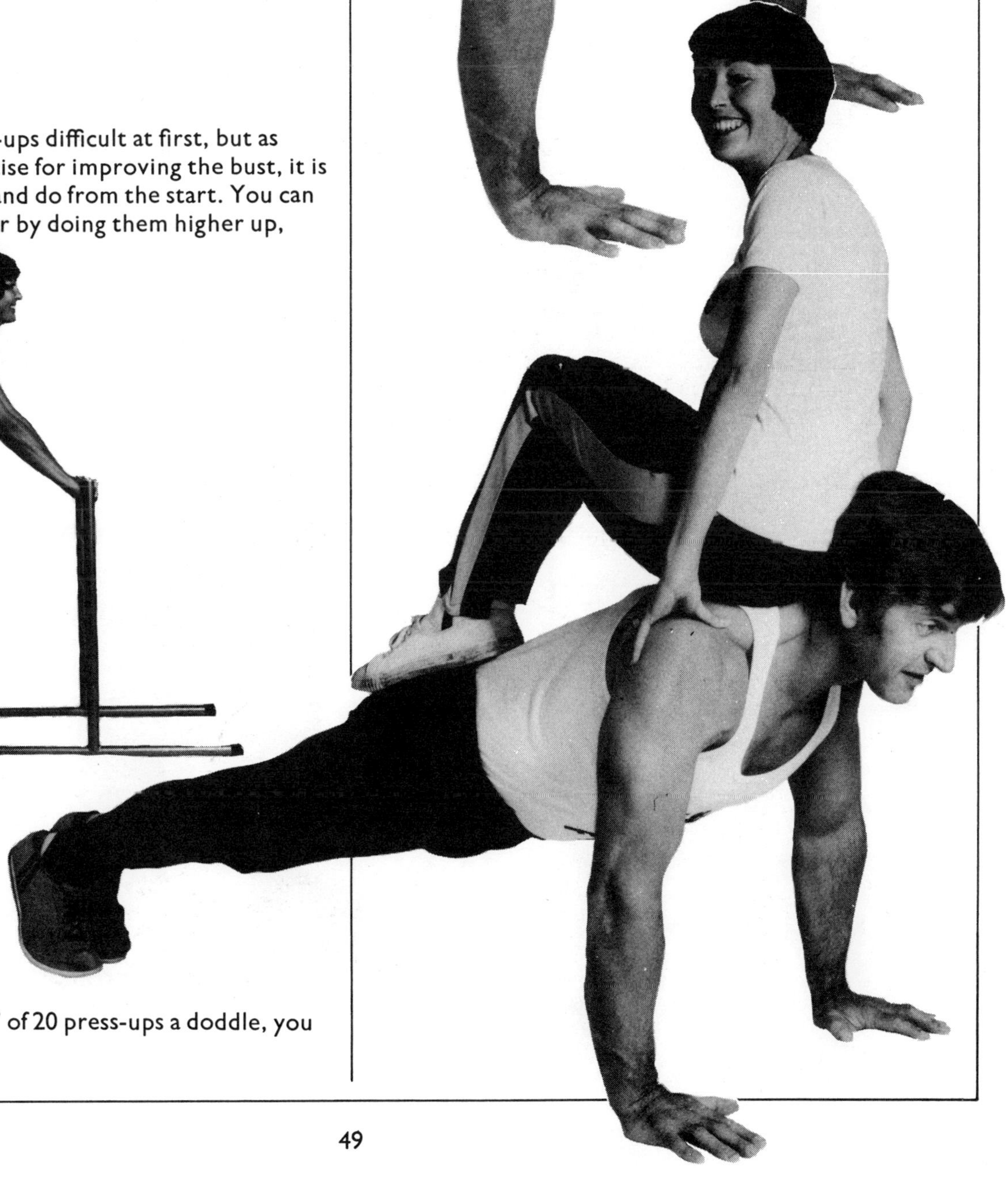

12. Flyers

Equipment: two light weights.

Stand with weight in each hand at arm's length at waist level.

Take deep breath and swing arms backwards and upwards to shoulder level, forcing the shoulders back. Repeat 20 times.

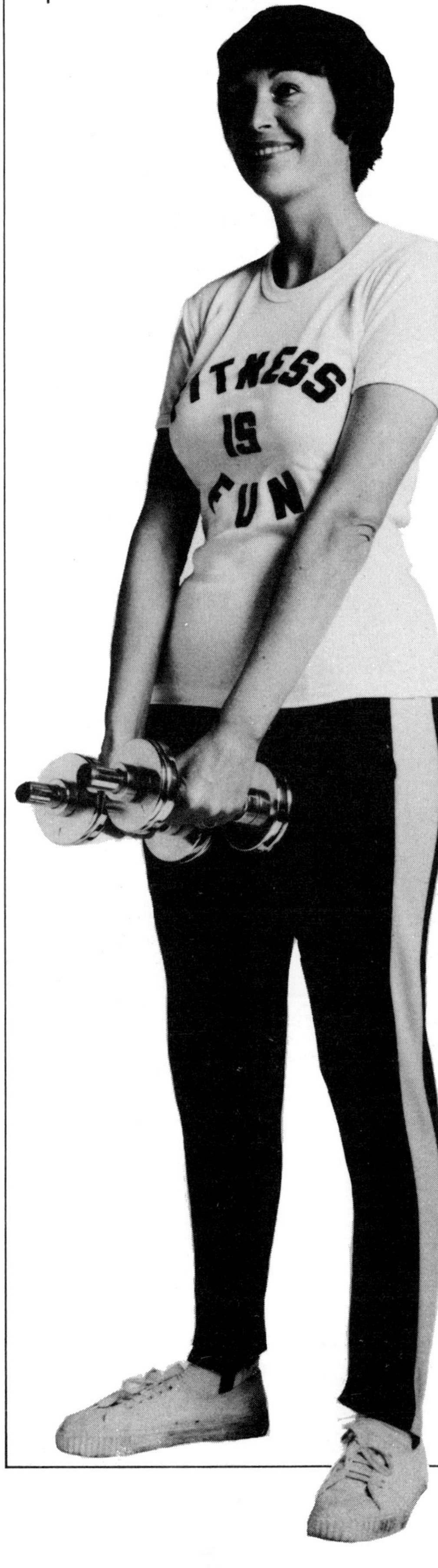

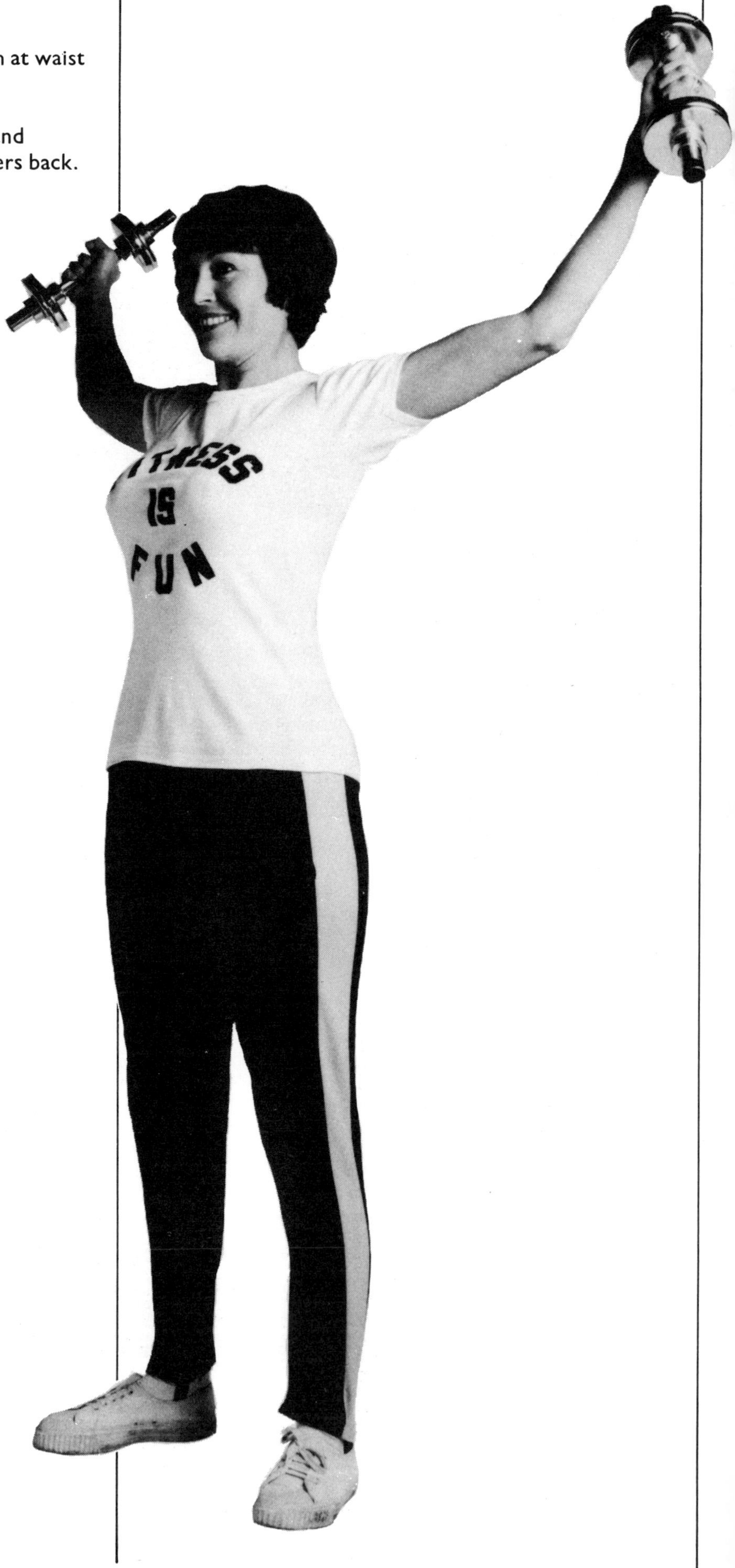

13. Lateral raises

Equipment: two light weights.

Stand upright, feet 15–20 ins apart, with weight in each hand held at hip height in front.

Take a deep breath then raise weights sideways to shoulder level or slightly higher with palms downwards.
Try to keep arms straight.
Lower weights under control to start position.
Repeat 15 times.

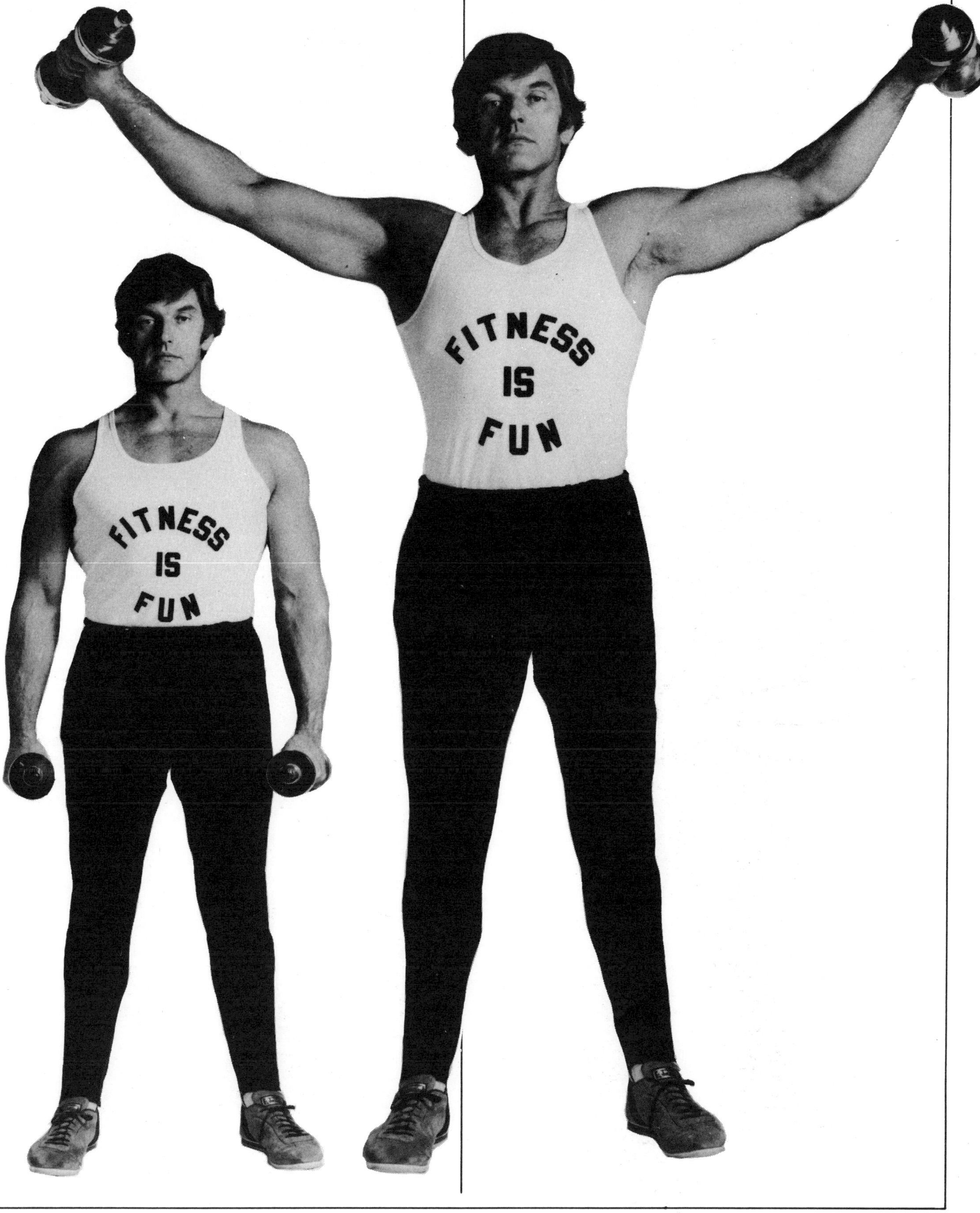

14. Curl and Press

Equipment: two light weights.

Stand upright, feet 15–20 ins apart, holding weight in each hand palms facing forwards.

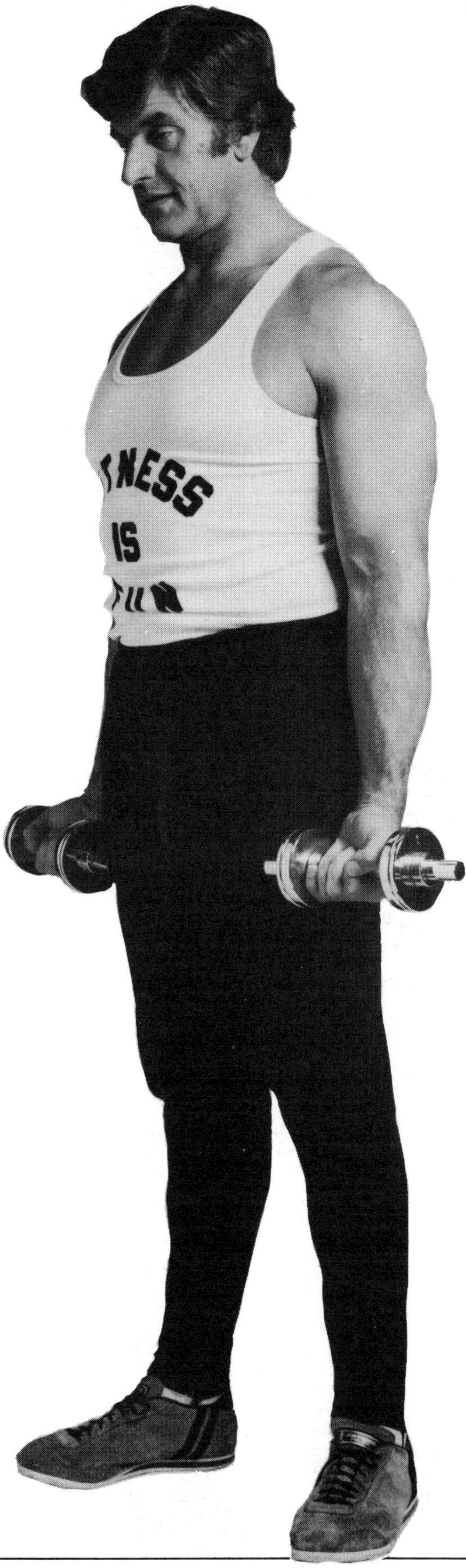

Bend arms at elbows and bring weights up to shoulder height, twisting weight at top so it faces end on.

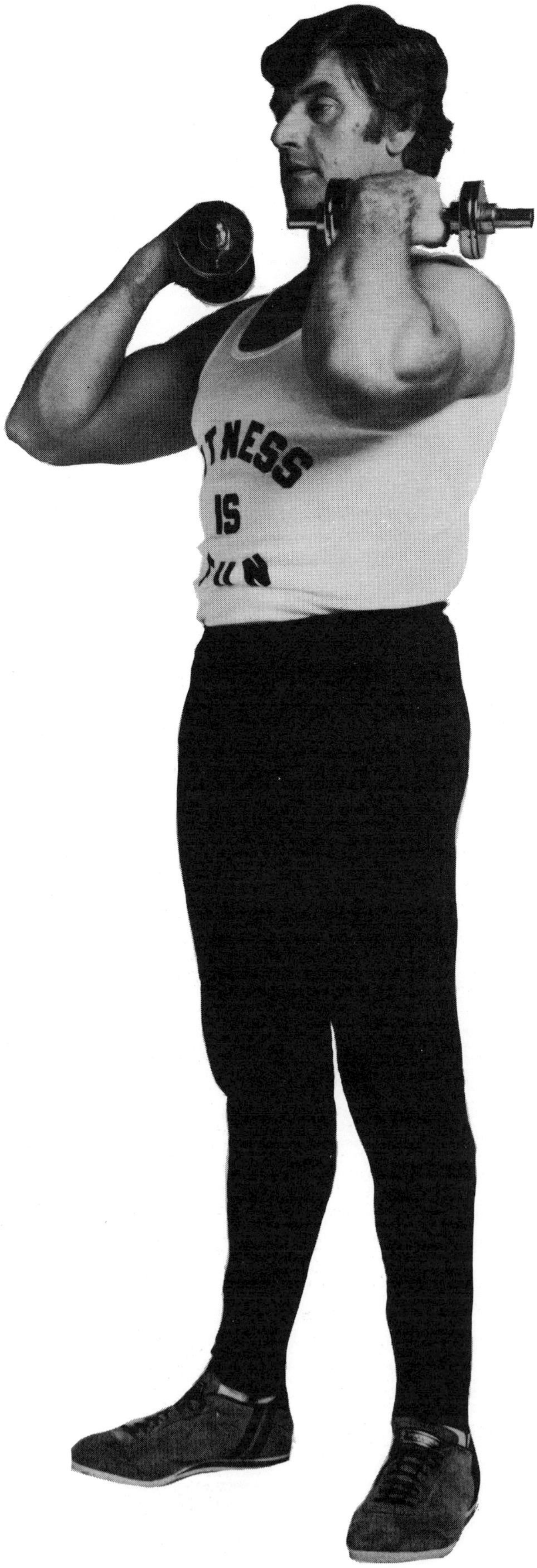

Push weight to arm's length over head.
Return weight to shoulders.
Turn weight so that knuckles point forwards.
Return weight to start position.
Repeat 15 times.

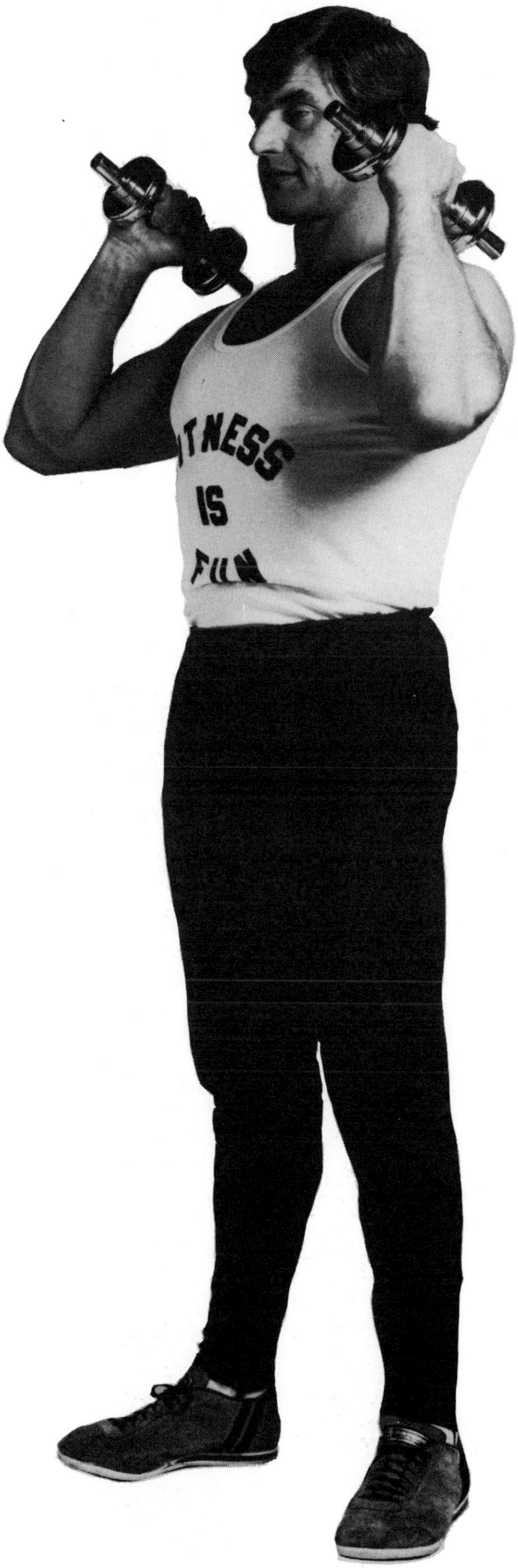

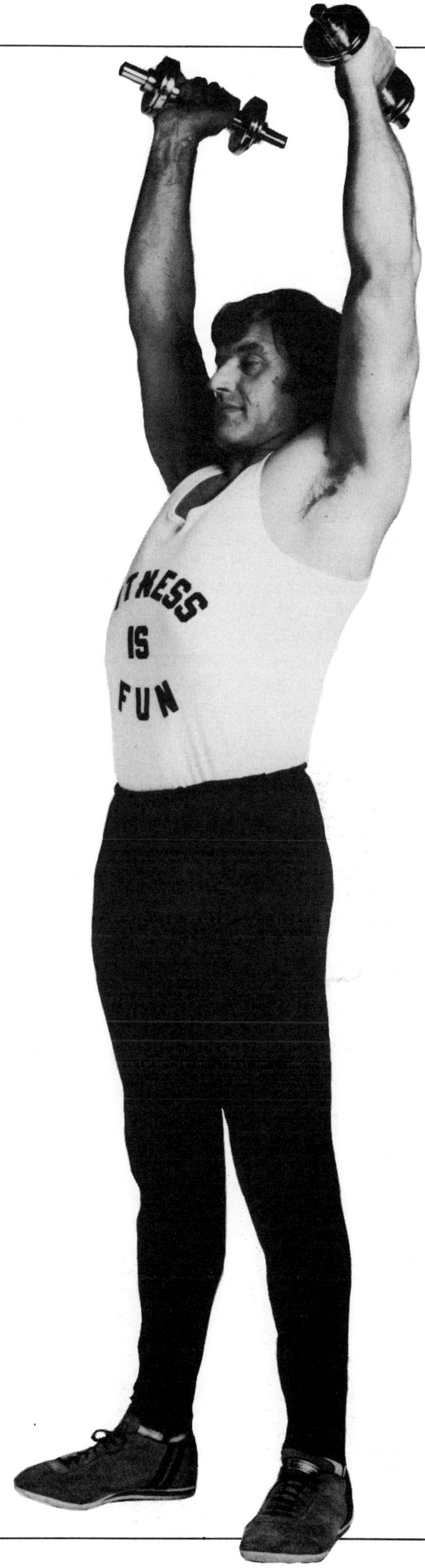

15. Free squats, or deep knee-bends

Stand with feet 15–20 ins apart. Fold arms across chest and lift elbows into Cossack dance position.

Bend knees to deep squat position, keeping elbows up to keep back straight.
Return to start position.
Start at 20 times and work up to 50. If you're not puffing and blowing and your heart's not thumping away, the exercise hasn't done you any good, so work up towards 100.

It's widely believed that muscle, when disused, turns to fat and that is why an ex-athlete is often flabby and out of condition. Muscle does *not* turn to fat. If you are a competitive athlete, you train like mad and you diet accordingly. You need the food to fuel your body. When you cease regular training, the usual thing is that you don't cut down on your diet accordingly. A footballer who retires and takes on a pub does three things. He stops training, carries on eating and starts drinking – and every whisky gives you more calories than a three-course meal. The formerly well-trained muscles atrophy (grow smaller) through under-use, and the fatty tissue develops around them. But athletes who control their diet and maintain their fitness after ceasing competition need never worry about their figures. Look at Dawn Fraser, the Australian wonder girl; or Sir Roger Bannister, the first four-minute miler. Or, if you like, me.

Muscle won't turn to fat; and fat won't turn to muscle.

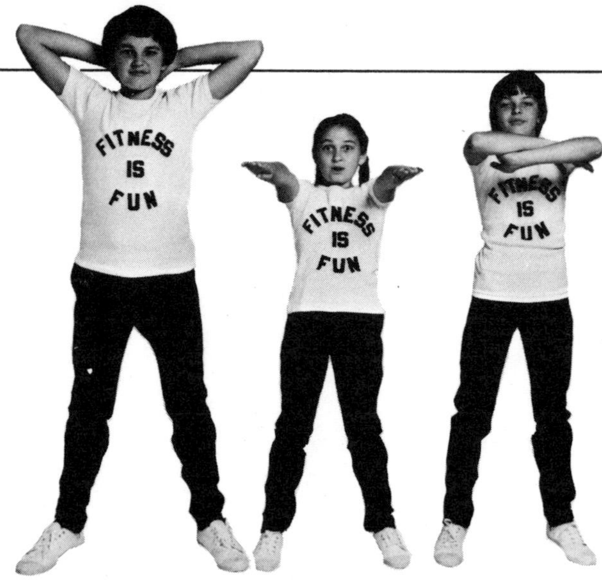

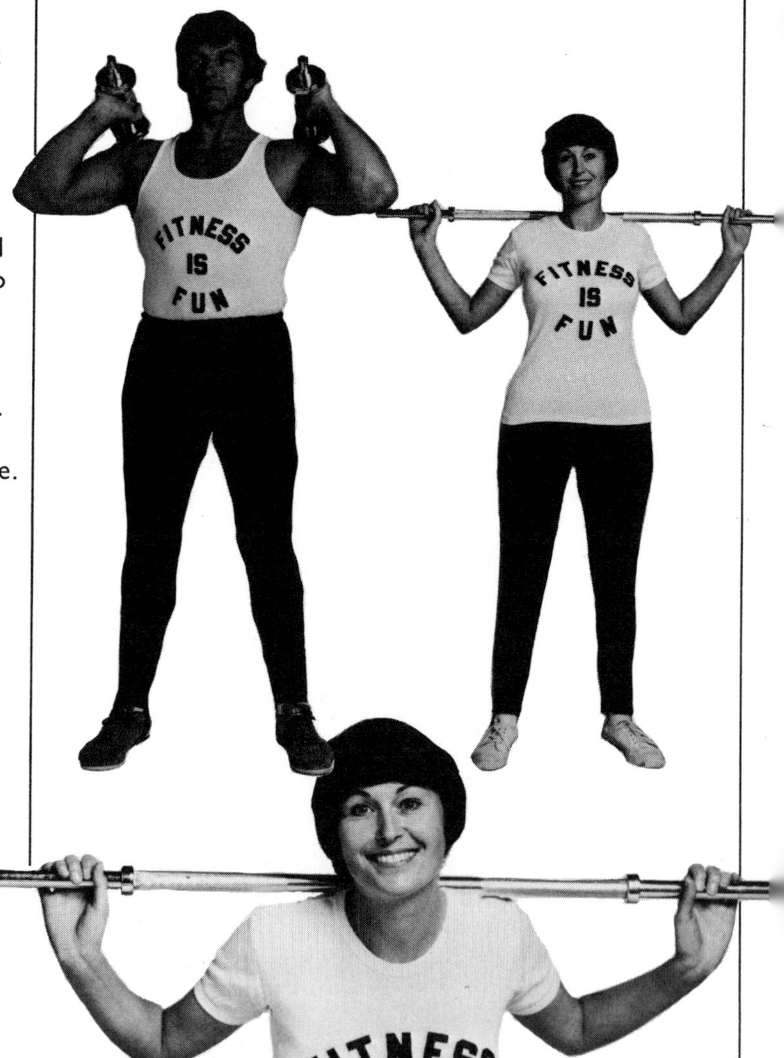

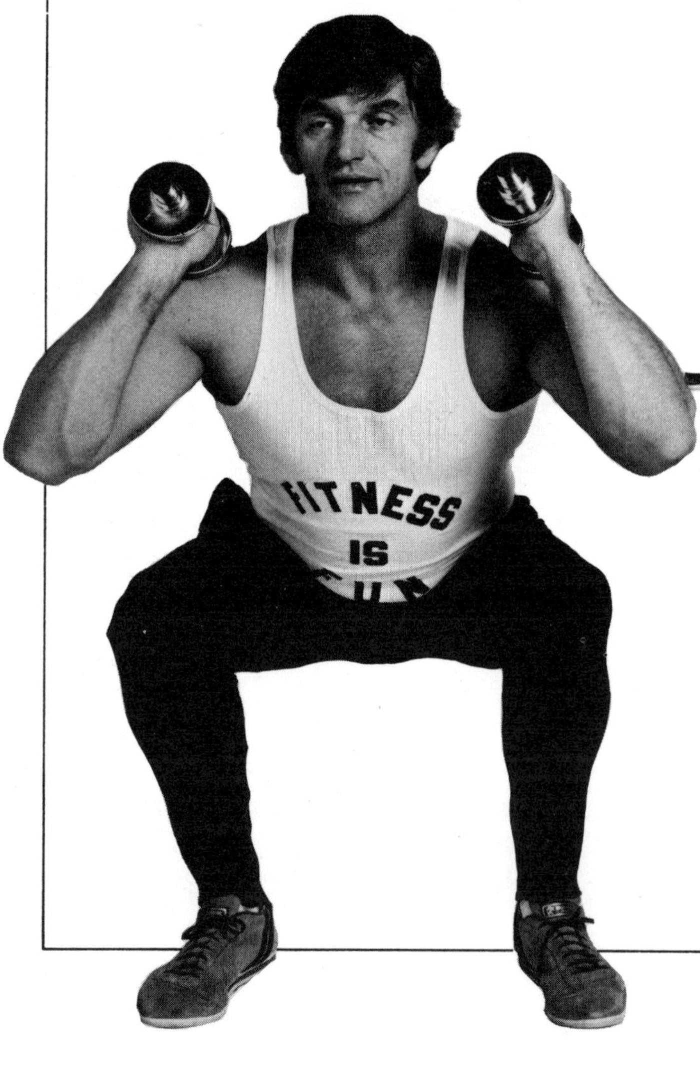

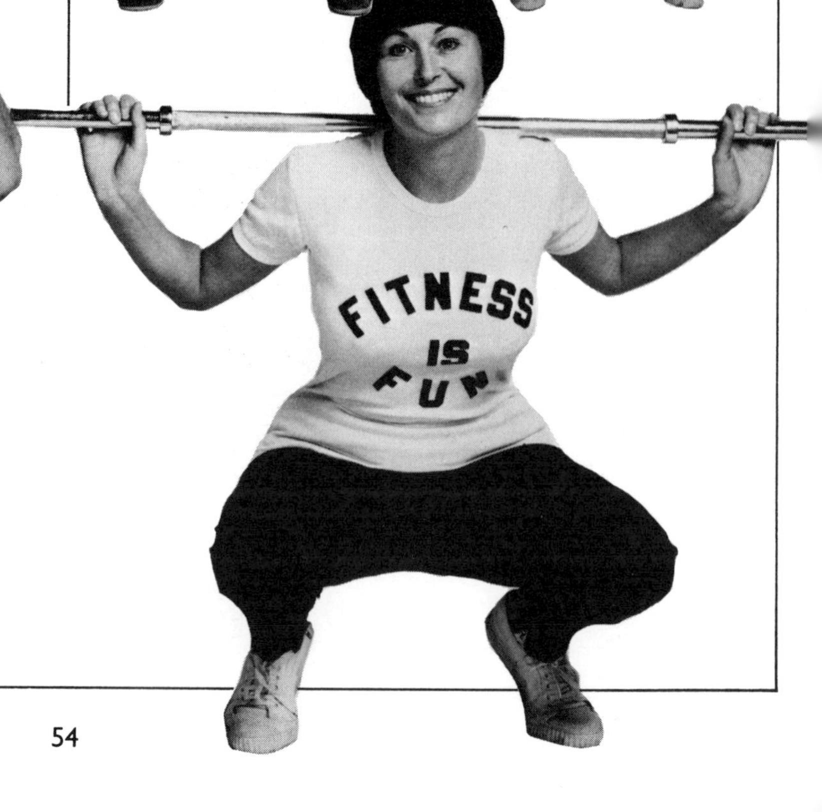

Family Exercise Programme No2

Let's try our second exercise programme, a little tougher this time. The first two exercises repeat Exercises 1 and 2 in Family Programme No 1
Then do Exercises 3 and 4 as follows;

3. Two-hands swing

Equipment: a heavy book, a house brick, or a 10 lb dumbell.

Stand up straight, feet comfortably astride, about 15–20 ins apart. Hold the weight with both hands, letting it hang at full arm's length.

Raise the weight to eye level with both hands.

As the weight descends, bend your knees into the deep squat position, keeping your back straight, feet flat on the floor.

Thrust upwards with legs and arms making weight travel through 180 degrees until it is above your head at full stretch, feet on tiptoe. Don't go too far.

NB If you do the exercise correctly, you will tend to overbalance forwards. This is counteracted by lowering the weight to the bottom squat position.

Repeat 20 times.

(That'll really get you at first! It is what we call a massive exercise, affecting every part of your body.)

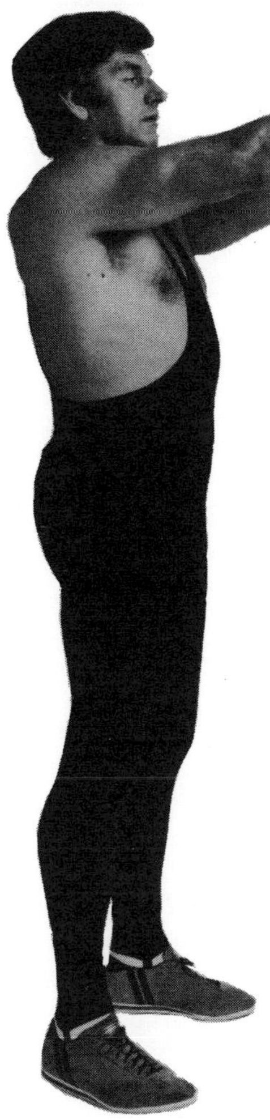

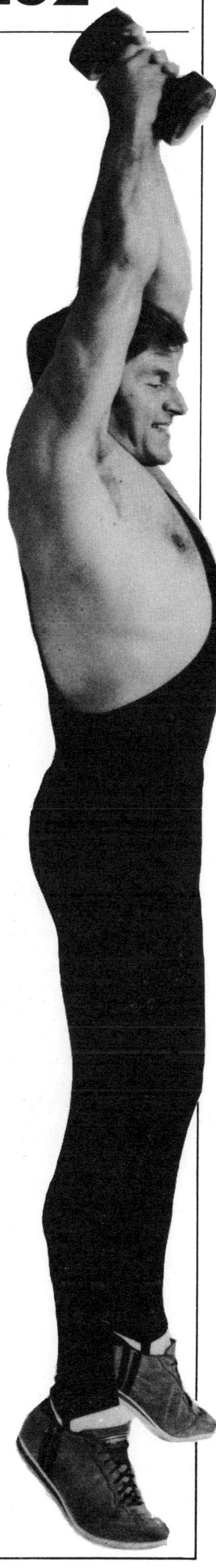

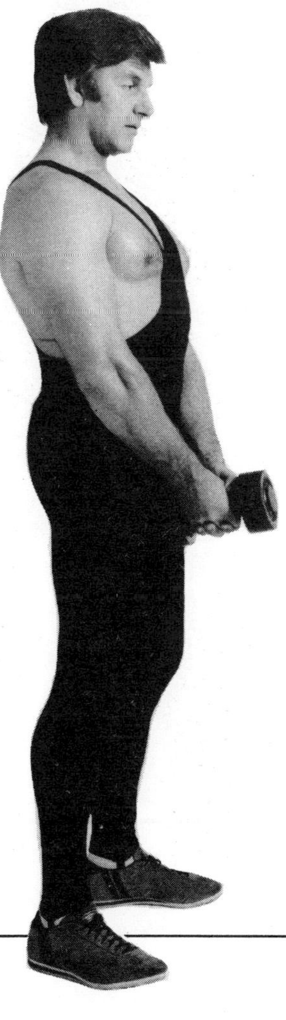

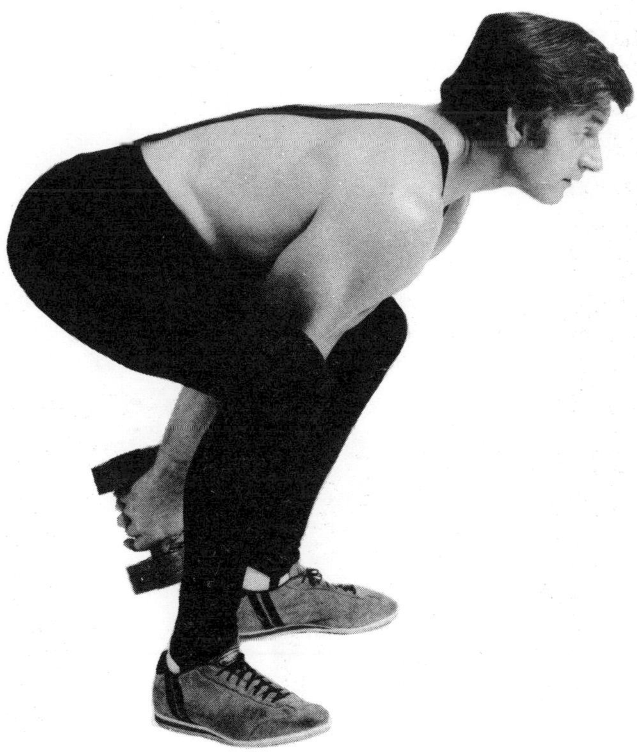

4. Squat and press

Equipment: two books, two bricks, or two dumbells.

Stand up straight, feet apart, holding a weight in each hand, resting one on each shoulder, with elbows forced upwards.

NB If you drop your elbows, the weight bends the back forwards into a bad exercising position.

Take a deep breath, sink into squat position, keeping elbows up.

Thrust upwards with knees. When you're three-quarters upright accelerate thrust and push both hands to arm's length above your head.

Steady. Lower arms slowly to shoulders and sink back into squat position, keeping elbows up.
Repeat 20 times.

If you never progress further than mastering these programmes and practising them regularly, I promise you will be a fitter, healthier, more active person.

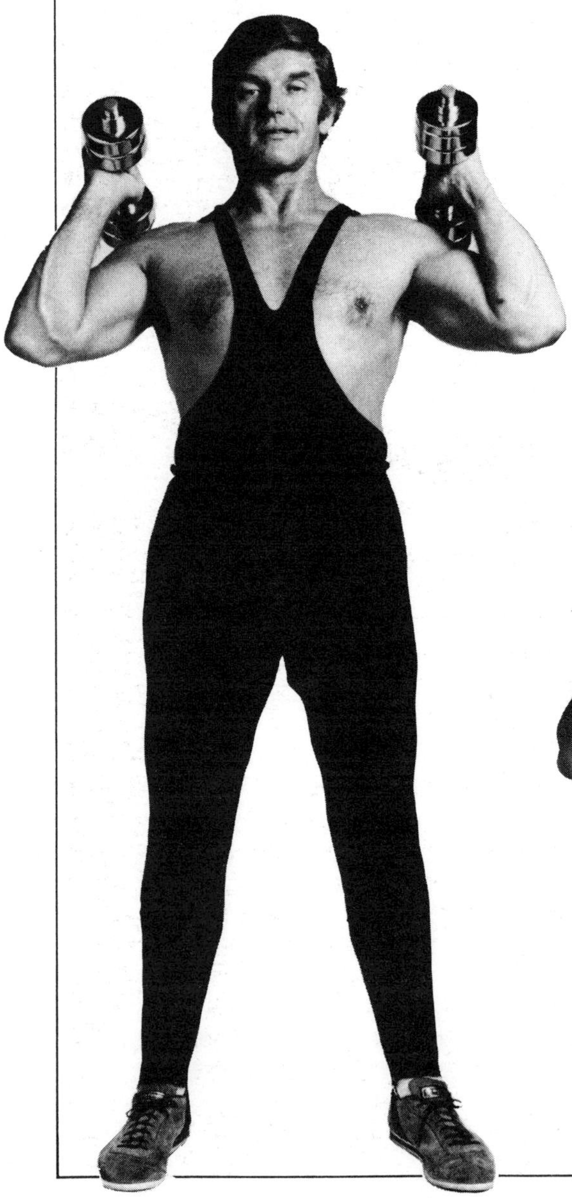

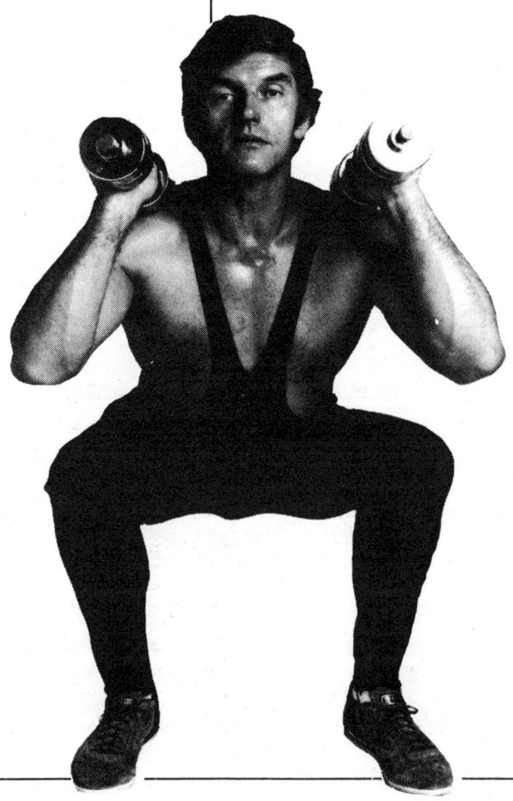

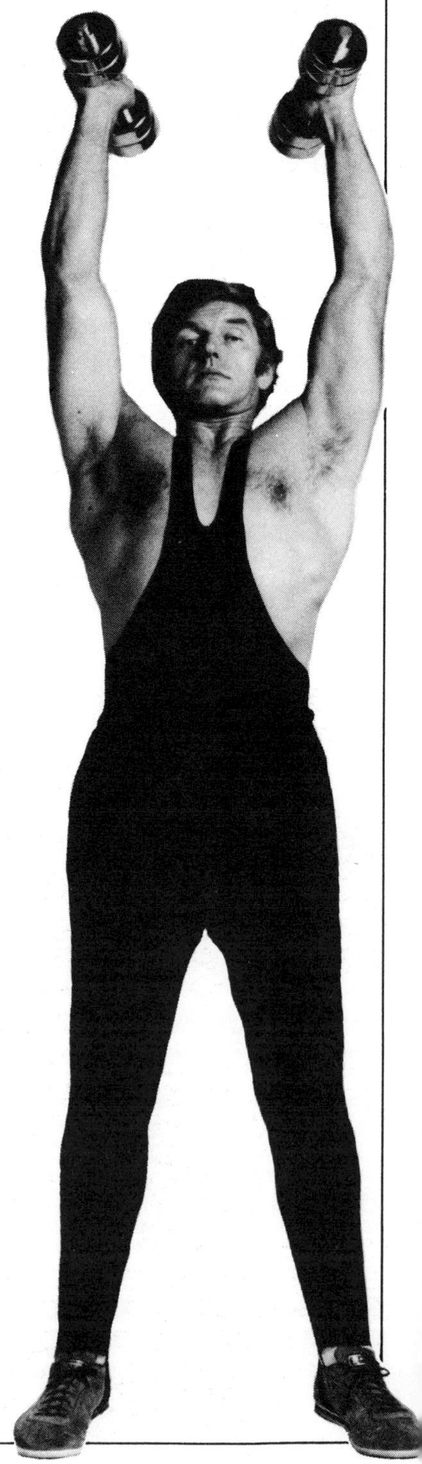

Chapter 7

HOW YOU FUNCTION

It's not much use messing about with your body if you don't know what you're doing. It would be like employing a bodger mechanic to tune your Maserati. But if you know the basic whys and wherefores you'll find that not only will you get more enjoyment out of your exercise programme but you'll also get a better understanding of your 'inner self'.

Everybody wants to improve himself. The fact that you're reading this book proves that you want to improve just that little bit more than the next person. The requirements for physical improvement are a desire to get fit and stay fit; proper training, a sound body to start with and the knowledge of how your body is going to set to work to convert your physical efforts into a new, physically improved person.

The SKELETON is the body framework on which we are formed. Within it the vital organs that make our bodies work are housed. Our skeleton enables us to stand up straight, and protects the vital organs such as the brain, heart and lungs.

JOINTS are where the bones meet so that the body may move this way or that; they are really like hinges but they cannot move of their own accord and need a motivating power, which is supplied by the MUSCLES and TENDONS.

MUSCLES are energy convertors – turning the nutrients from the food we eat into energy for our use. Muscles are attached to the bones by means of the TENDONS (which are nothing more than the gristly end of the muscle). The attachment to the bone is called the 'origin'. The muscle then crosses over a joint and ends up attached to another bone by its other tendon; this attachment is known as the 'insertion'. The body has over 600 muscles, each of which has its own function.

With every joint movement you have various sets of muscles working together. Some move to contract the joint, others move to relax it and return it to the 'rest' position. The muscles which perform the initial movements are the 'agonists'; those with the opposing action are the 'antagonists'. Take the simple example of the upper arm. The 'agonist' is the biceps muscle whose action is to flex the elbow joint to bring the wrist towards the shoulder and also to rotate the lower arm. The 'antagonist' is the triceps muscle, at the back of the upper arm, whose function is to straighten the arm at the elbow joint and return it to the normal position. This is oversimplified, I know, but I think you will realise that whenever there is a joint movement of any sort it is not just a matter of agonist and antagonist reaction, but a whole set of muscles move together to make the body function smoothly.

The BRAIN is the mechanism which directs all the functions. It sends out impulses to the muscles to which they respond. The brain channels these impulses through a system of nerve tissues, either via the brain itself or via the spinal cord, ending directly in the muscle itself. Every fibre of every muscle has its chain of command to the brain. But the muscle itself consists of 70 per cent water, 20 per cent protein and 10 per cent chemicals. It requires an adequate supply of chemical energy to make it work efficiently. Glucose and oxygen are the two most important muscle foods, and these are brought to the muscles via the blood vessels.

The CIRCULATORY SYSTEM consists of HEART, LUNGS and BLOOD. At the centre is the heart, which is nothing more than a muscular pump. It is very like the other muscles of the body and differs only in that its function is purely to pump blood. The heart pushes out blood via the blood vessels; first to the arteries; diminishing to the arterioles and lastly to the capillaries. Fluids escape from the capillaries into the surrounding tissue thus feeding the muscle fibres with the chemical energy (oxygen and glucose) they need to process into energy. Then the reverse system begins with the blood flowing in from the capillaries to a system of veins that increase gradually in size until the blood is carried back to the heart. The heart then pumps the blood into the lungs to receive its oxygen supply and the re-oxygenated blood is then returned to the heart to be pumped out to the rest of the body.

Oxygen is essential to life. The brain dies within seconds of losing its oxygen supply. The air we breathe is our source of oxygen and just over 20 per cent is pure oxygen. Breathing carries oxygen to the lungs with the rib cage acting as bellows. The muscles expand the rib cage to drag air into the lungs and then contract to expel it. While the air is in the lungs the blood is taking the oxygen it needs; at the same time carbon dioxide which has been carried away from the muscles is being removed. During exercise we need up to 20 times more oxygen than when we are at rest.

All this is merely meant to give you a brief insight into how your body works. There are many publications which go into the subject more deeply. But at this stage this is all you need to know to get that little extra from your training programme and give you a better understanding of how it all works.

Having a well-trained, efficiently working body need be no accident in these days of knowledge, scientific training and expert nutritional advice. But good health is still a thing of privilege, to be used, not abused. George Hackenschmidt, the famous wrestler of olden times, coined the expression: 'Life is Movement.' Nothing could be more true in this modern-day, sedentary society.

To go back to our metaphor of the expensive car. You can't spend a fortune on it, bring it home, store it in the garage for months, and then expect it to run immaculately the moment you try to start it up again. The battery is flat; even if it does start it will not run smoothly because the timing is wrong, the vital oil and petrol and water are not circulating correctly, and the tyres may well be flat as well.

To function well at all times your body should be kept working, like your car. Even the Old Crocks still manage the Brighton Run!

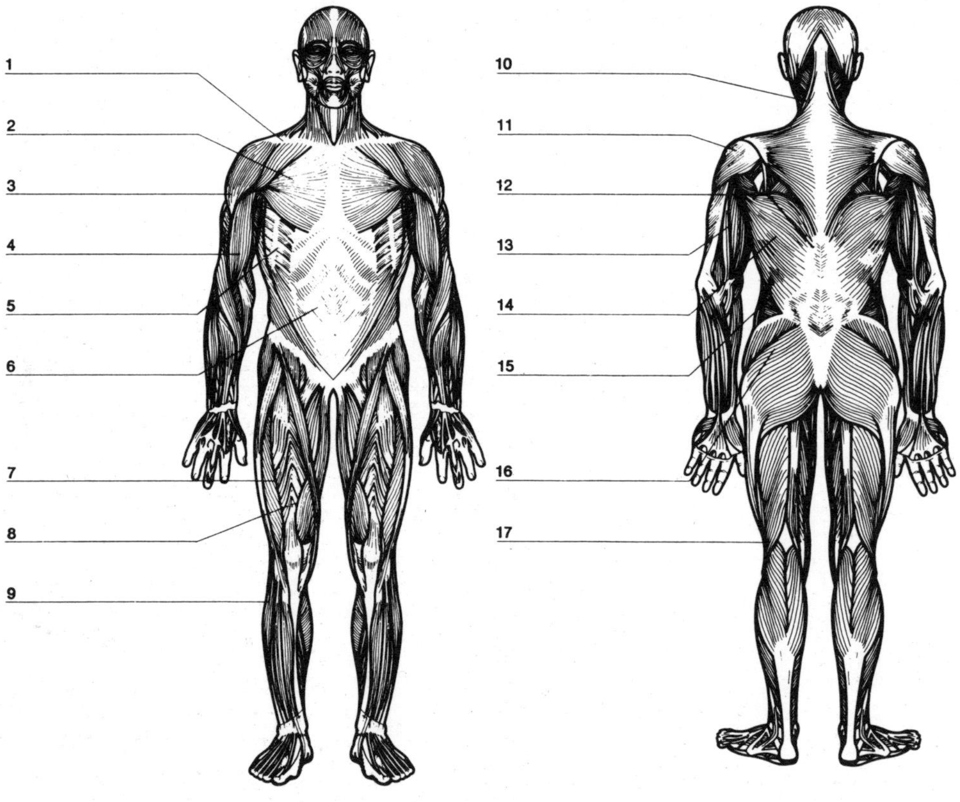

MUSCLE CHART
1. PECTORALIS MINOR, 2. PECTORALIS MAJOR: THE BIG FLAT CHEST MUSCLES. **3. DELTOID:** SIDE (LATERAL) FRONT (ANTERIOR) BACK (POSTERIOR). **4. BICEPS:** TWO HEADED MUSCLE AT FRONT OF UPPER ARM. **5. SERRATUS:** RIB LIKE MUSCLES ON THE SIDE OF THE CHEST. **6. ABDOMINALS:** THE MUSCLES OF THE STOMACH. **7. QUADRACEPS:** AN 'ALL IN' TERM FOR THE MUSCLES AT THE FRONT OF THE THIGH. **8. VASTUS INTERNUS:** THE MUSCLE THAT CONTROLS THE FLEXING OF THE KNEE. **9. GASTROCNEMIUS:** THE MUSCLES OF THE CALF. **10. TRAPEZIUS:** A DIAMOND SHAPED MUSCLE OF THE UPPER BACK AND NECK. **11. DELTOID:** (POSTERIOR). **12. ERECTOR SPINAE:** THE STRONGEST MUSCLES IN THE BODY. THE BIG TRUNK SUPPORTING MUSCLES. **13. TRICEPS:** THE THREE HEADED MUSCLE AT THE BACK OF THE ARM, USED IN ALL ARM STRAIGHTENING MOVEMENTS. **14. LATISSIMUS DORSI:** THE MUSCLES WHICH GIVE THE V SHAPE TO THE UPPER TORSO. **15. EXTERNAL OBLIQUES:** THE SIDE WAIST MUSCLES. **16. GLUTEUS MAXIMUS:** YOUR BACKSIDE. **17. BICEPS FEMORIS:** (HAMSTRING GROUP).

Chapter 8

SKIP THE JOGGING

Once you've got the hang of these introductory exercises, it's time to begin thinking more seriously about exercising, what it's for and how far one should progress. Not so long ago I appeared on a platform with several doctors, all of us talking about the nature of exercise and its uses; and the doctors made the point that heart disease is one of the major killers in today's society. Three factors contributed towards it; 1. Lack of *quality* exercise; 2. an excess of animal fats in the modern diet; and 3. smoking.

My concern is with the first point: quality exercise. Any exercise programme, to do you any good, has to be progressive. That means it has to grow progressively more difficult as your body grows fitter and stronger and more able to cope.

I'm not a great believer in exercise programmes such as 'jogging'. I think they're grossly over-rated. If you go out for a jog regularly your body soon becomes accustomed to the degree of effort needed; after that your jog does you no further good. Either you have to jog faster, in order to increase the effort, in which case it isn't a jog any more, or you have to adjust your route to take in various gradients. If you're jogging, your heart and respiration soon accustom themselves to the optimum level needed, and you won't increase that level, whether you jog for one mile or ten. Quite often a jog will not increase your heartbeat even to an acceptable work level. It's the same with golf. The best thing a game of golf does is to get you out for a walk in the fresh air. You don't stretch your heart or your respiration one iota by following that little white ball around the countryside. After all, your body is accustomed to walking about the place anyway. Frankly, I feel that all the good the walk in the fresh air is likely to do you is just as likely to be undone by the frustrations the ordinary golfer experiences in playing the game at all.

Quality exercise not only works your heart and respiratory system; it brings into play your whole muscular system. Once your appetite has been whetted (as I hope it has been) by the introductory exercises, it's time to consider where we go from here. Now you'll have found that most of these introductory exercises are what we call 'free' – that is they don't use any equipment or, if they do, it is of the simplest kind that you can find almost anywhere. Now I hope that you're feeling like going into something a little more serious. So at this stage I'd like to set out for you the various commercial appliances for keeping fit there are on the market; to give you some idea of what you can spend compared with what you need to; and to give you some idea of how these appliances work and what they do for you. I must add here that these are my own considered opinions, formed by more than 20 years of experience.

The first and cheapest method of keeping fit is by means of free exercising, largely as described in our first two programmes. You don't need any equipment, so the lay-out is confined to your own clothing. You don't need much space, so you can perform the programme in the convenience of your own bedroom, hotel room, living room, or even office. You don't have to have anyone helping you and it's simple to gauge your progress. On the other hand, a free exercise programme can be time-consuming, because you'll find as you get fitter and stronger, you'll have to do more and more difficult exercises in order for them to have a beneficial effect on your heart, lungs and physique.

The logical progression is to go into exercises using some form of resistance, using household objects or some form of weight or equipment training. Boredom is one of the dangers of a free exercise programme, and you find that if you've a piece of equipment to train with (or against) your interest does not tend to flag so readily. It was a Charles Atlas course of free exercise which in fact started me out on the physical culture scene. The Charles Atlas course has a registered name for its exercising – 'Dynamic Tension' – but that's purely what we in the business call contractions, using your own body as resistance. To put it more technically, it's a form of isometric training. You don't have to worry too much about the names of these forms of exercise. All that will concern you is the repetitiveness of the exercise and the possibility of accompanying boredom.

Possibly the first step in graduating from free exercising to equipment exercising is the chest expander. This can be made either from steel springs or rubber cables fastened to a pair of handles. Besides being used in body development and strength training, chest expanders are also used in official competition; they're called 'strand-pullers' and there's an international strand-pullers' association. A chest expander set can cost anything from about £1.50p to £10, depending on the number of strands or cables used; and also the strength of the cables. The cables are usually graduated in five pound measurements from 10 to 40 pounds. You'll have either three-strand or five-strand handles.

Expanders are a good form of resistance training and an excellent means of starting. But they do have drawbacks; their programmes are primarily geared for upper body work, and the major argument against them is that the 'push' part of the programme, when you stretch the resistance, is the only part of it that does you much good. (When the cables contract to their normal position, it can be quite dangerous if the trainee doesn't exercise considerable care and attention. If you're 'stretching behind neck', for example, the springs can catch the short hairs at the back of the neck and give you quite a painful haircut into the bargain.) They're sometimes difficult to adjust, too, with a complicated series of clips at the handle.

There are a number of different brand names on the market, all in roughly the same price range, but the firm of Terry, of Redditch, in Worcestershire, probably have the best reputation for expanders.

Next in the price ladder is probably the largest selling piece of physical training equipment in the world – the Bullworker. I have been involved with the Bullworker in differing degrees since it was first introduced in Britain in 1963. The Bullworker was invented by a German, Gert Kolbell, as a training aid for the German Olympic team of 1964. It's virtually the opposite of the chest-expander – instead of stretching the equipment you compress it. Kolbell intended his machine purely and simply as a strength training aid and never as a physique developer, which it subsequently became. After I turned professional in 1964, I became associated with the firm marketing the Bullworker in Britain and in fact I re-wrote the Bullworker training course for the company and my version of it is still in use today. I also photographed the current wall-chart used by the company and laid out the text. For five years I acted as consultant to the company, dealing with training correspondence and although I no longer act as training consultant, I still have a loose (but warm) consultant connection with the Bullworker.

In my opinion the Bullworker is one of the major physical culture happenings of the past 60 years. It has made more people aware of physical exercise than ever before and it has given the public a most convenient, relatively simple system of exercising at a price most people can afford. The Bullworker works on a system of

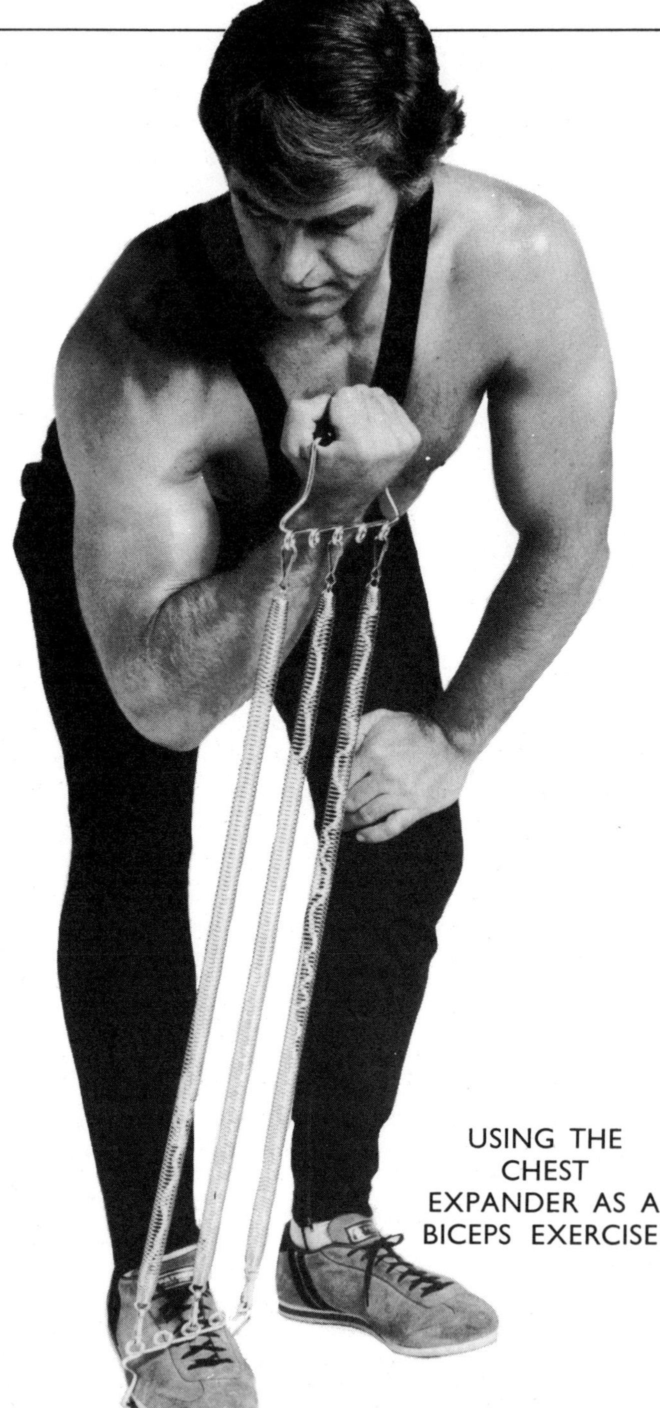

USING THE CHEST EXPANDER AS A BICEPS EXERCISE.

isotonic contractions – sometimes the contractions are called isometric, but really a contraction can only be described as isometric when the muscles contract statically – when there is no muscle movement – and you'd have to be very weak indeed for the exercise with Bullworker to become isometric. The Bullworker course is a 25-exercise course although only 24 are shown on the wall-chart. The 25th is included in the booklet and was left off the wall-chart because it was too difficult to photograph. However, Exercise No 25 is probably the most important of the whole series, for it's the only one which can be described as a cardio-vascular fitness exercise. So don't leave out Exercise 25.

The isotonic contractions consist of breathing in deeply and compressing the Bullworker appliance in various positions using various muscle groups. The time that you spend holding the contraction is usually around seven seconds, and the effort you put into it is as near to dammit seventy per cent of your maximum effort. Seventy per cent is a bit difficult to gauge, but if you strain as hard as you possibly can that'll be around seventy per cent of your true maximum.

I've said, and I still believe, that the Bullworker is a remarkable and most successful appliance; but having said that I must issue a warning. Don't be misled by all the colourful and encouraging publicity put out by the proprietors . . . 'Let me make you a new man in 49 seconds a day' type of thing. It will take a lot more effort than the seven second contractions, or even the seven contractions of seven seconds each to make a new man of you. My own research has shown that the Bullworker will give its best results if used for training twice or even three times a day. You're now talking about spending as much as an hour a day on your physique; which is just as time-consuming as any other method.

Another thing to remember is that although Bullworker was designed as a strength apparatus, it is now sold largely as a body-building piece of equipment. But in fact use of the Bullworker will, first, improve your fitness and strength; any improvements in physique and building up of the body will be incidental.

But if you use Bullworker sensibly, taking the claims for it with a pinch of salt, you'll get some very good results. And as the machine sells at between £16 and £18, that's pretty good value for money.

Next up the financial scale in exercise training appliances is the rowing machine. There are various types on the market, of which three need concern us. The first is the spring-operated type, which is relatively cheap, ranging from £20 to about £50. The second have what look like genuine oars on which the resistance occurs on a brake pad, with two clutch plates rubbing together; and thirdly there are the hydraulically operated machines, which are the best, and which go up to £115 to £120 each. With a rowing machine, the benefits come *literally all the way round*: in one piece of apparatus, you exercise your cardio-vascular system, your waist, your back, your thigh and calf muscles, the chest, arms and shoulders. The second main benefit is that you only need to spend about ten minutes a day on it to get the absolutely maximum result. They're adjustable, so the whole family can use them.

I have considerable problems persuading girls to use rowing machines. It's the old fallacy – they think they're going to look like the Oxford and Cambridge Boat Race teams. But really, if more women were to use the rowing machine judiciously, we would soon notice, as a nation, a vast improvement in figures. So much depends on diet; it's a bit difficult to explain that a woman can use a rowing machine to reduce her weight (while taking the correct diet) while a man may use the same machine actually to increase weight at the same time as improving his physical fitness. (Ten minutes rowing training a day is very serious training. When you consider the exhausted state of those very fit young men at the end of the Boat Race you must remember that they've been rowing for only 18 minutes or so!)

Now we come to exercise bicycles and with them some of the biggest misconceptions in the field of fitness training. Ninety per cent of those who buy exercise bicycles do so to reduce their waistlines. Now the bike's good for a great many things, but one of the areas where it has no effect is around the waist. The exercise bicycle is first and foremost a heart and lung trainer; apart from that it really only works your hips, thighs, knees, calves and ankles and has little or no effect on the muscles of your upper body.

It's a most convenient form of exercising, of course. It

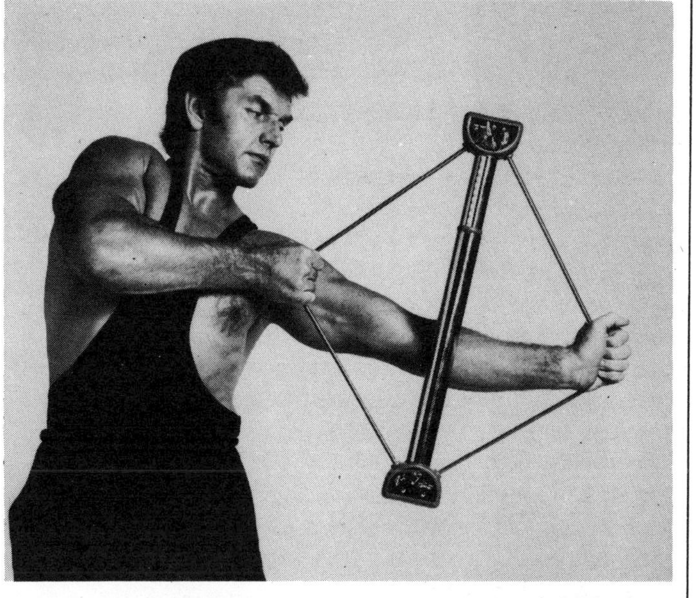

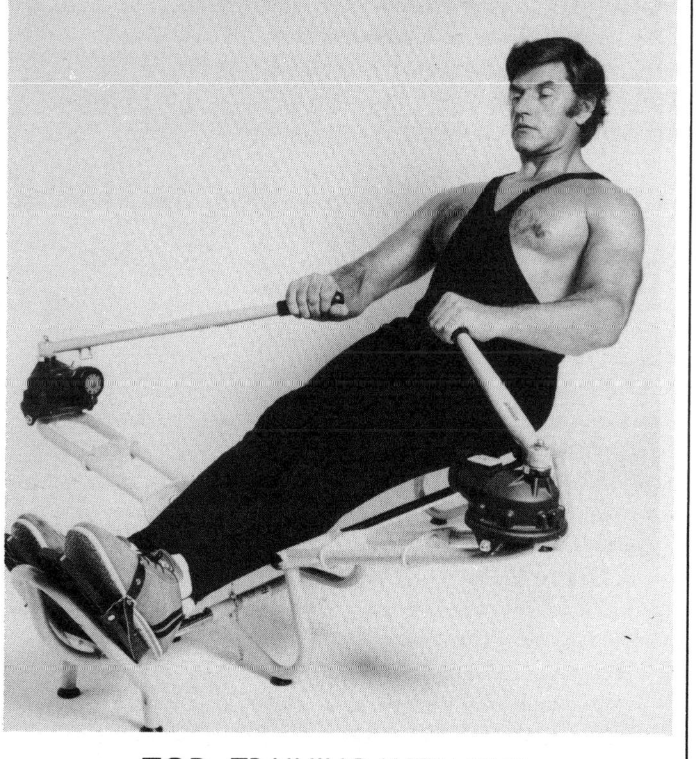

TOP: TRAINING WITH THE BULLWORKER. **ABOVE:** THE ITALIAN ROWING-MACHINE FROM CARNIELLI.

doesn't take too long, you don't have to go out in all winds and weathers you can sit the bike in front of the telly if you want to and pedal away while you watch. Lots of people love them – Mr Heath was a case in point; he'd pedal away for hours. He was pretty fit too, but nobody could pretend that the cycling actually improved his waistline.

The best cycling machines on the market will cost around £130–£140 (cheaper ones from £70) which sounds a lot, but in terms of the fitness benefit, is it really that expensive? If you can combine an exercise cycle with a rowing machine you've got very nearly the ideal combination. As in everything else, you get what you pay for, and in the matter of exercise cycles and rowing machines the more you can afford the better the equipment.

There's nothing in the jogging machine line I feel able to recommend for private use. Any machine that's worth its sale will cost well over a thousand pounds and will be found only in hospitals or big gymnasia.

So we come to the system of weights, or, as it is known, progressive resistance training. The weights are probably the simplest form of exercising, and because of this have developed as the most versatile system of training over the years. There has never been a world-class physique that has not been developed with weights, no matter what other system has been employed in addition. So if you wish to develop to the ultimate you've eventually got to go into some form of weight training.

Weights come in two forms; barbells and dumbells. The barbell is the two-handed piece of equipment which normally consists of a bar, covered by a sleeve. The weights go on either end of the bar, and there are two collars to hold the weights on the bar. Of course you can add on as many weights as you like.

The dumbell consists of a much shorter bar, 15–16 ins long, with a smaller sleeve, weights on either side of the sleeve and the retaining collars. These are for single-handed or separate-handed exercise.

The weights themselves are nothing more than steel or cast-iron discs with a one-inch diameter hole, which is virtually standard. Some little time ago a famous body-builder decided to go into the business and produced a set of weights on a different diameter bar (about 1⅛ inch) just to be different. It sounded okay, but he soon discovered that while his weights would fit anyone's bar, albeit a bit loosely, nobody else's weights would fit on his bars; he soon went out of business.

Costs, of course, are always on the increase; but at the time of writing the cost of the barbell sleeve and collars will be about £12; for the dumbell about £14 and the weights are added on top of that. As near as you can reckon, they work out at between 20 and 25 pence a pound; roughly 50 pence per kilo. A reasonable set for a beginner – barbell set; dumbell set and weights will cost £60 – £70 and will probably weigh around 50 kilos. As you progress, so you can add weights as you wish. It's advisable to begin by buying four of everything; which means you can load up both barbells and dumbells.

One of my most prized possessions is one of the oldest relics in weightlifting, the Thomas Inch Unliftable

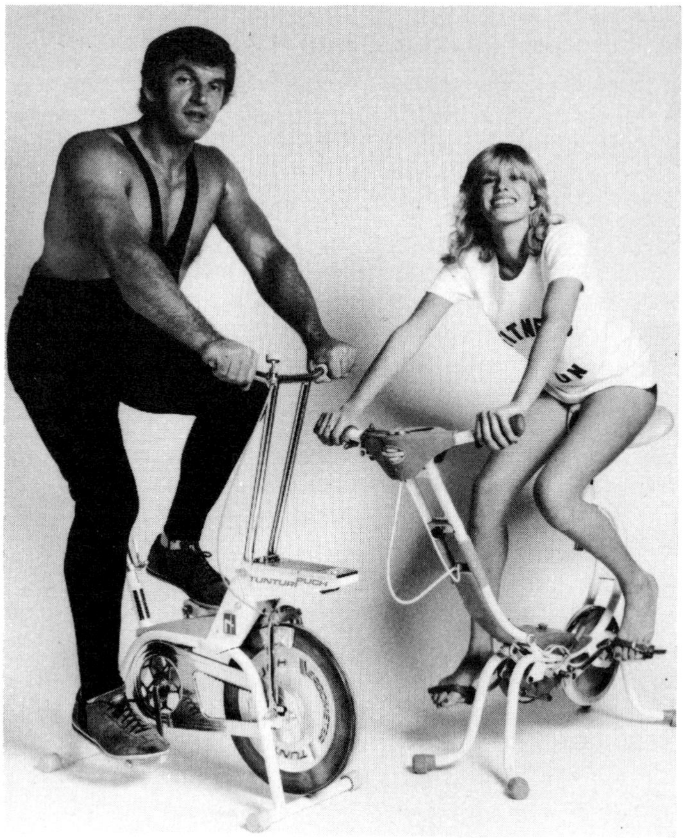

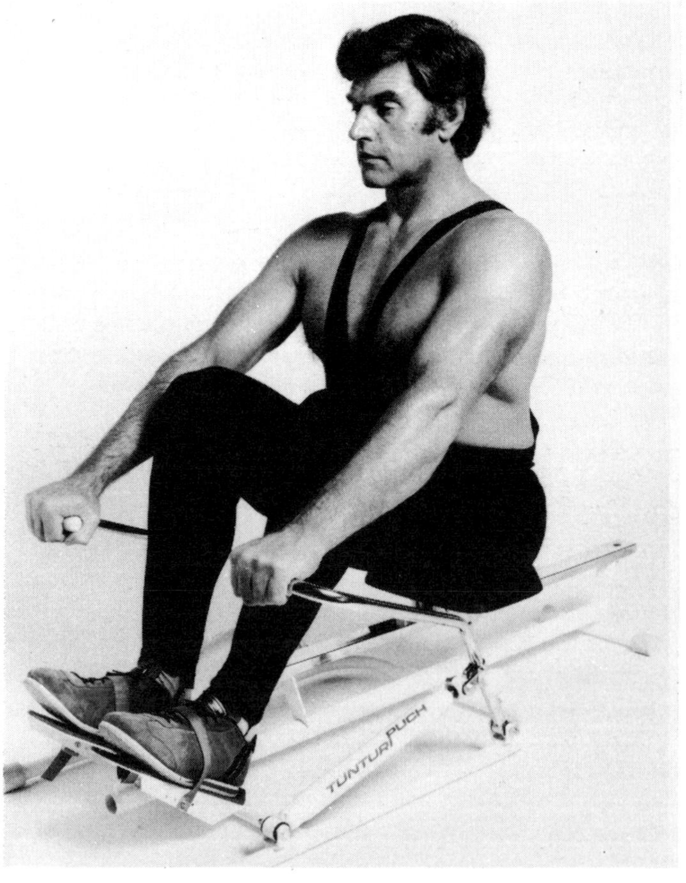

TOP: EXERCISE BIKES CAN BE FUN TOO. **ABOVE:** THE FINNISH TUNTURI ROWING MACHINE. **OPPOSITE:** NORMA DOES THE WORK WHILE I LOOK ON. **INSET:** TRAINING EQUIPMENT.

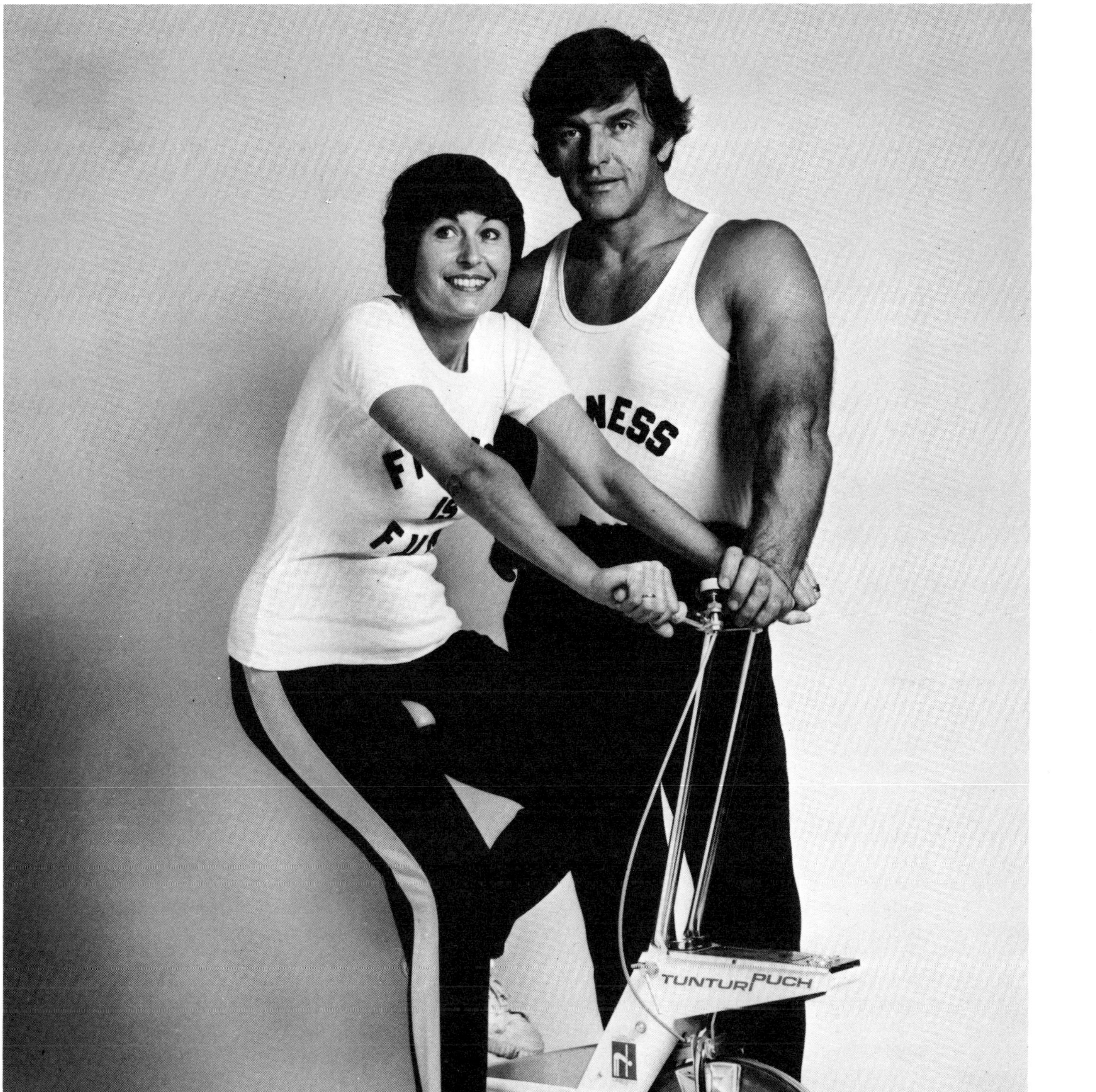
TUNTURI PUCH
ERGOMETER
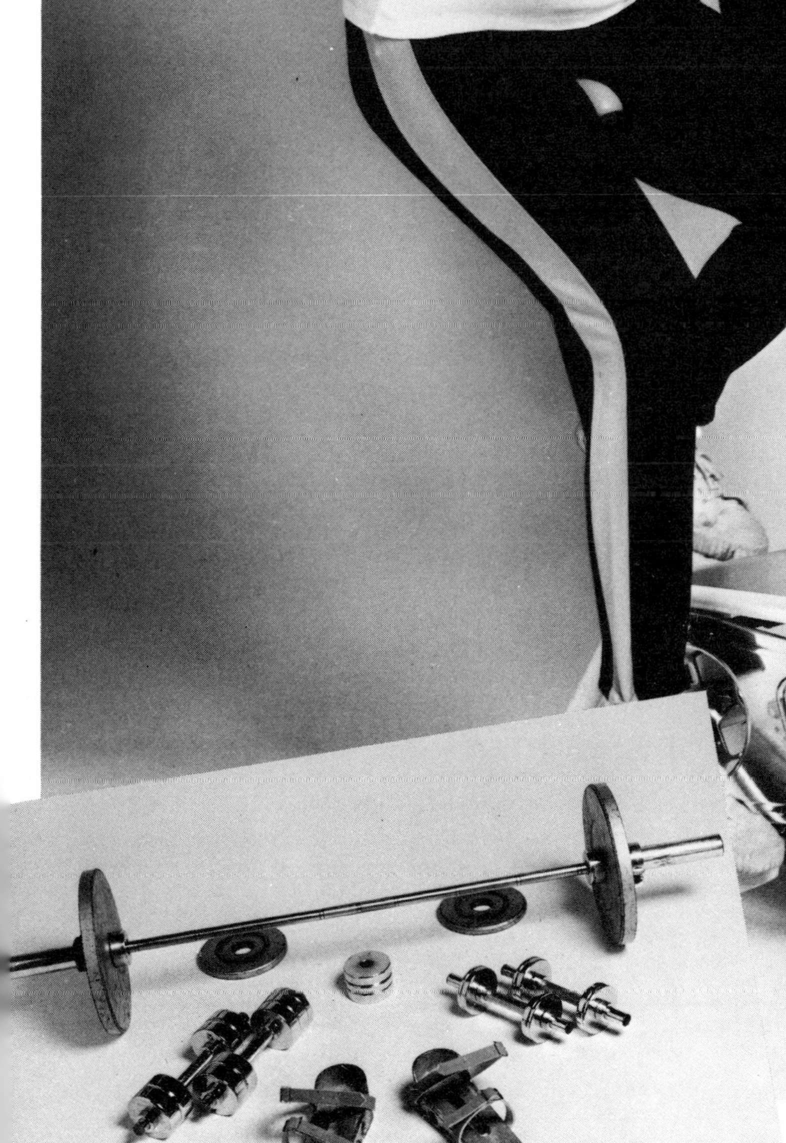

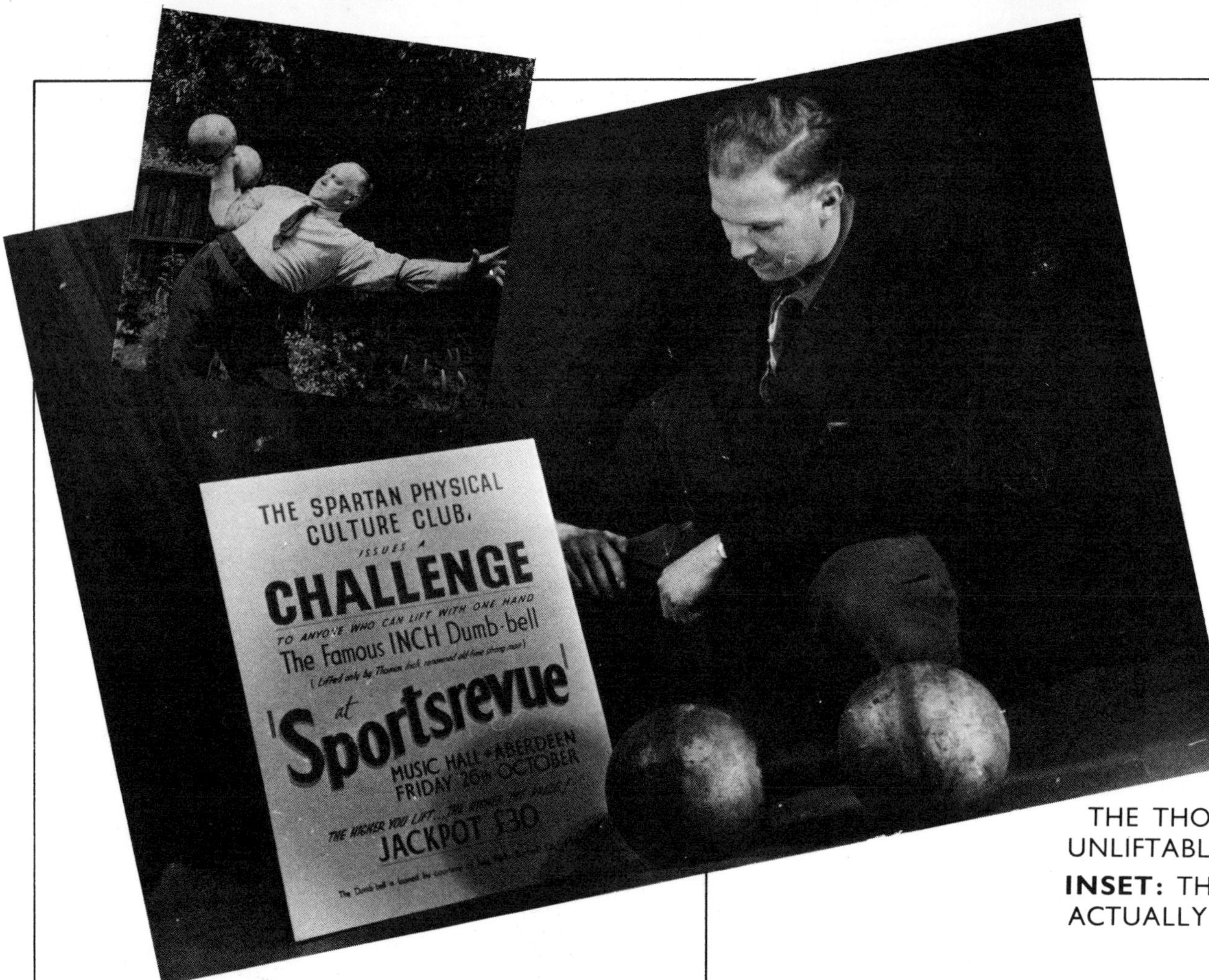

THE THOMAS INCH UNLIFTABLE DUMBELL.
INSET: THOMAS INCH ACTUALLY LIFTING IT.

Dumbell. Thomas Inch was a famous English strong man in the early part of this century, and he had three dumbells made specially for exhibitions. One weighed 130, the second 150 lbs and he gave the foundry carte blanche to cast another, roughly 170 lbs. They did so, but failed to tell him that they had made the handle as big as a milk bottle. Well, 170 lbs is fairly easy to lift if you're reasonably strong, but with a thick handle like that it's virtually impossible. Anyway, Thomas Inch couldn't lift it, until he'd practised for months, and after he died it passed down through many hands. Reg Park, the greatest physique in the world, owned it once, and after him it belonged to Bert Lightfoot, who kept it in a shed on a caravan site, and offered it to me. I went along to see it, and between us we dragged it out of the shed. It was in its own very heavy box, and I bent down and picked it up, box and all, quite easily. I've never been able to manage that since. . . .

One aid which has been on the American market for a long time, but hasn't been seen in Britain much yet, is a form of weighted straps. In America they're called Voight weights. The system has now arrived in Britain under the name of Portabelles. The company do two straps – three pounds and five pounds. The three-pounder is intended for girls, five pounds for fellows; but I personally believe that three pounds is too light except for the slightest of girls; and I never recommend anything other than the five-pounder. I have three pairs of the five-pound Portabelles, so I can if I need put 15 pounds around each wrist or ankle – a total of 30 in all. They're nothing more than weighted straps, Velcro ended so you just touch them together and they hold fast.

Finally, under the heading of weights comes the weighted shoe or boot, which we in the trade call the 'iron shoe'. These shoes come in two different weights, 3 lbs and 5 lbs although they're so made that you can insert an inch dumbell rod through the shoe for additional weights should you require them. It is obviously an easy way of increasing resistance for various leg exercises, ideal for leg extension work and used a great deal in hospitals for remedial purposes. A pair of iron shoes, to fit over your usual training shoes, would be about £10.

From time to time various fads and fancies enjoy passing fame. Yoga, for example is one of the most persistent of practices. I've nothing against Yoga – many of the exercises are excellent for suppleness and improvement of mobility, but Yoga plays no real part in any modern fitness programme. Exercise wheels enjoyed a short season of popularity until people began to do themselves quite a lot of harm by mis-using them. They were followed by spin-a-disc, where you stood on a sort of record turntable and twisted yourself round. That died a death – deservedly so. Hula-hooping, was fun, but you'd have to do a devil of a lot of it to reduce your waistline.

The alternative to home training, if you don't think for one reason or another that you can manage it, is of course to go to a gymnasium or exercise and health studio. If you know what training is all about, and if you are fully aware of what you're going into, health studios are probably the best value for money you can get anywhere. But once again, health studios are (usually) guilty of making fitness training look both easy and fantastically effective. So many people join expecting the maximum results for the minimum of effort; and when it doesn't happen like that they become easily discouraged. The fact that to make dramatic improvements no matter what method you use you'll have to work pretty hard and go on a fairly rigid diet at the same time takes a bit of getting used to.

So many health studios make the bulk of their money from people who begin with the best intentions in the world and then pack up. The cost of a good course of training will be £70 to £150 a year – say three or four pounds per week. That's a great deal of money – and yet when you realise what you *can* get for this, it is really one of the bargains of the century. Your £3 per week gives you unlimited access to the health studio, its equipment and its enthusiasm and its tuition. It's a very personal thing, this individual tuition, and if you're paying that sort of money you can insist on getting it; so it's as well to ensure that you're going to get on well with your instructors before you undertake the expense.

The amount of machinery in gymnasia has increased enormously in the past ten years. As well as all we've been talking about above, there will be leg-extension, thigh-curl machines, another machine which is used exclusively for doing bench presses for developing the chest, altering your body position to perform all forms of pressing movements. There's a leg-press machine, which takes the grind out of doing squats – instead of going up and down with a barbell on your back, a fairly uncomfortable way of exercising to say the least, you lie under the machine and push weights up and down with your feet. It's very popular with weightlifters, because it develops basic driving power with the legs.

One marvellous piece of equipment in gymnasia these days, which I'm not too fond of although it does save space and enable a great deal of exercise to be done without supervision, is the jungle machine, or multi-purpose gym. This is a basic framework on which a team of exercisers (footballers, cricketers, tennis players) can exercise individually at a separate station, moving round the machine to vary the exercises. Not only are these very expensive, but they weigh a great deal. They're being promoted as the be-all-and-end-all in exercising, but I have my reservations, because they don't necessarily work the muscles over their full range of movement. They're ideal for local authorities, sports clubs and so on where there may not be adequate supervision, because they're safe and easy to use, but they are really only *strength* machines, not body-building or physical fitness machines. So they're right and proper for athletes looking for additional strength. They cost between £2000 and £5000, depending on the number of stations. To avoid the weight problem, you can have the individual stations separate – I've got several in my own gymnasium, which is on the first floor and wouldn't take the couple of tons of a complete 'jungle gym'. But really they're *not* a replacement for barbell work.

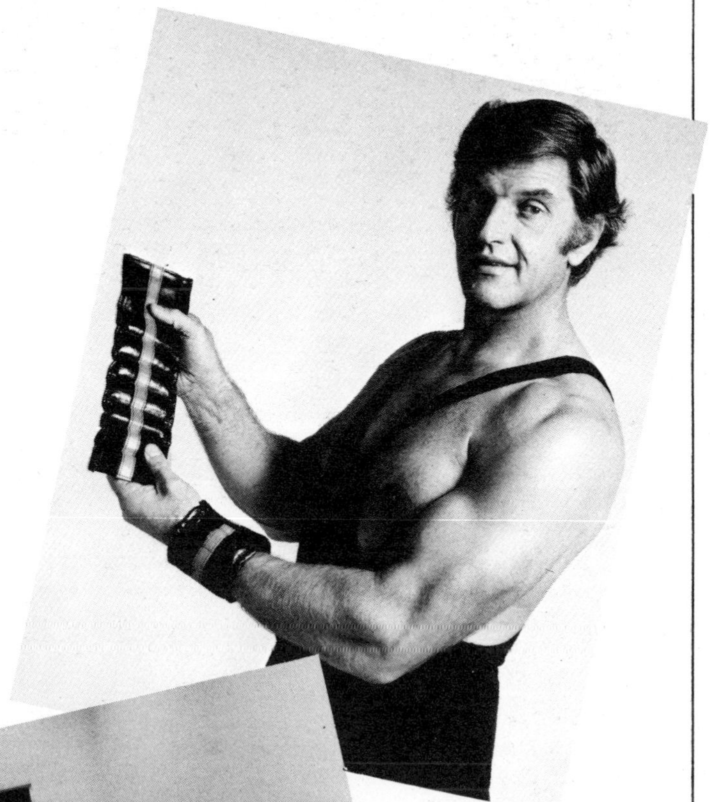

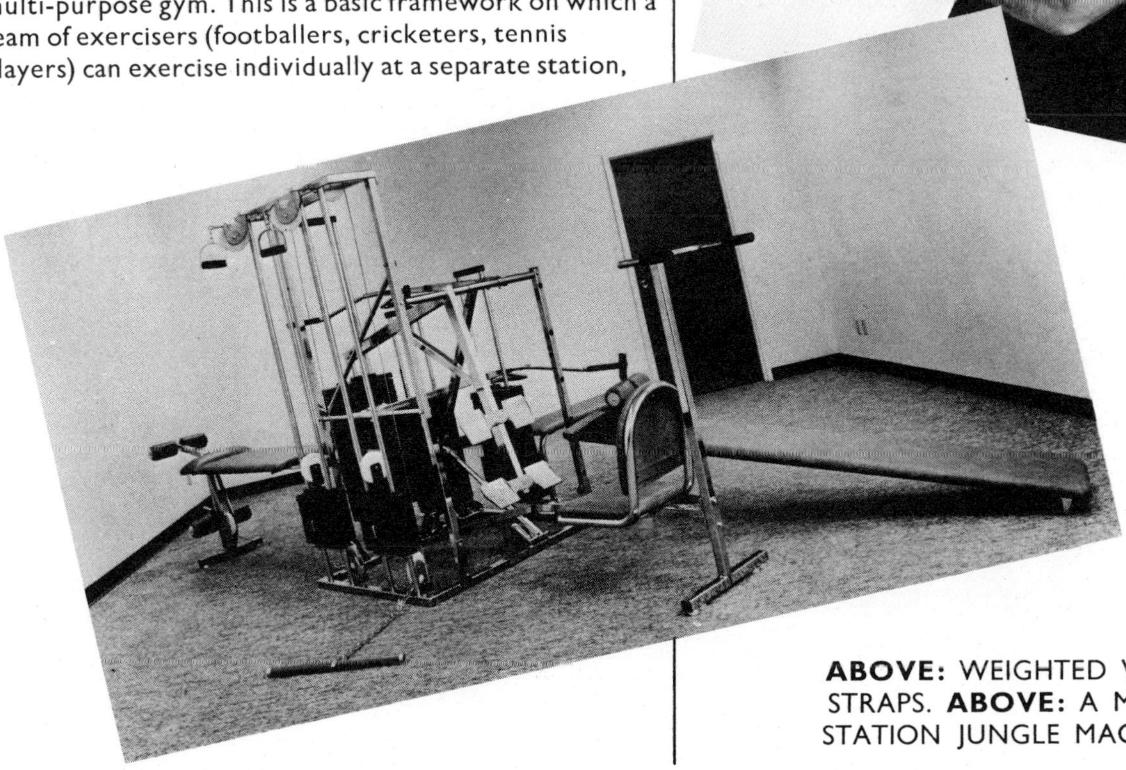

ABOVE: WEIGHTED WRIST STRAPS. **ABOVE:** A MULTI-STATION JUNGLE MACHINE.

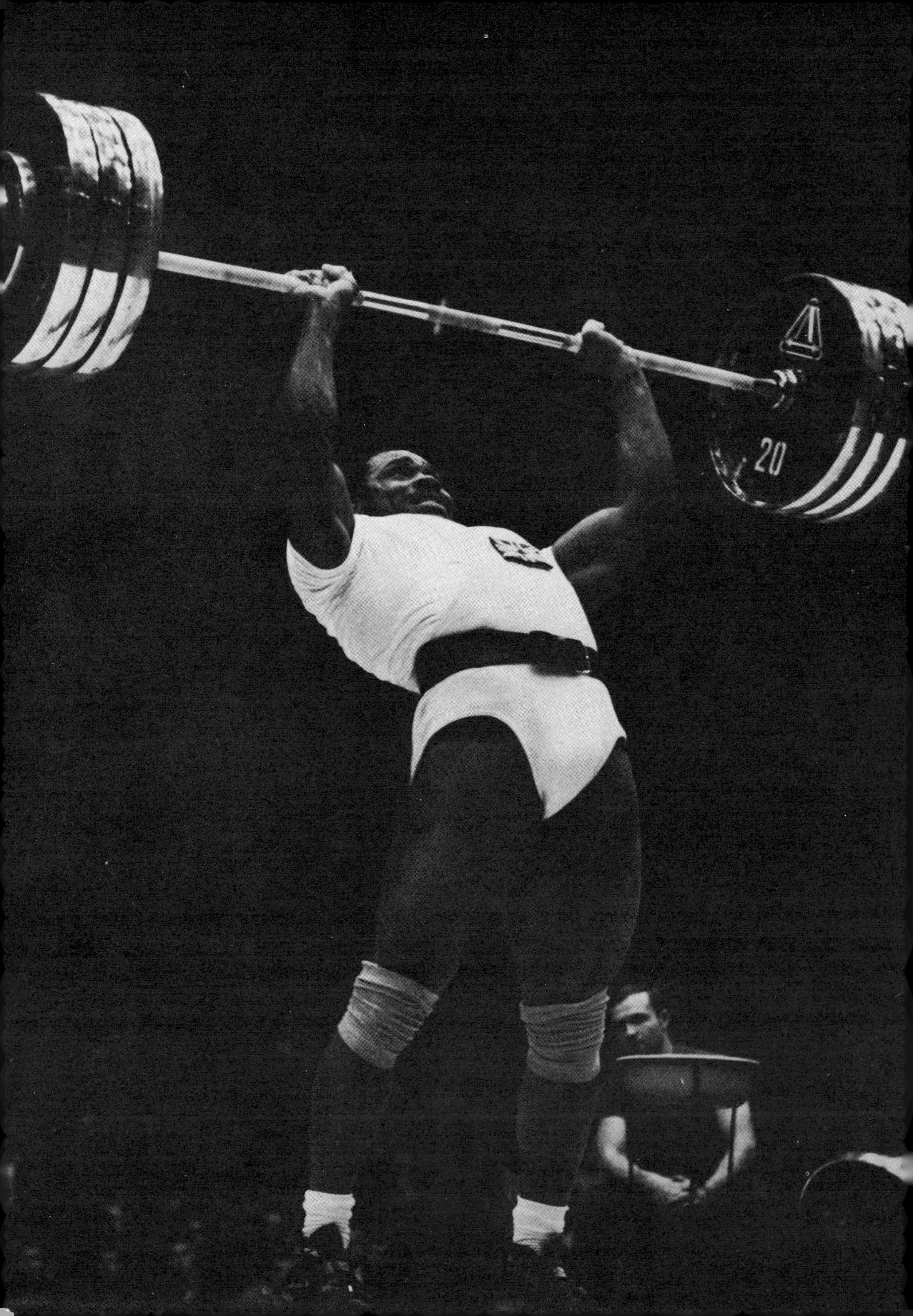
20

Chapter 9

GETTING THE WORDS RIGHT

Exercising, like every other form of human activity, has its own jargon, and I think it would be helpful to explain just what the various terms mean that we commonly use in the gymnasium and health studio.

An EXERCISE is a prescribed series of movements designed to work a specific muscle or part of a muscle group. It comprises SETS of REPETITIONS.

A REPETITION is one complete movement of the prescribed exercise; i.e. in the two hands press the bar has to go from the shoulder to arm's length and back to the shoulder again.

A SET is a group of repetitions. You will have noted the maximum prescribed for beginners is three sets in any one exercise.

You'll also have noticed that the number of sets and repetitions are laid out for each exercise, usually three sets of eight to ten repetitions. However these may vary with the type of training you're doing. If the exercise is to become a cardio-vascular fitness one, to improve your heart and lungs, the number of repetitions in each set is increased, for it's the number of repetitions you do that gets you breathing deeply and your heart pumping. But if you want to do an exercise for strength, you decrease the number of repetitions, increase the resistance – the weight, and increase the number of sets. As a rough guide, it's usual to decrease the repetitions from ten to six in each set; and increase the number of sets from three to six or even ten.

When I was lifting competitively, I found it best to establish a kind of pyramid system – starting with six repetitions per set, then five, then four, and so on; working up to the maximum weight on number one. Then I'd come down on an odd poundage, so if I'd worked up, say 250 lbs, 260 lbs, 270 lbs, up to 300 lbs; then I'd 'come downhill' 295 lbs, 285 lbs, 275 lbs and so on.

Real body-building, in advance of anything in this book, invariably means doing six to eight sets of repetitions per exercise, and six to eight repetitions per set. You can work up to doing 16 to 20 sets if you wish, as some fanatics do.

A SCHEDULE or PROGRAMME is a block of exercises prescribed either for oneself or by oneself to work out all or as many of the body's muscle groups as desired.

SUPER-SETTING is an advanced body-building term used when you take two specific related muscle groups and exercise them alternately. – i.e. biceps and triceps.

OPPOSITE: WORLD MID-HEAVYWEIGHT CHAMPION LOUIS MARTIN, MBE.

FLUSHING is practically the same sort of thing, but taking two or three exercises to work the same muscle group – for example you might do a biceps exercise with a dumbell, followed by a barbell, followed by chest expanders.

POWER is a combination of strength and speed. This was the name I chose for my magazine, which dealt with both weightlifting and body-building. Geoff Capes, the shot-putter, is a fine example of a 'powerful' man – the body explodes into action from nil to full speed and strength in a distance of seven feet.

ISOTONICS are muscular contractions with movement.

ISOMETRICS are muscular contractions without movement.

DYNAMIC TENSION, the phrase coined by Charles Atlas for 'isometrics', is really a system, as ancient as the Greeks who knew all about it, of isometric training using the body as its own resistance.

Isometrics were all the rage at one time, but research has disproved many of the more extravagant claims made for this type of exercising.

Some competitive weightlifting terms need to be explained.

The CURL is bending the arm at the elbow or the leg at the knee, against resistance.

The CLEAN is lifting the barbell from the floor to the shoulders.

The PRESS means straightening the arms against resistance, no matter what position you do it in.

The JERK is lifting a weight from the shoulders to arm's length in any way you like, usually with some form of leg drive.

In general terms, the pushing muscles of the body are much stronger than the pulling muscles. When you are 'cleaning' – lifting a weight from the floor, your arms and big back muscles will pull the weights up to around waist level, no further. At that stage, the weightlifter must use his technique to get underneath the weight, to bring the massive thrusting muscles of the thighs and arms into play to drive the weight upwards at arm's length.

SPLITTING is one of the two methods of getting the body under the bar. As the pull brings the bar up to the waist, the front leg goes forward about a foot, simultaneously the other leg goes two to three feet backwards. Ideally the line of the back from the back foot through to the shoulders forms an arc. The back knee must not touch the floor. It is a most beautiful movement when performed smoothly and correctly. Its one drawback is that the line of balance is very narrow indeed, which makes it less stable and therefore slightly less powerful than the second method.

SQUATTING. In this movement the feet travel in a small jump sideways and outwards, from 12 inches apart to about 15 inches apart, and slightly forward of the starting line. The difference is that in the squat, the lifter recovers on both legs; whereas in the split, the back leg is used solely as a prop, which is limiting in both power and balance.

THE SNATCH is sometimes used as an exercise, as in the power snatch, where the bar has to go from the floor to arm's length in one direct movement with no stopping. The lifter will have to split, or squat, to perform the snatch, but this time, because the weight is not so great and the hand grip farther apart, the weight tends to come up as far as the bottom of the lifter's chest. At this stage he has to get underneath it at arm's length without the weight dropping back. It's a very technical lift, and we refer to being 'in the groove'. If you're not 'in the groove' by as little as an inch, you can feel it at once, and there's no holding it. So you just let it go, and abandon that try.

Newspaper reports of weightlifting are misleading. When you read that so and so has lifted 500 kilos, you must remember that in fact he hasn't – in one go. He in fact does two different lifts, the Snatch and the Jerk with three attempts at each; and the best in each are added together to give him his 'total'.

Chapter 10

IF YOU CAN DO IT, IT'S WRONG

Now it's time to move on to basic resistance training and what I'd like to do first is to take you on a tour of your own body; showing the basic exercises which will affect the basic groups of muscles over the whole range of their actions. We'll show you how to do them, and what you are doing to your body when you do them. After that, we'll suggest a series of programmes designed for different purposes.

There are a number of important points to remember

1. Always warm up before you begin serious training. Take the 'good mornings' and 'side bends' from Chapter Six and the 'seated stretch' exercises, do a few 'squats' and swing your arms around to warm them up over the full range of their activity. Use an exercise bike, if you have access to one; run on the spot. Warm yourself up first to avoid any danger of stretching and straining when your muscles are cold.

2. In all these exercises, unless I stipulate otherwise, try for three sets of ten repetitions (10–10–10). Oddly, if you can do this, the exercise is too easy and you should increase the 'resistance' i.e. the weight, until you can accomplish something like 10–8–6. As soon as you can do 10–10–10 you increase the weight again.

3. While the exercises must be a struggle, don't deviate from the exercise position. If you do, you are trying for too heavy a weight; and if you do alter the position, you will find yourself not exercising the correct muscle group; or exercising the correct group incorrectly; you may actually be harming yourself.

4. You breathe *in* at the start of the exercise; breathe *out* when you're over the hard bit.

5. There's no set weight to start with; it will vary with each person. Roughly speaking a youngster of 18 to 20 can 'clean', that is to say, lift to his shoulders, about 60 to 70 pounds; if you're over 40 drop to 40 to 50 pounds to start with.

So, let's start with the SHOULDERS; in particular the DELTOID MUSCLES; and the basic exercises; the CLEAN and standing PRESS. This used to be the Olympic event until the early sixties, when the theorists and the experts ruined it between them by making it all too complicated. It's simply lifting a weight to your shoulders and then hoisting it aloft above your head. At my best I used to be able to 'clean' and 'press' around 325 pounds.

The shoulder girdle for a man is one of the most showy areas, if he wishes to develop an impressive physique. The girls aren't so interested in shoulders, and they'll probably pass over this one. The shoulders consist primarily of two quite large muscles, known as the shoulder caps, which are in fact the deltoid muscles. They are directly tied in to the chest muscles (pectorals) and the biceps and triceps, and the trapezius, the big neck muscles. If you work your deltoid muscles, you invariably exercise your arms, neck and chest at the same time. The action of the deltoid is to raise the arm to the level of the shoulders and then to raise it overhead as well. Therefore, any exercise to be of use must work over the full range of the muscle action.

So, probably the most important exercise of all for the deltoid muscles is the two hands press; which can be done with barbells (two-handed) or dumbells (single-hand weights; both hands at once or one at a time); and the exercise is merely to push the weight from the shoulder position to the full arms stretch position over head. But, of course, you've got to get the bar or the dumbells up to your shoulder first; so we start with the clean.

Two-handed clean

This in itself is one of the best exercises for all-round development; it works on your whole body.

1. Select a barbell which is within your capabilities.

2. Stand central to the barbell, with your feet 18 to 20 ins apart with the bar touching your ankle.

3. Crouch down, grasp hold of the bar, wrists on top, with your hands equidistant from the weights and your hands just outside your foot placing, and fractionally wider than your shoulders. Your shoulders should be in front of your knees which are in front of the bar; and your back must be straight. Your head is up. Breathe *in*.

4. Drive vigorously with your legs. The bar should come off the floor immediately. You pull the bar up purely by the straightening of your legs until it starts to pass your thighs. You then bring your arm and shoulders into play and continue the movement smoothly until the bar moves up and into your shoulders. Breathe *out*.

5. Your elbows should be well up to lock the bar into position. (If you're doing the clean purely as an exercise, you then lower the bar to your thighs, crouch back down and return the bar to the floor into the starting position).

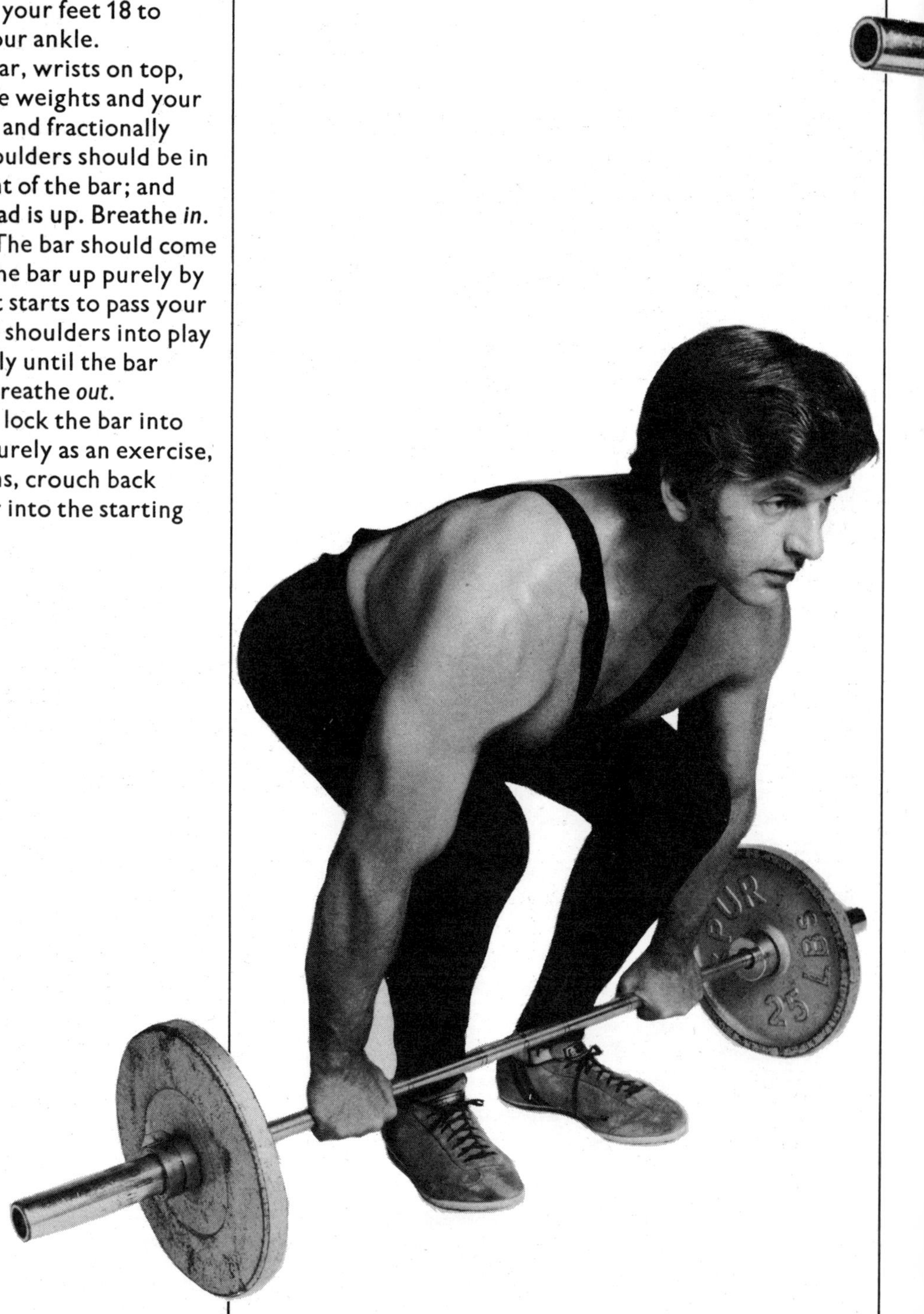

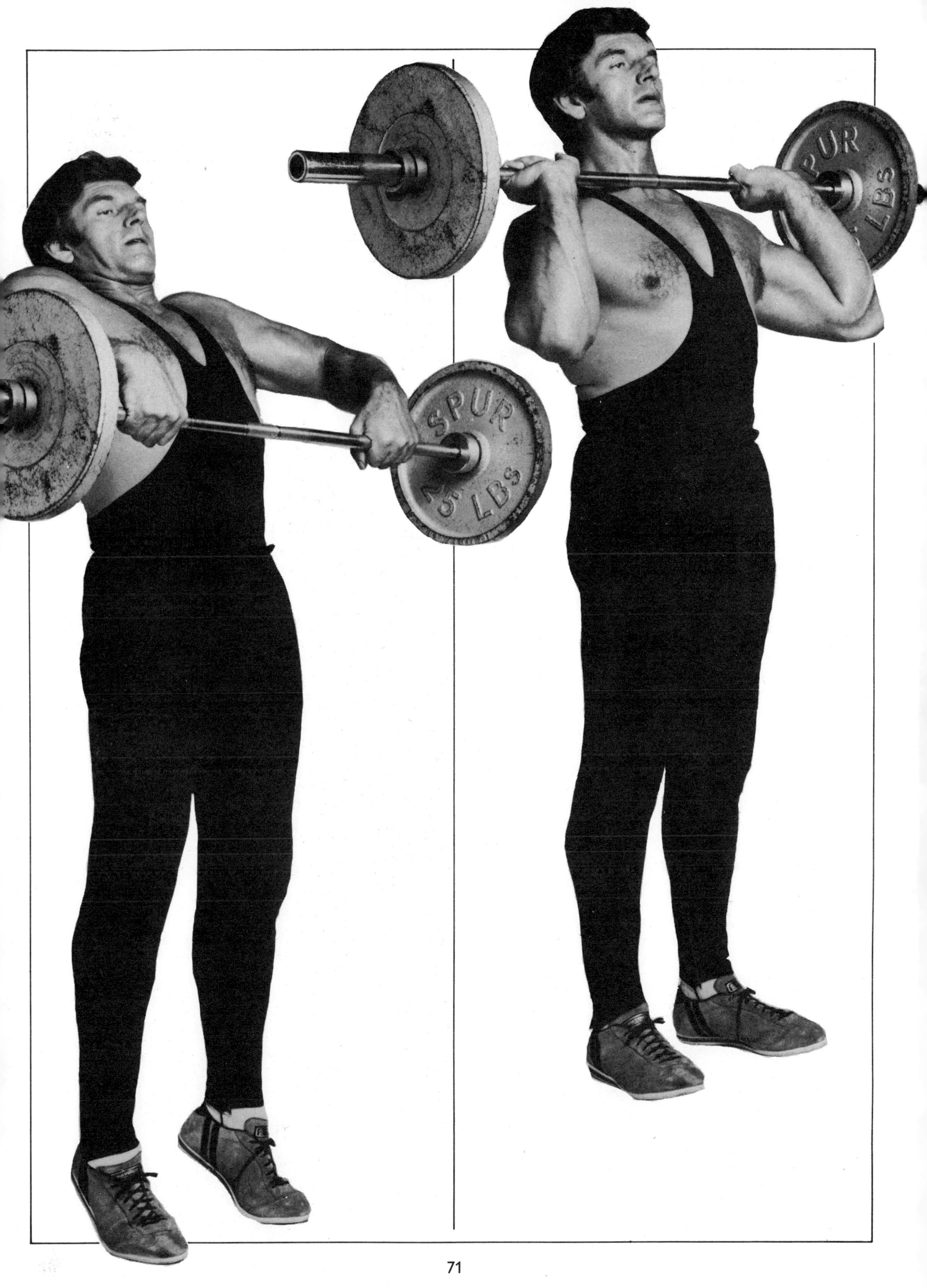
SPUR
25 LBS
SPUR
LBS

Two Hands Press

1. Stand with barbell across the front of your chest as at end of the clean. Breathe *in*.
2. Press the bar above your head, using only your arms and shoulder muscles.
3. Breathe *out* after the hard bit – that's after it passes above your head – and lock your arms at full stretch above your head.
4. This is really the starting position of the exercise.

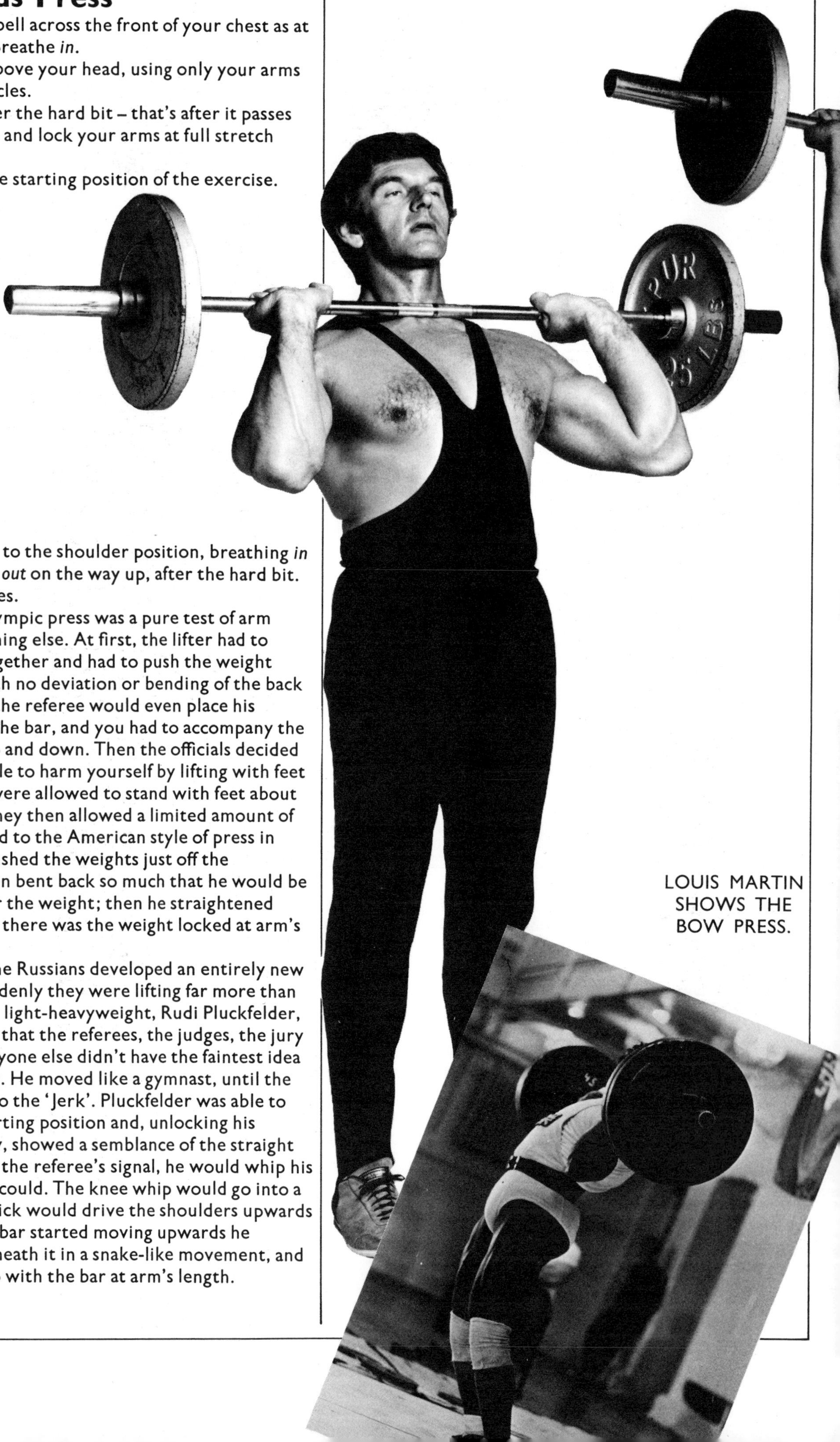

Lower the barbell to the shoulder position, breathing *in* on the way down; *out* on the way up, after the hard bit.
5. Repeat ten times.

The original Olympic press was a pure test of arm strength, and nothing else. At first, the lifter had to stand with feet together and had to push the weight above his head with no deviation or bending of the back at all. Sometimes the referee would even place his finger on or near the bar, and you had to accompany the referee's finger up and down. Then the officials decided that you were liable to harm yourself by lifting with feet together, so you were allowed to stand with feet about 16 inches apart. They then allowed a limited amount of back-bend. This led to the American style of press in which the lifter pushed the weights just off the shoulders, and then bent back so much that he would be almost lying under the weight; then he straightened everything up and there was the weight locked at arm's length.

Around 1960, the Russians developed an entirely new technique and suddenly they were lifting far more than ever before. Their light-heavyweight, Rudi Pluckfelder, was so fast in 1961 that the referees, the judges, the jury of appeal and everyone else didn't have the faintest idea what he was doing. He moved like a gymnast, until the 'Press' merged into the 'Jerk'. Pluckfelder was able to get into a bow starting position and, unlocking his knees very slightly, showed a semblance of the straight position; then, on the referee's signal, he would whip his knees as fast as he could. The knee whip would go into a hip kick, the hip kick would drive the shoulders upwards and as soon as the bar started moving upwards he would sink underneath it in a snake-like movement, and then he'd stand up with the bar at arm's length.

LOUIS MARTIN SHOWS THE BOW PRESS.

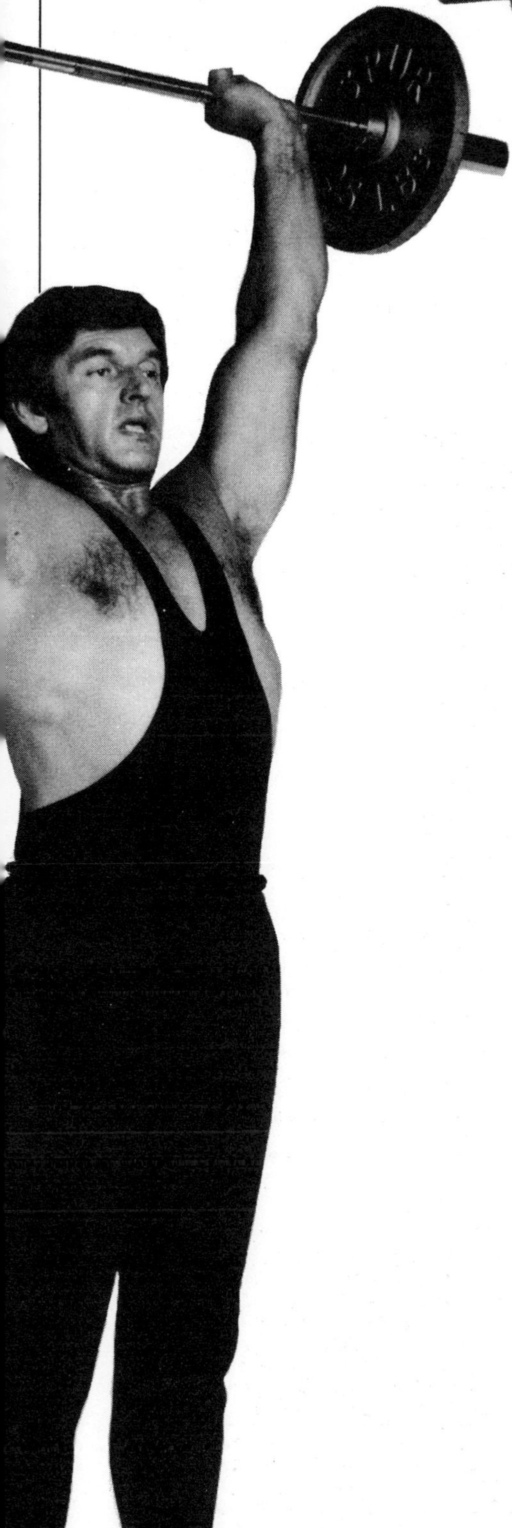

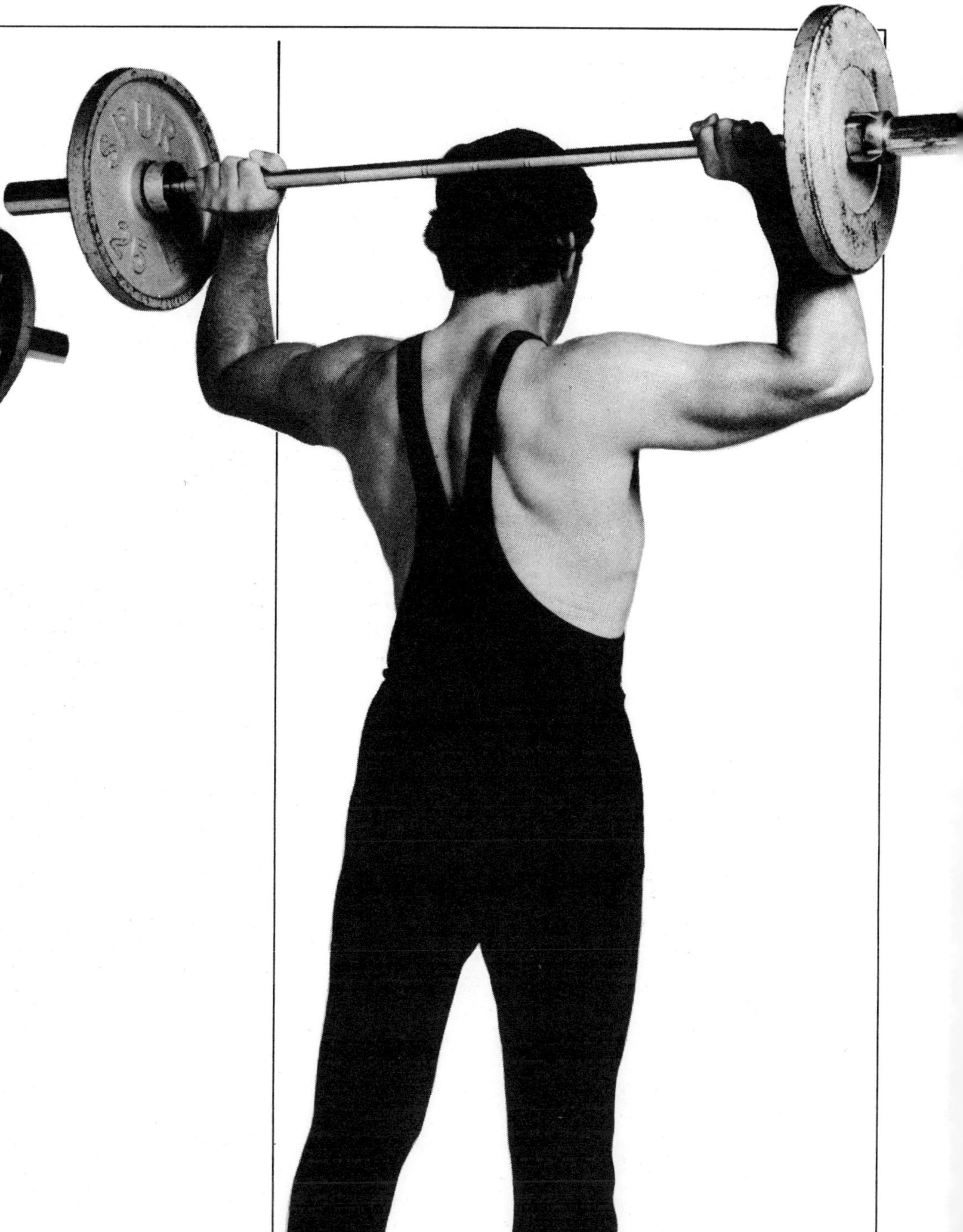

The two hands press can be done from the seated position, which makes it that much more disciplined an exercise; it may also be performed as the two hands press behind neck, which is popular with body-builders as it not only brings into play the deltoids, but also makes more use of the trapezius muscles and triceps.

Lateral Raise

This is an exercise which can be done with either barbell or dumbell. It is done in three different ways to affect the three different areas of the deltoid muscle group. There is the lateral, or side deltoid, the anterior, or front deltoid and the posterior, or rear deltoid. The lateral raise exercise used in most exercise programmes is the side lateral raise in which two dumbells are used.

Side Lateral Raise

1. Select a reasonable pair of weights (10–15 pounds).
2. Stand upright with the dumbells hanging at arm's length, the weights resting at the side of your thighs.
3. Breathe *in*. Keeping your arms as straight as possible, raise the dumbells to the side until they are above shoulder level.
4. Lower, keeping arms straight, breathing *out* on way down.
5. Repeat 10–15 times (up to three sets).

This is a shaping exercise, more than a strict building exercise and most physique contestants include plenty of this in their routines.

The lateral raise for the anterior, or front, part of the deltoid is done almost in the same way, with a slight difference.

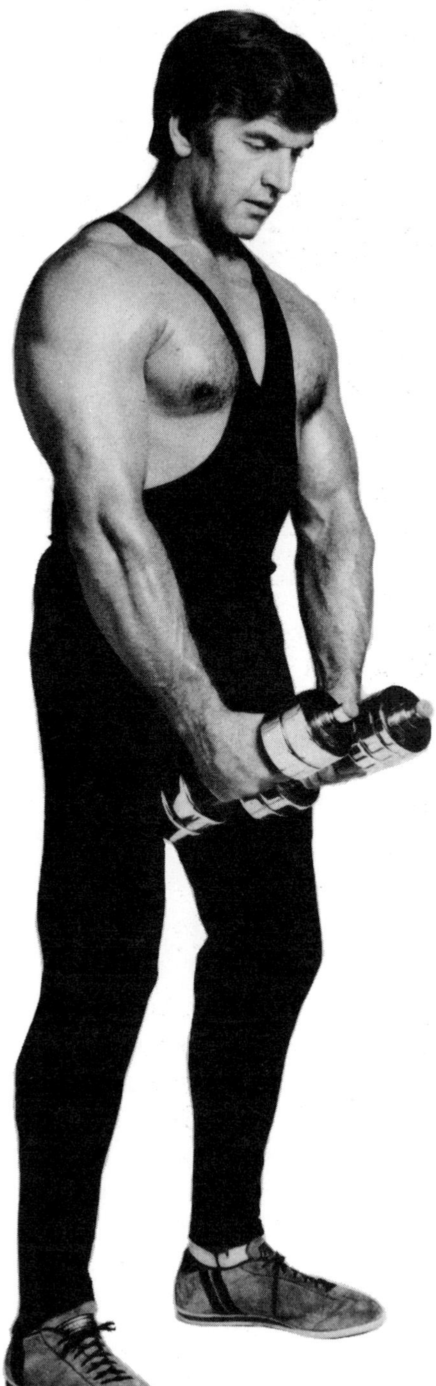

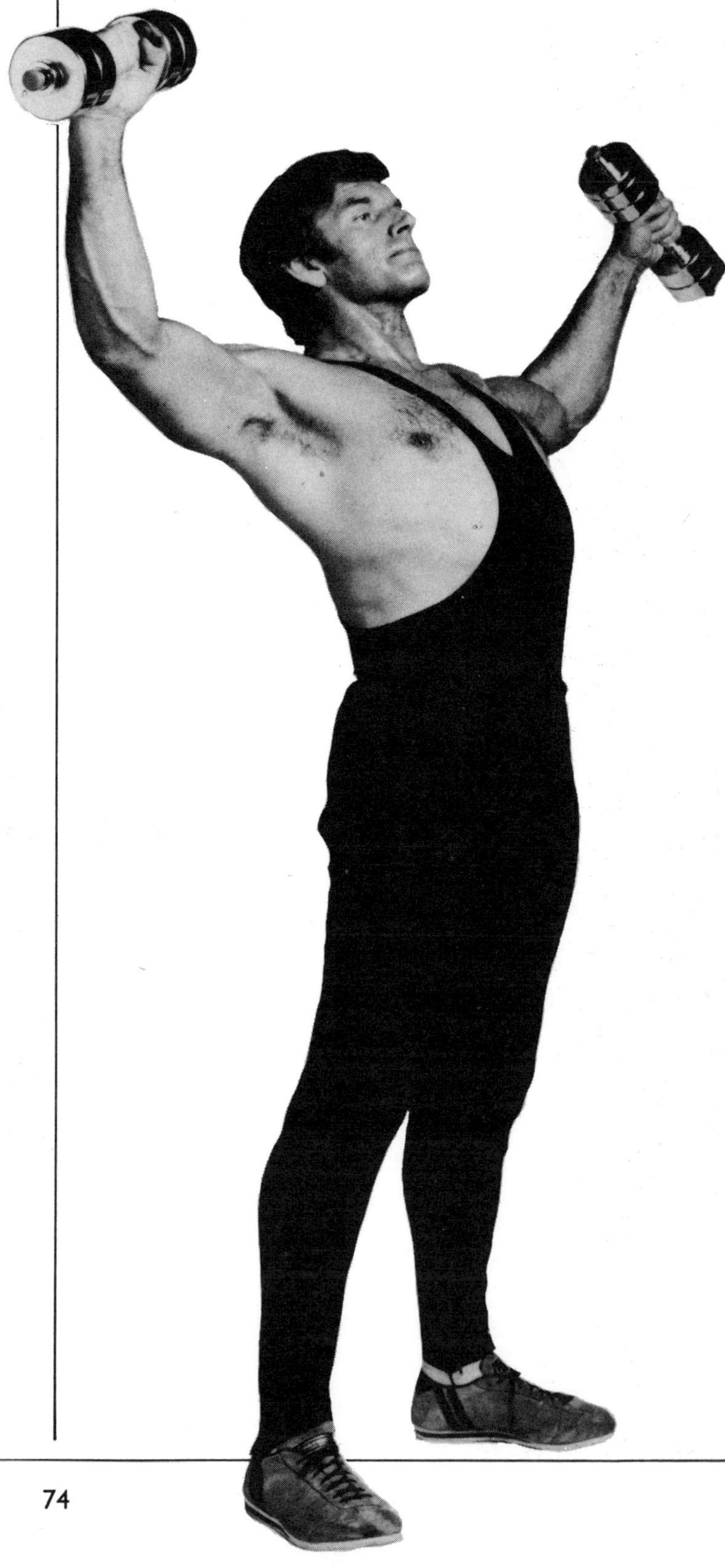

Front Lateral Raise

1. Hold the dumbells so they are resting at front of thigh.
2. Breathe *in*. Keeping your arms straight, raise them *in front* of you to just above shoulder level.
3. Lower, keeping arms straight. Breathe *out* on way down.
4. Repeat 10–15 times (up to 3 sets).

Incidentally, this exercise can be done alternately with dumbells one arm at a time, so you get a sort of see-saw effect.

For the rear, or posterior section of the deltoid, you have to alter your body position to enable you to work this particular area of the muscle group. The exercise is called the bent-over laterals.

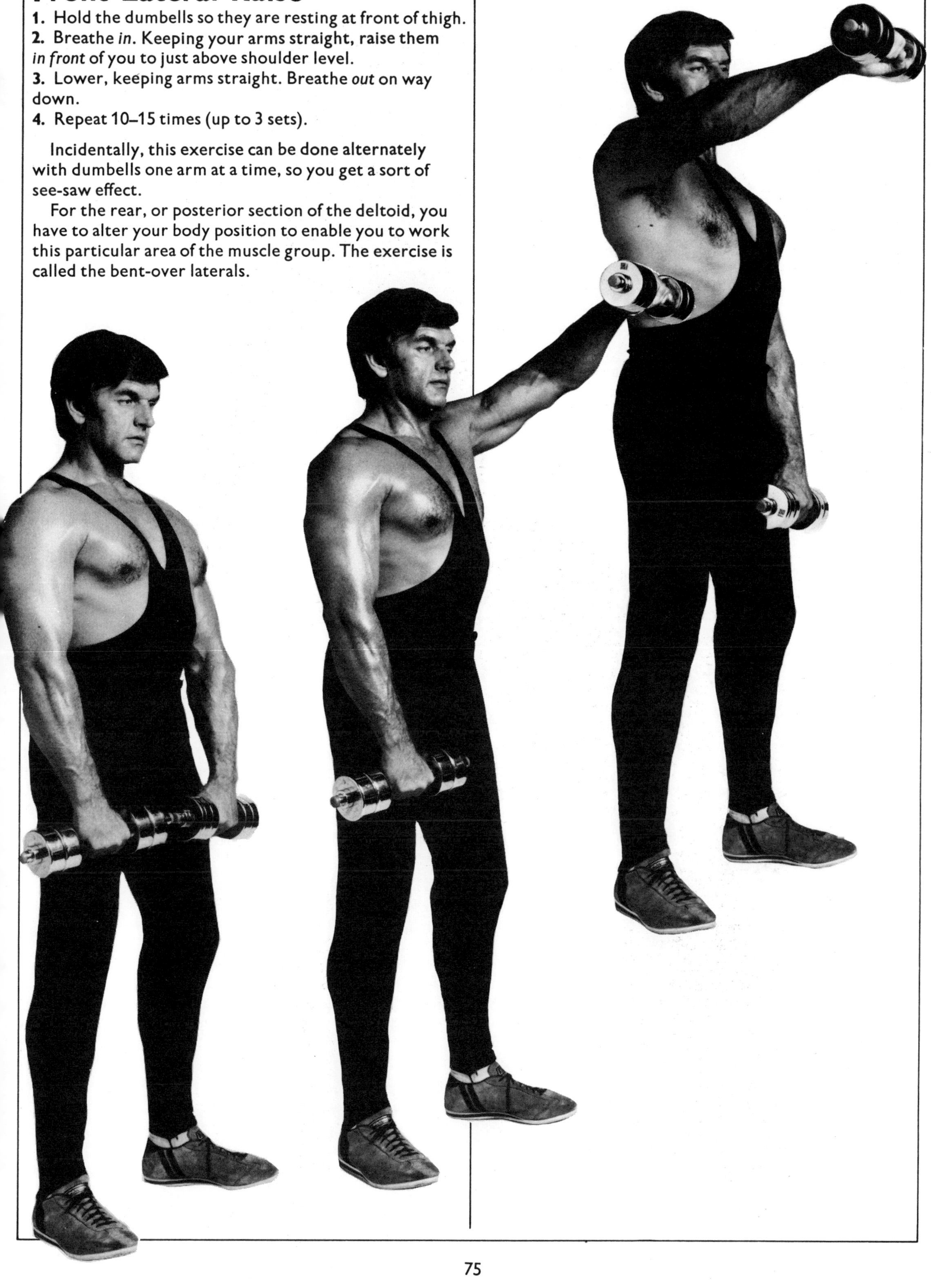

The Bent-over Laterals

1. Select a much lighter weight (maybe 5–10 lbs).
2. Stand feet astride. Bend forward so your back is straight, parallel to the floor, and with the dumbells hanging at arm's length nearly touching the floor.
3. Stay in this position, trying not to get any back movement at all. Breathe *in*. Raise your arms out sideways level with your shoulders, keeping your arms straight.
4. Return to Position No 1. Breathe *out* on way down.
5. Repeat 10–15 times (up to 3 sets).
NB This is a most important part of physique development, and one which is most commonly neglected.

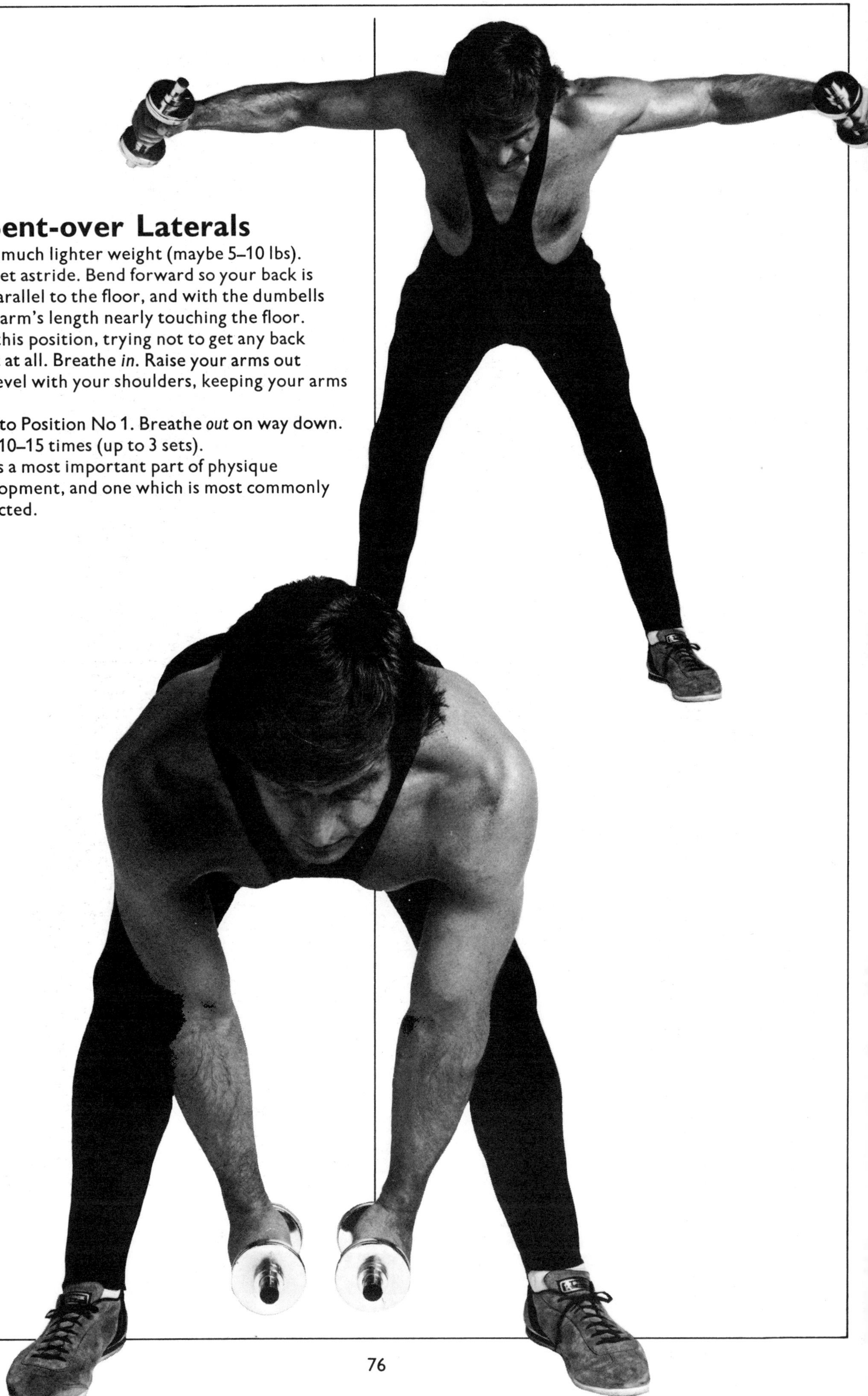

Upright Rowing

This is another super exercise for your shoulders, and it also affects your trapezius muscles. Once again, you can do this either with barbell or dumbells, but it is most commonly done with barbells.

1. Select a suitable weight (for a beginner, about 40 pounds).

2. Pick up the barbell with a central hand grip.

NB It is essential to grip the exact centre of the bar. If you don't, the bar is going to wobble all over the place.

3. Stand up with the bar so that it is resting across the front of your thighs.

4. Breathe *in*. Bring your thumbs up to your chin, keeping your elbows up all the time (NB This is most important).

5. Repeat 10 times (up to 3 sets).

A reminder: in all these exercises, *maintain your exercise position*. This will ensure you're working the correct muscle group over the full range. That's enough for the time being about shoulders. Let's move on to arms.

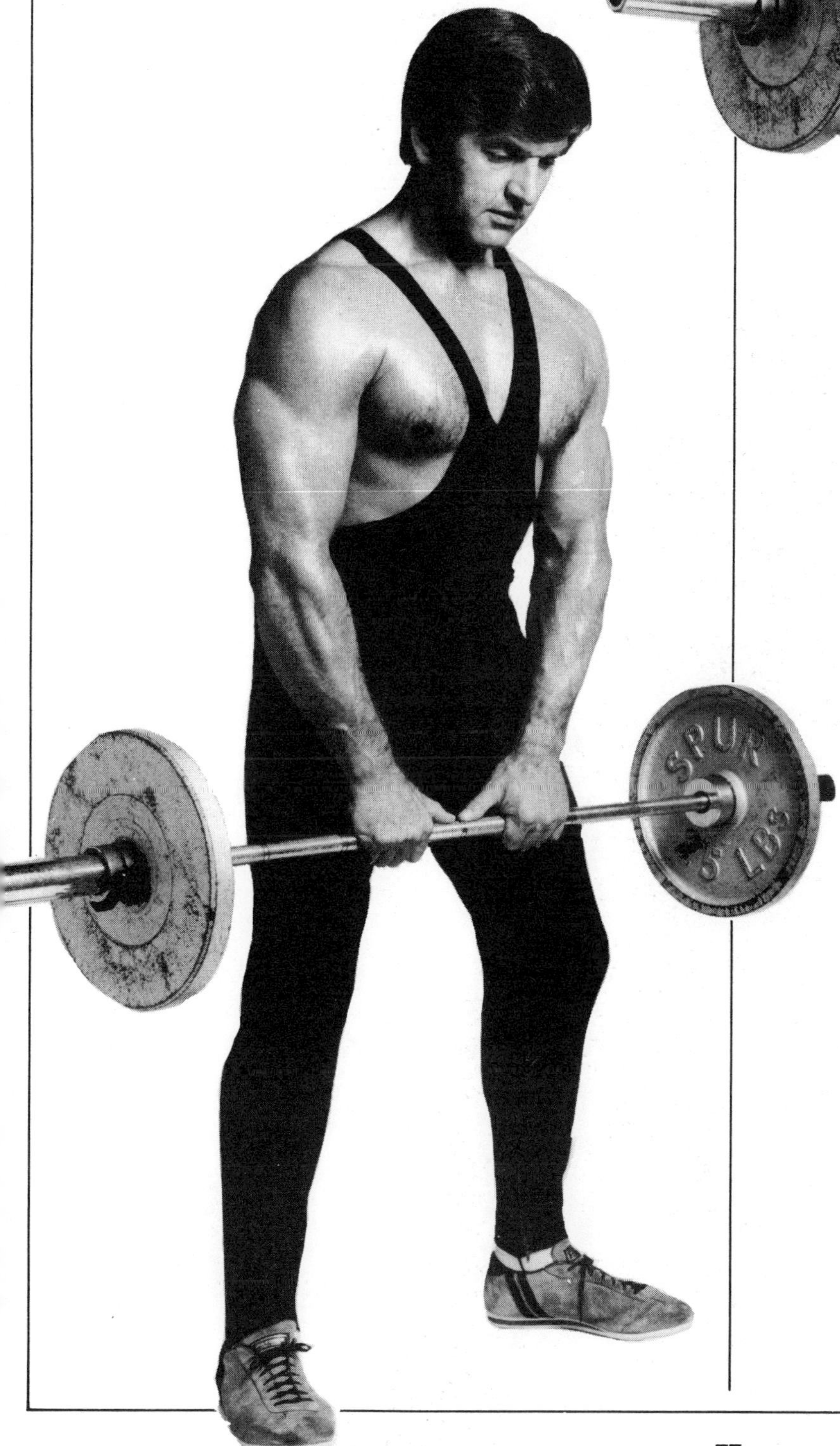

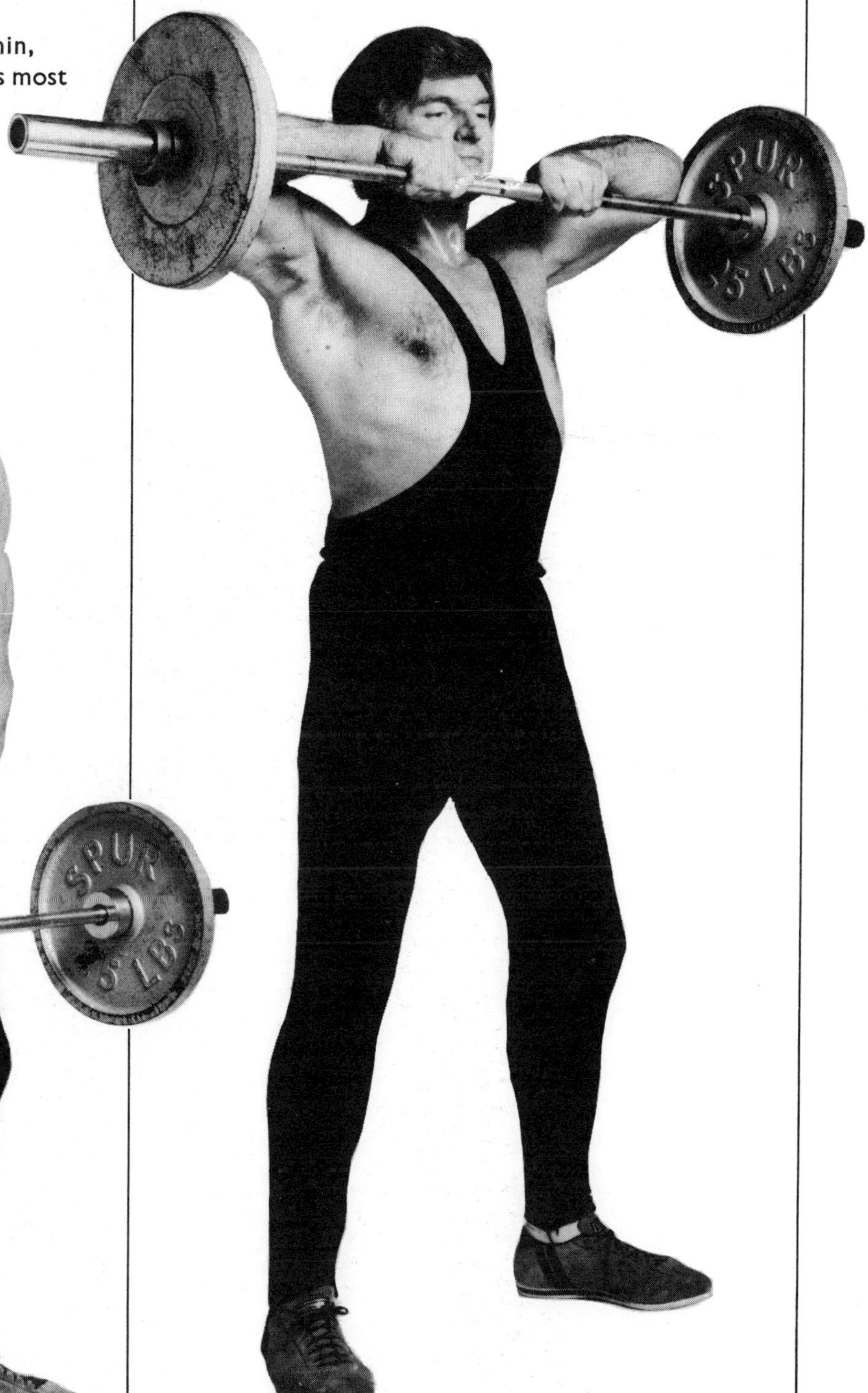

UPRIGHT ROWING AS A DUMBELL EXERCISE.

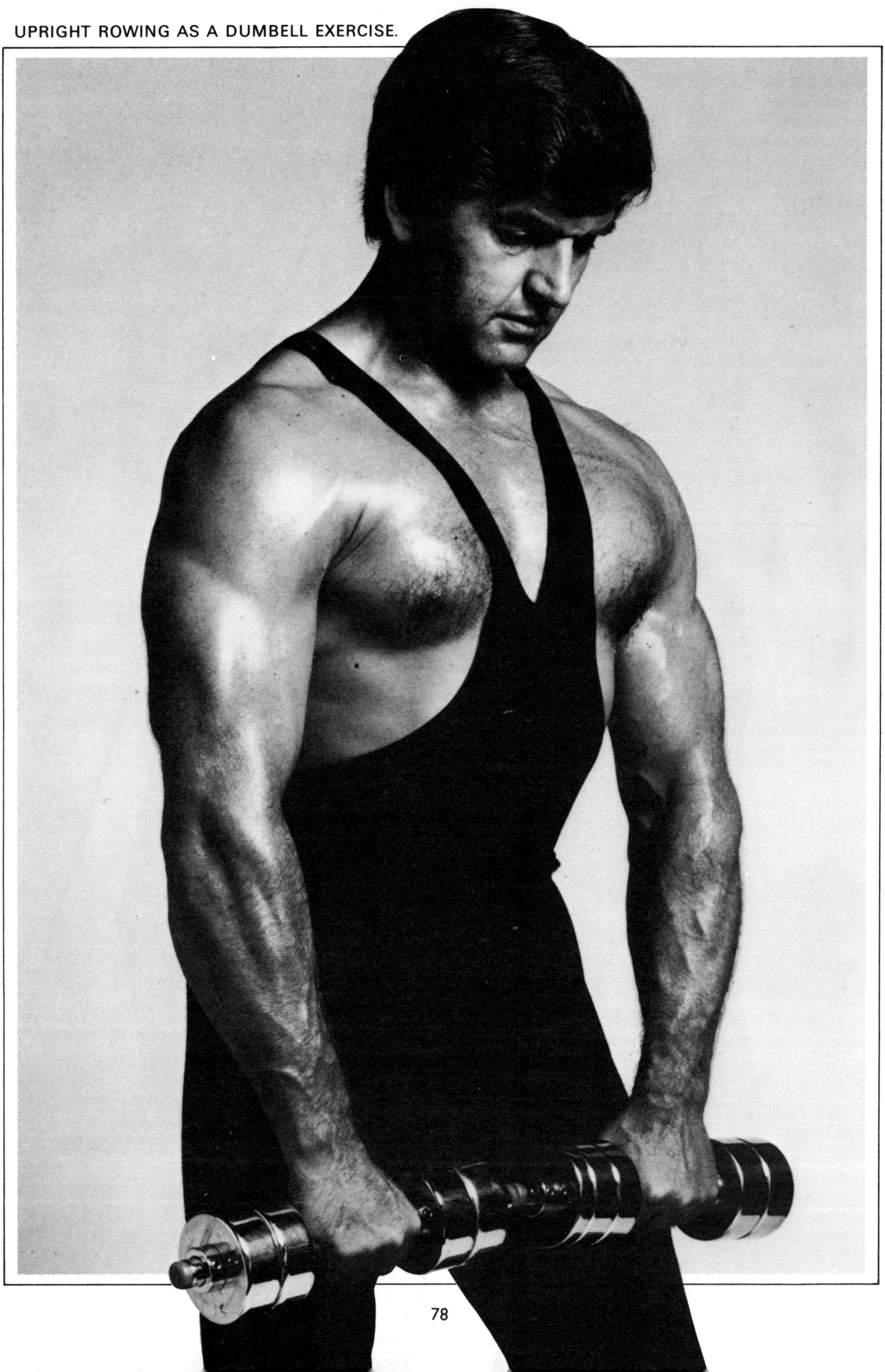

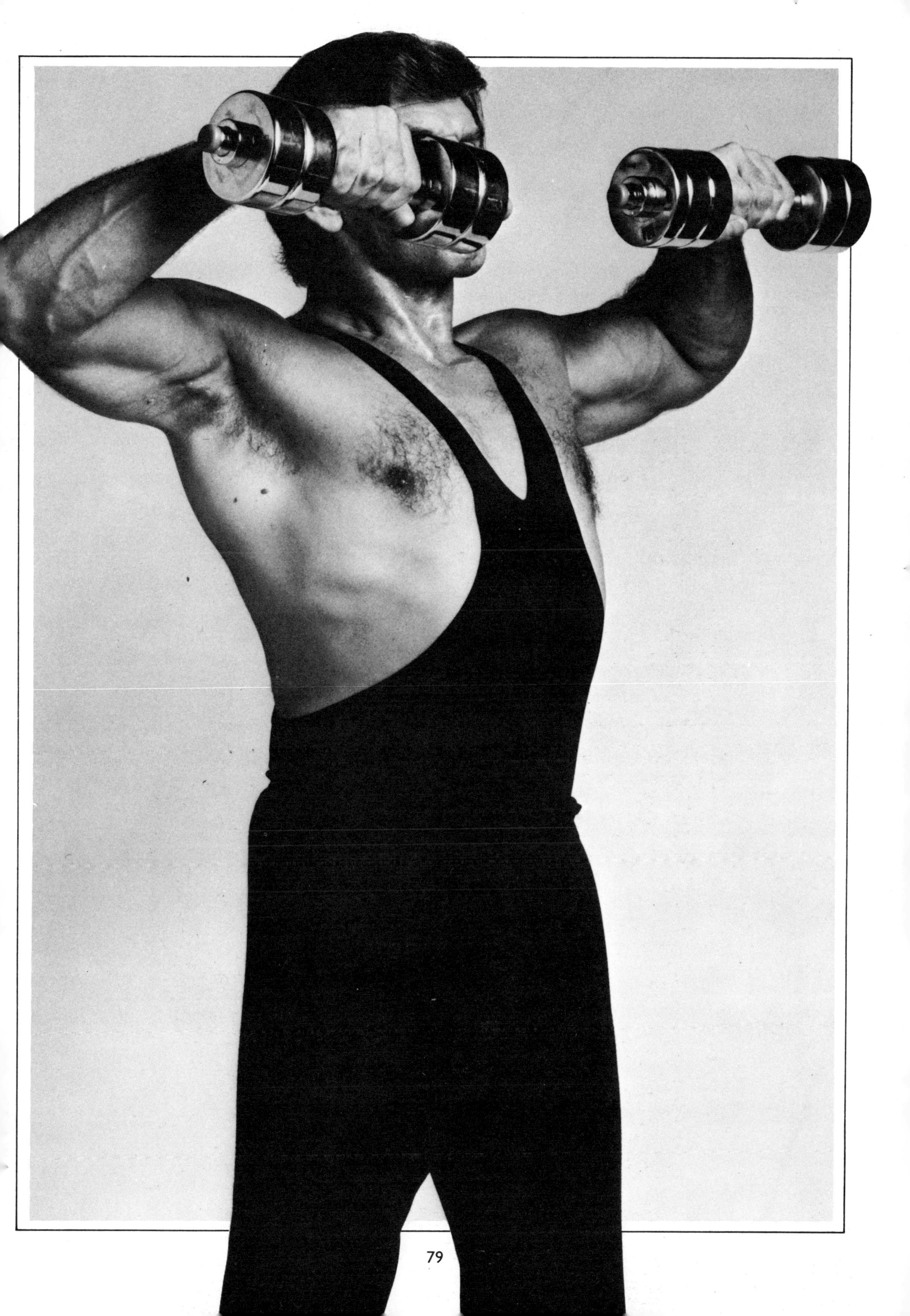

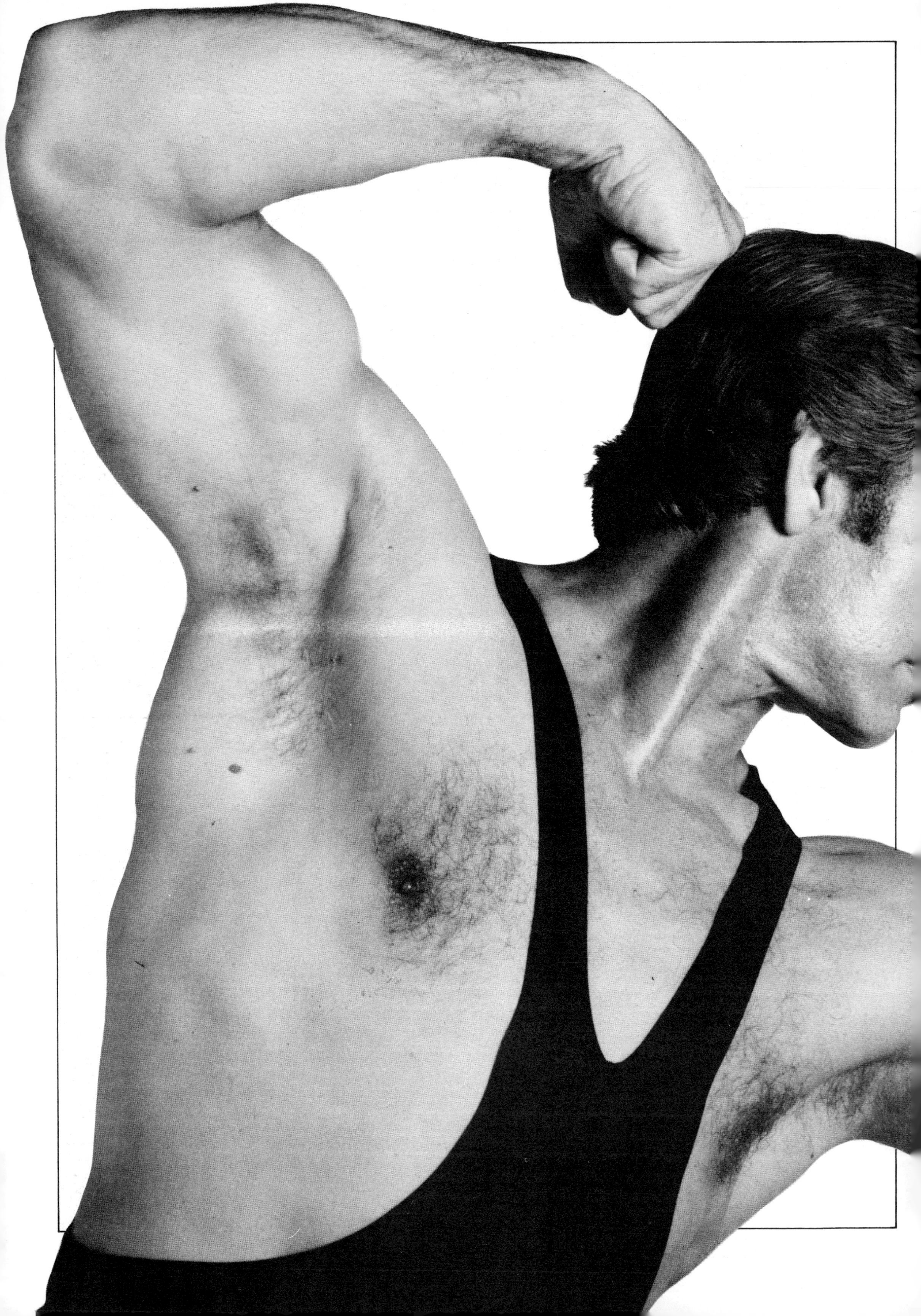

Chapter II

DO IT THE DAVE PROWSE WAY

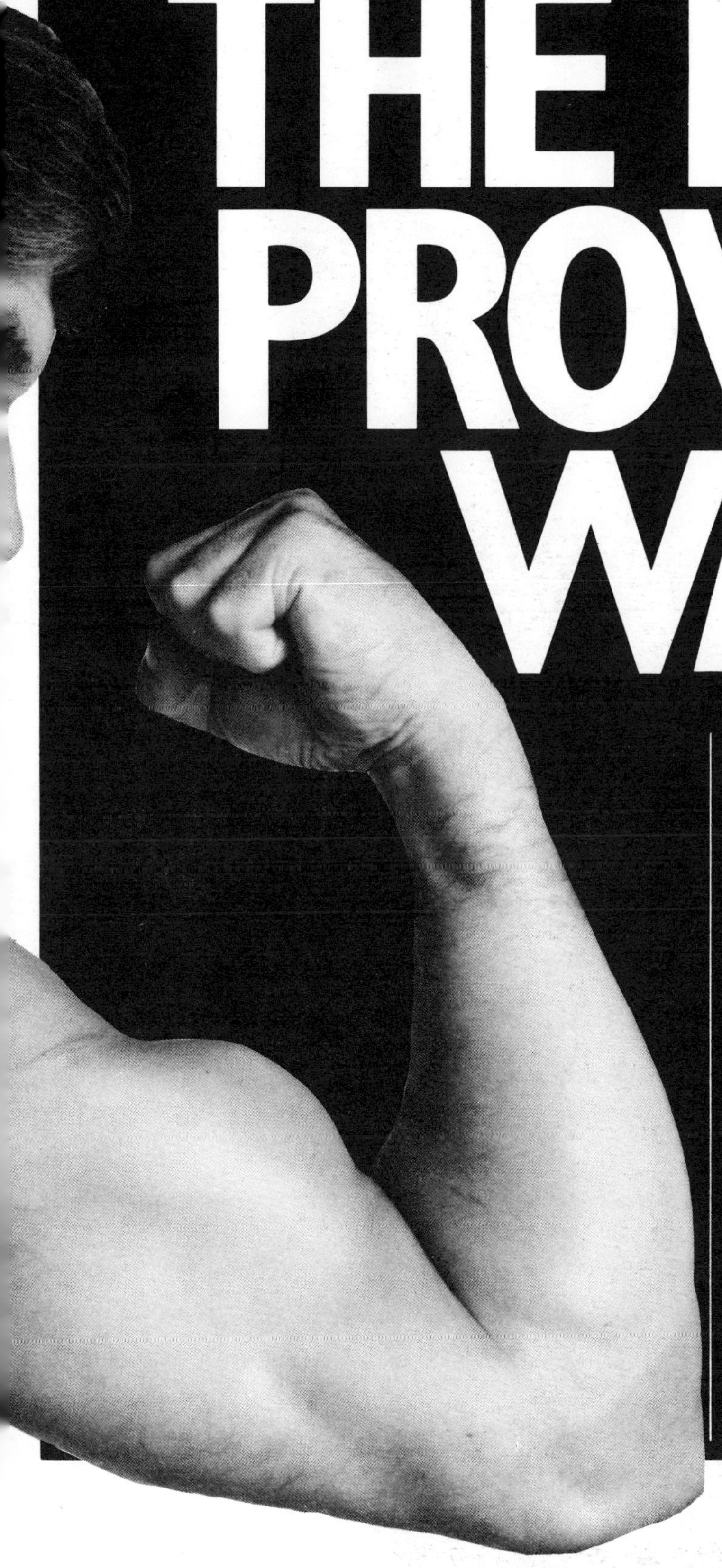

At this stage, I think we'll content ourselves with the two important muscle groups of the upper arm, the biceps and triceps.

The BICEPS is a two-headed muscle whose action is to bend the arm at the elbow (almost through 180 degrees) and at the same time to supenate (twist) it slightly. The TRICEPS muscle is the antagonist, or opposite muscle, whose function it is to straighten the arm.

The 180 degrees of the arm action is in fact split into three distinct areas. From the arm stretched position to about 60 degrees is the OUTER RANGE; the middle 60 degrees is called the MIDDLE RANGE; and the final 60 degrees to where the wrist comes in to the shoulder is called the INNER RANGE. Whenever you do biceps exercises, the exercise you're doing affects either one or two of those parts – very seldom do you find an exercise which works over all three parts. So if you want your exercise programme to be complete, you have to do several different exercises to cover the full range of movement, altering your body position to gain the maximum effect. This is why I have developed my own technique with the two hands barbell curl, to get as much work over the full range of movement as possible. Let's do it the Dave Prowse Way.

Two Hands Barbell Curl

1. Stand with your feet astride directly over the bar.
2. Grasp the bar with a slightly narrower grip (hands 12 ins apart) than usual, using an undergrip.
3. Stand up so barbell is resting across your thighs in front of you.
4. Bend your knees. Incline body forward about 30 degrees so your shoulders are in front of the bar. Keep body in this position throughout exercise.
5. Bend your arms, bringing the barbell up so your hands touch your chin.
6. Repeat 10 times (up to 3 sets).

Doing the exercise this way, you get very little effect over the OUTER range of muscle movement; as you go through the MIDDLE RANGE it gets progressively harder; and it's a positive struggle to get through the INNER RANGE. If you do this exercise properly, what we call the peak contraction part (i.e. the inner range muscle movement) is particularly taken care of. (That's the bit that makes the biceps bulge . . .).

Once more, don't deviate from or distort the exercise position prescribed. Choose a weight with which you can perform the exercise at the start. I've lost count of the times that people have come to me from health and exercise gymnasia, and complained they're having great difficulty in developing this muscle or that. The moment you see them exercise you know why – they're not maintaining the right positions and so aren't getting the benefit they're working so hard for.

This Dave Prowse two hands curl can be done either with the barbell or with two dumbells, both hands together or alternately. It can also be done as a seated exercise; seated with dumbells it becomes a complete range exercise but with barbell you're only working through half the range of movement.

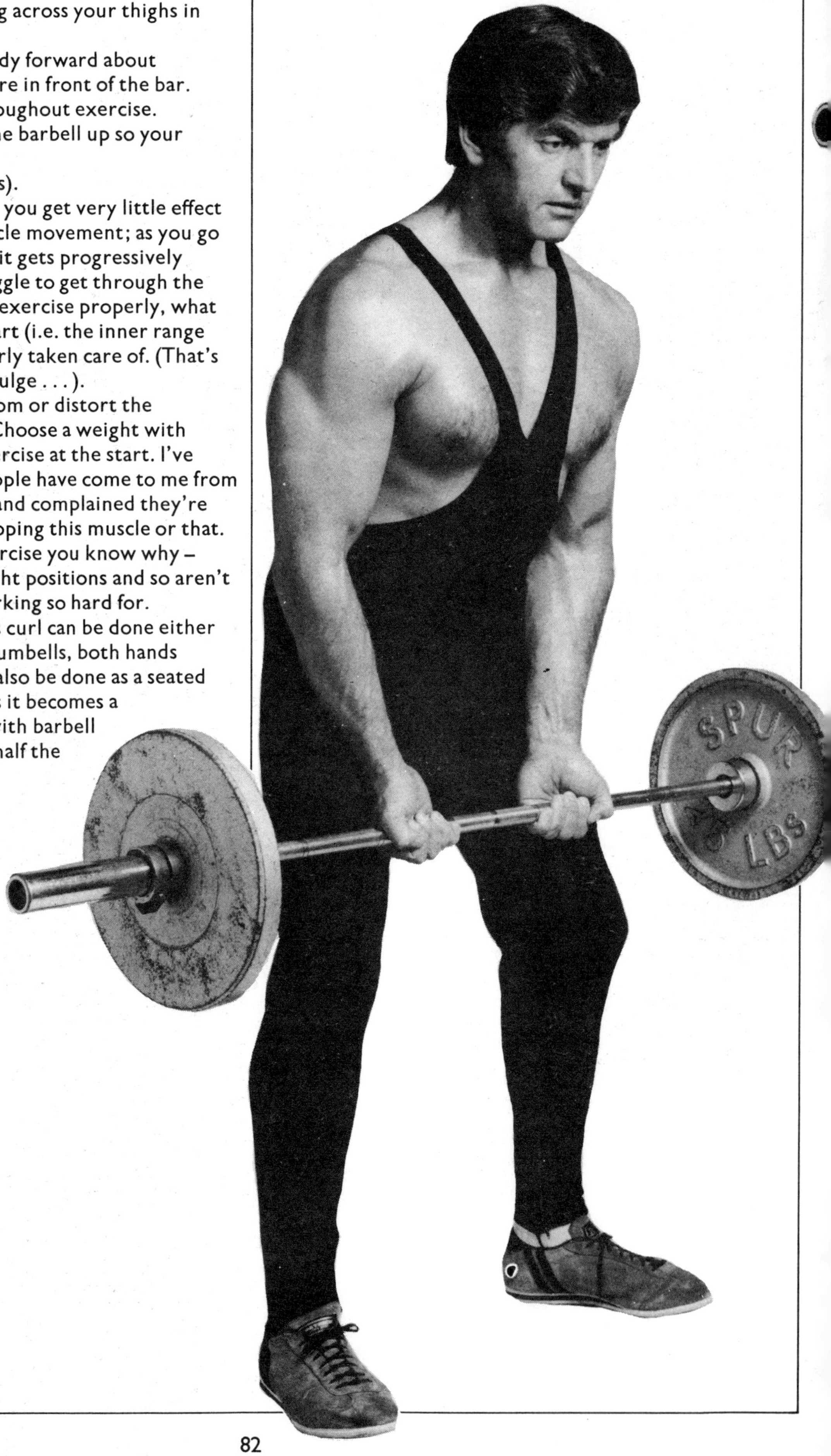

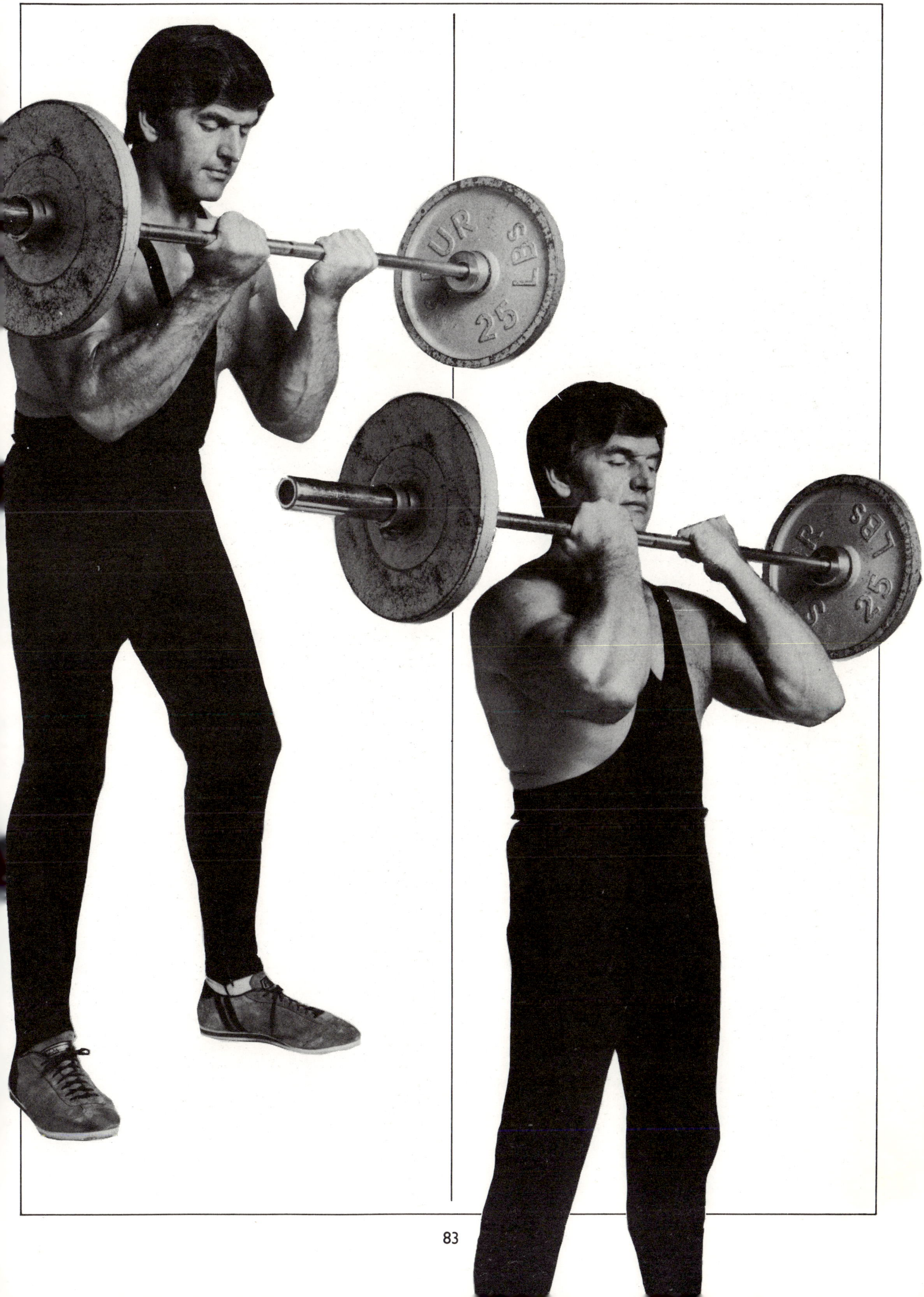
UR
25 LBS
UR
LBS
25

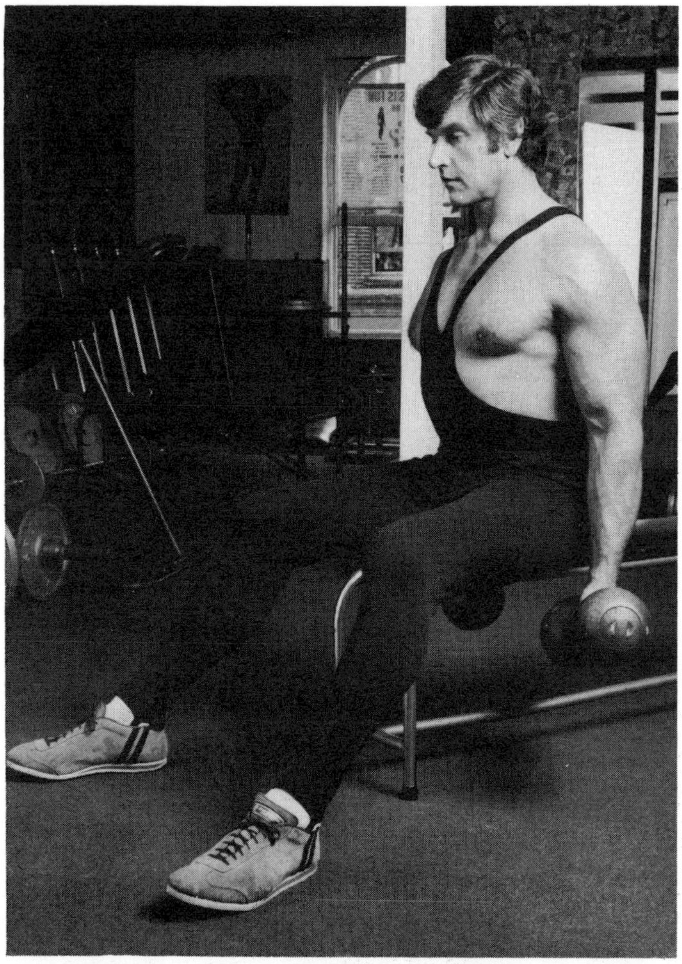

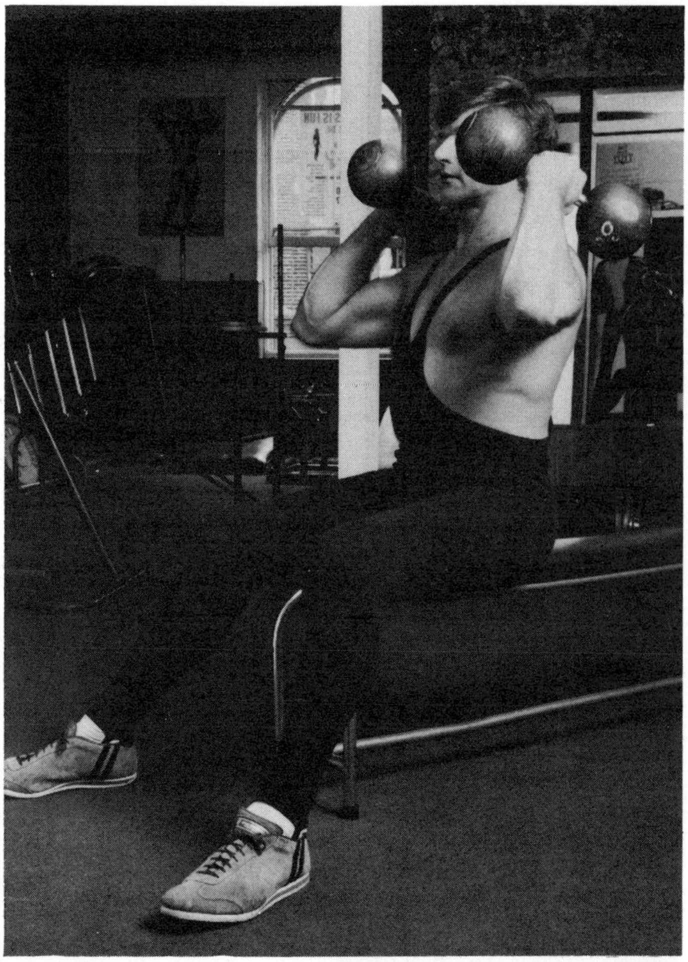

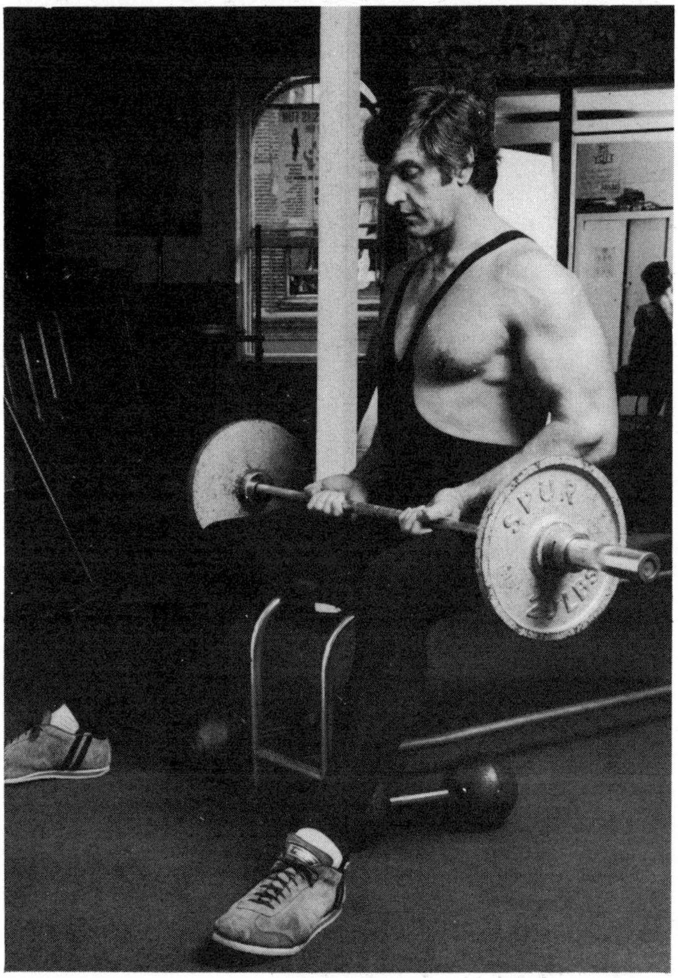
SPUR

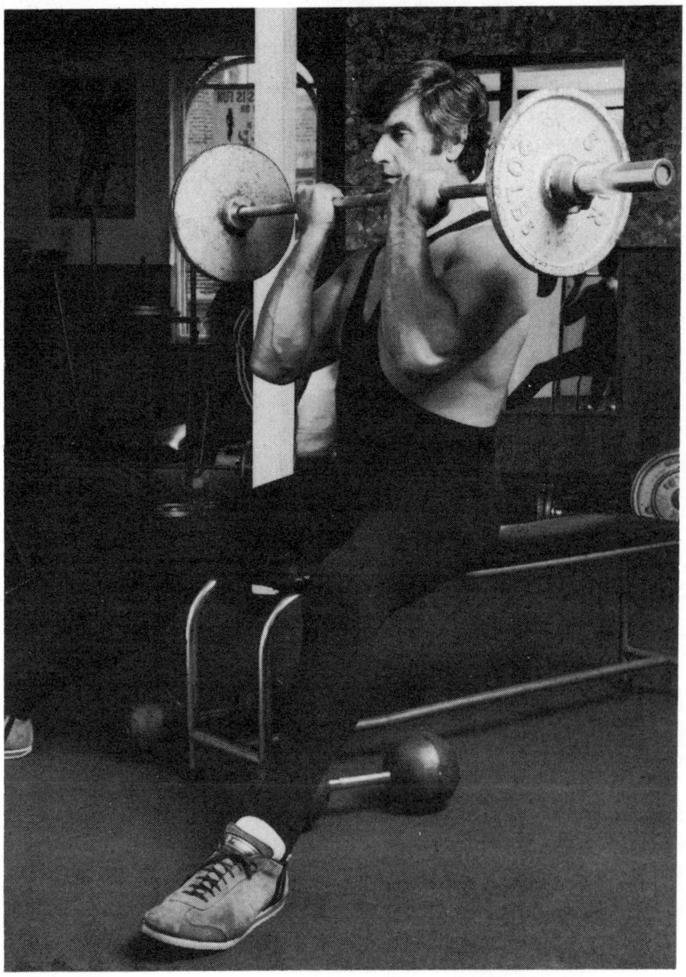

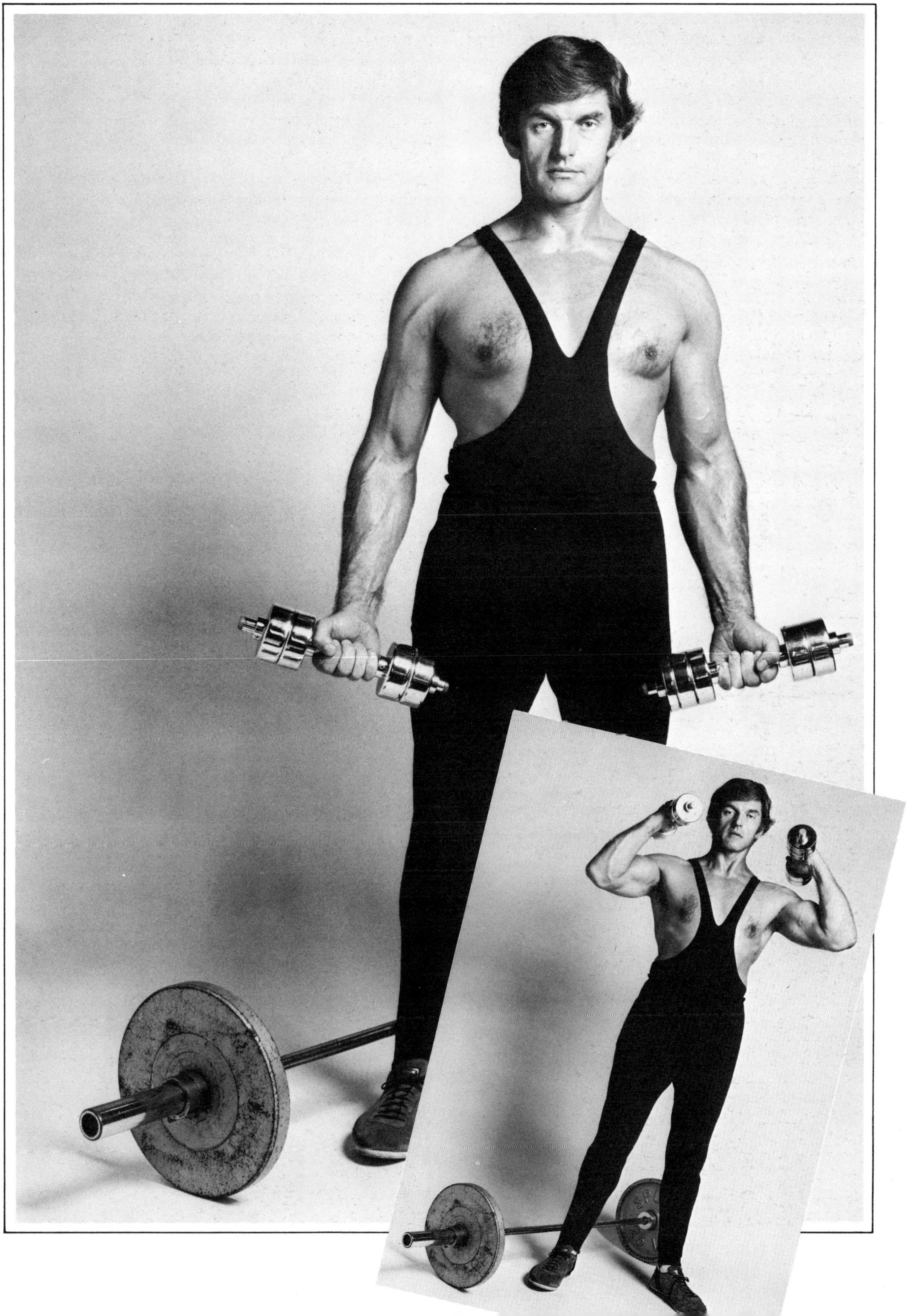

Bent-over Concentrated Curl

The theory of this exercise is that if you work hard at the top, or inner range of biceps movement, it tends to 'peak' the biceps and give you a nice-looking lump when you flex your arm muscles. Normally speaking, one would do this exercise with a dumbell.

1. Sit in a chair or on a bench. Select a weight you can handle fairly comfortably at the beginning, in order to get the position exactly right.
2. Place the hand you're not exercising on your knee; let the dumbell hang down between the legs with the elbow resting against the thigh.
3. Lean forward so that your shoulder is forward of the weight.
4. Keeping the shoulder in the same position, bring the dumbell up until it touches the shoulder. Do not lean back at all – you'll lose the whole point of the exercise.
5. Repeat 10 times with each hand (up to 3 sets).

There are other more advanced exercises for the biceps muscles, all of which have to involve the bending of the elbow; depending on the upper arm positioning, the exercises will affect different parts of the range of movement.

Most people don't realise that the triceps muscle is twice the size of the biceps; therefore, if you want to enlarge the size of your upper arm, you'll be much better off doing triceps exercises rather than biceps, even though the biceps muscle is the more showy one.

All triceps muscle exercises involve straightening your arm against resistance – it's an action you perform without thinking a hundred times a day – just pushing yourself away from the table, for instance, or putting something on a shelf above your head. Even pushing the bedclothes off while you're lying in bed is a triceps exercise. What I like to do when I work the triceps is to bring other correlated muscle groups into play. One of the best triceps exercises is in fact one of the best chest exercisers too. It's the parallel bar dip.

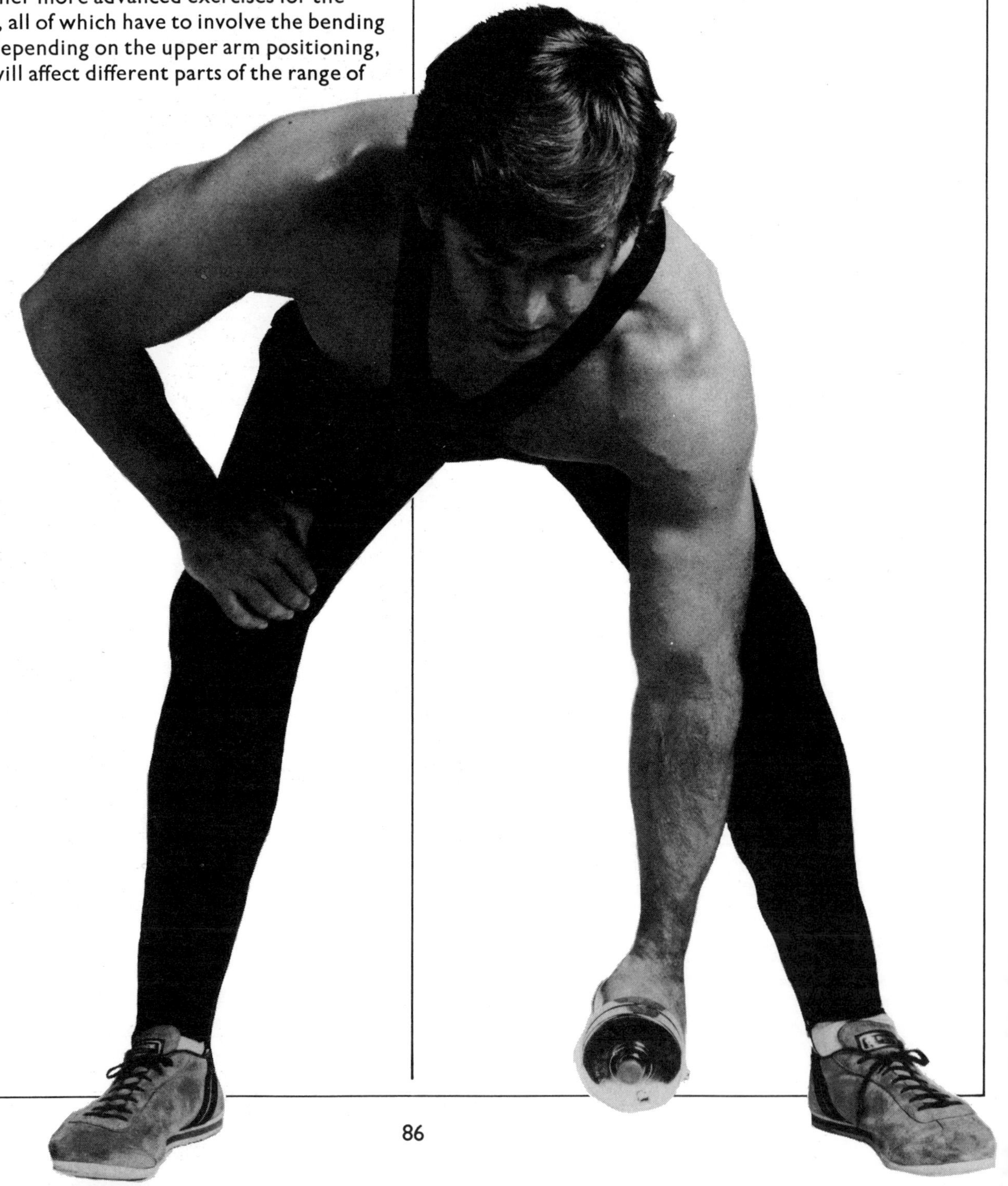

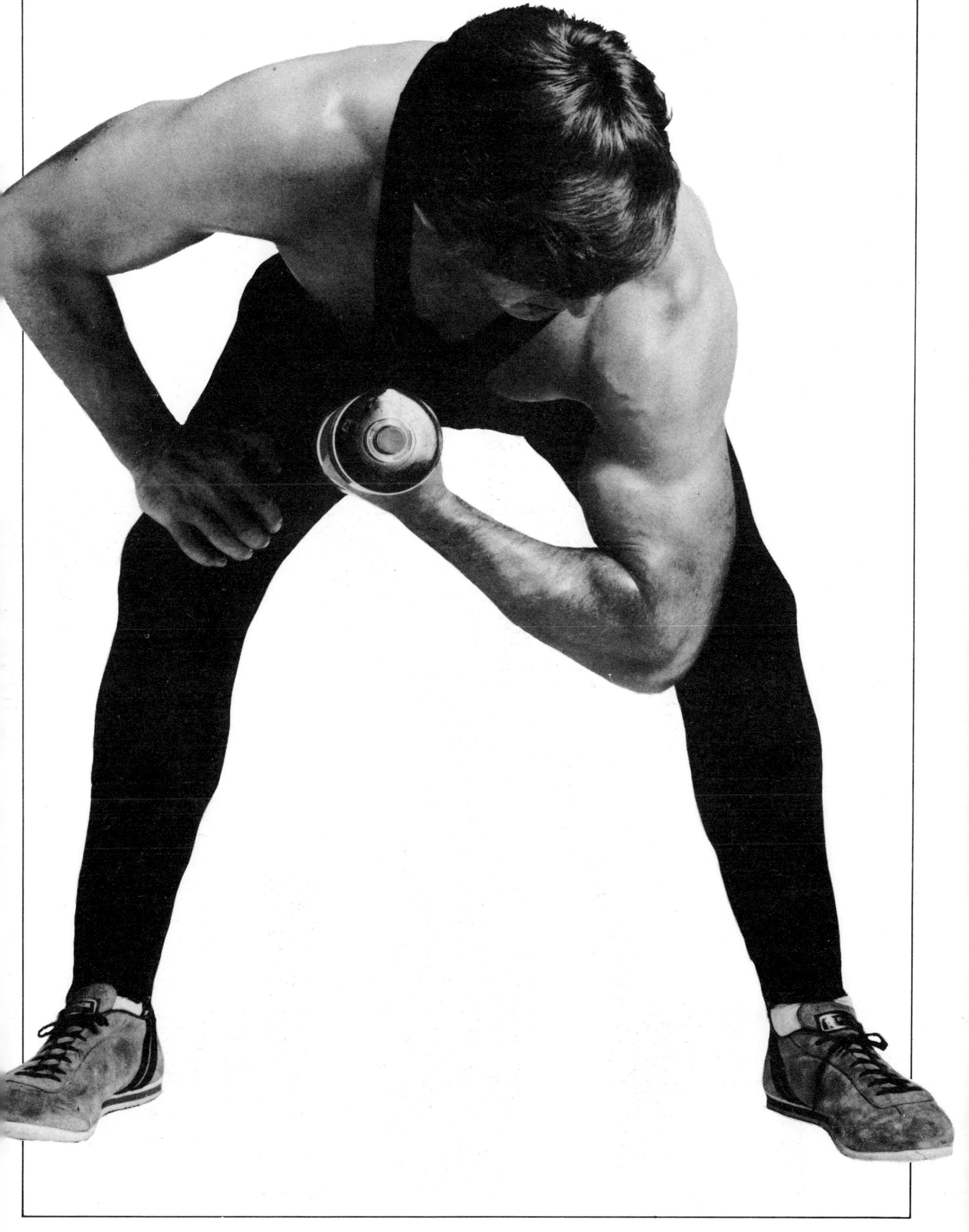

Parallel Bar Dip

It can be done on parallel bars, or equally well on the backs of two chairs, provided they're well anchored.

1. Place the chairs a little wider than shoulder width apart. Stand between them, grasping the tops of the chairs with each hand.

2. Lever yourself up into an arms straight position. Alternatively get into an arms straight position and lift your knees behind you, taking the weight on your arms.

3. Breathe *in*. Lower yourself until your shoulders practically touch your hands.

4. Straighten your arms.

5. Repeat 10 times (up to 3 sets). But this is such a marvellous chest exercise as well you can increase the repetitions to 20 or 30.

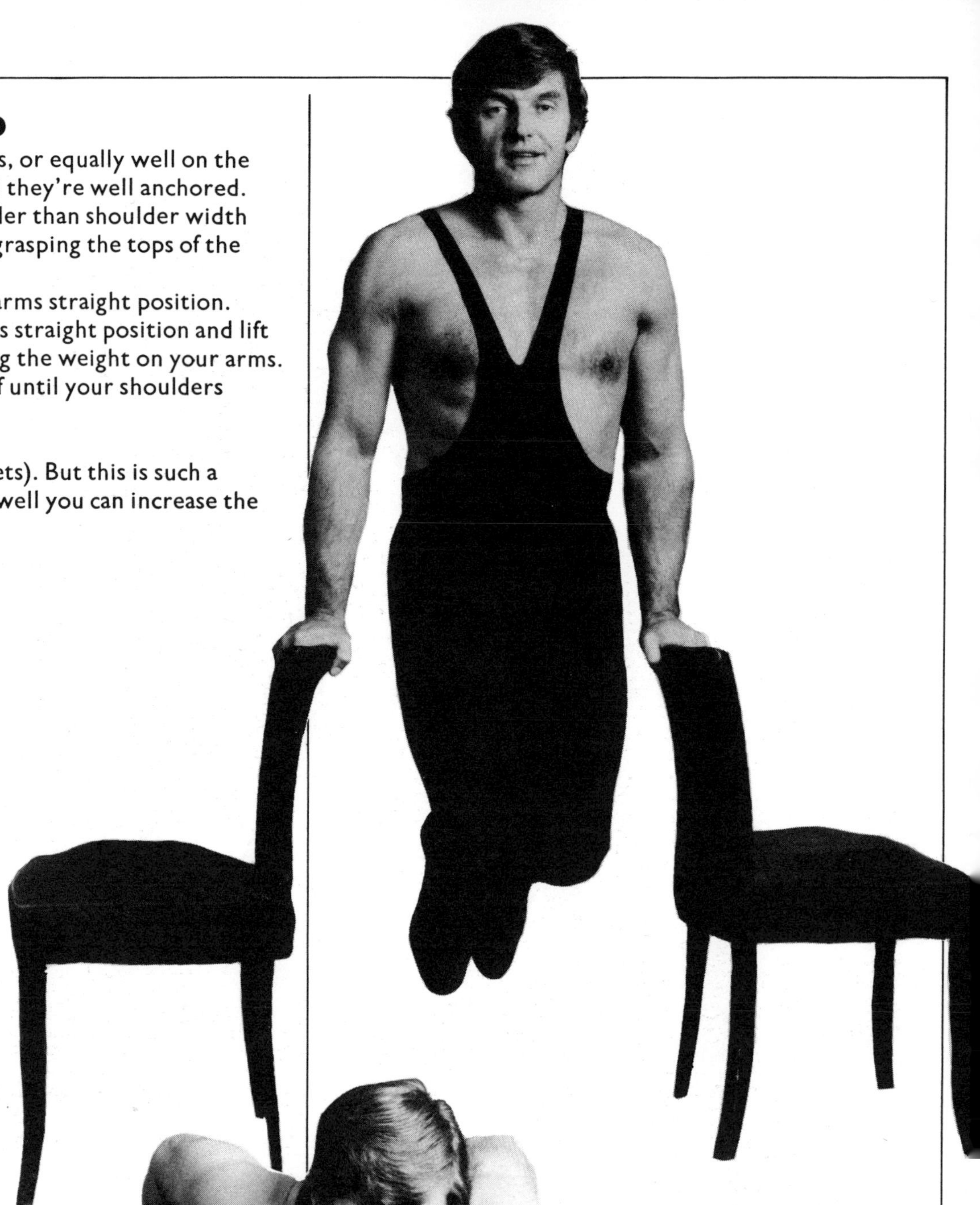

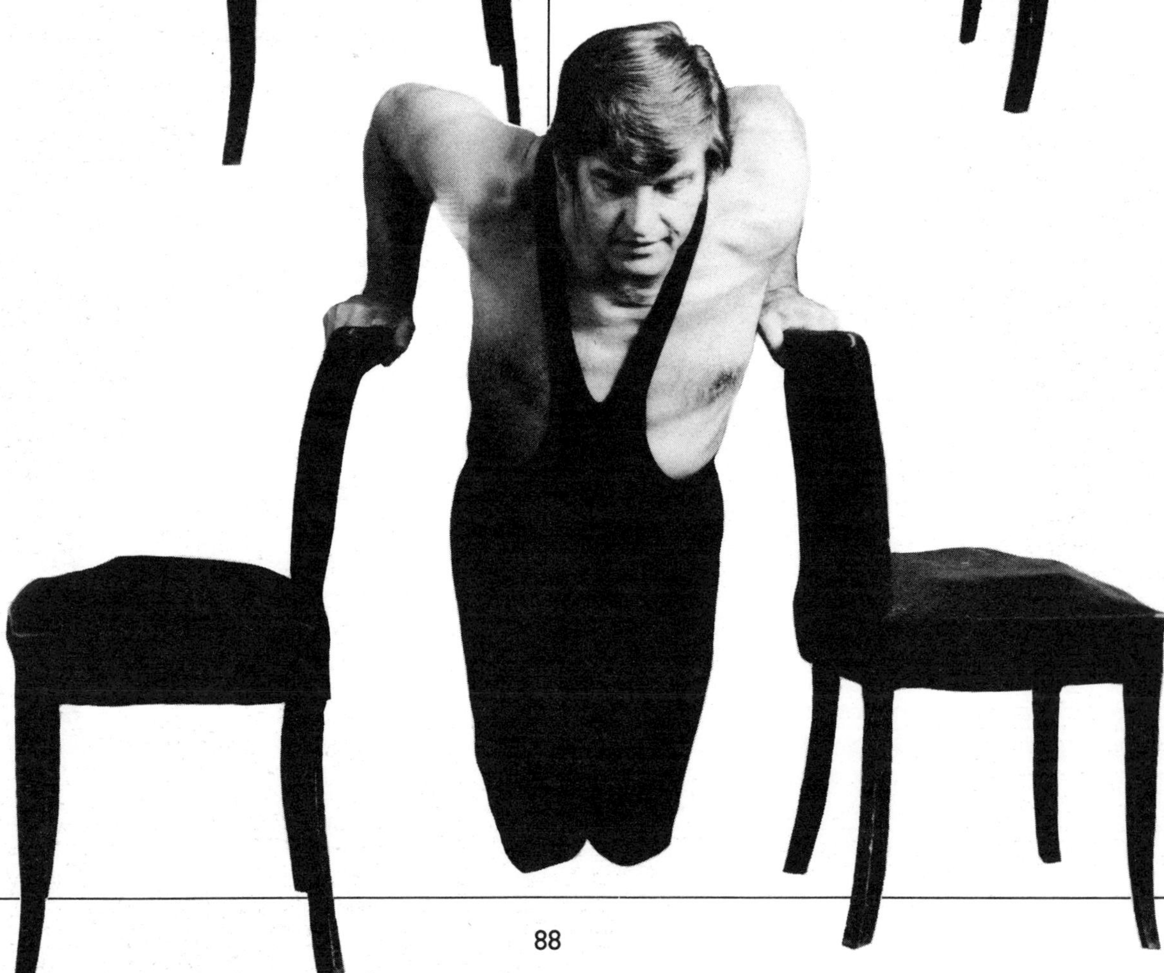

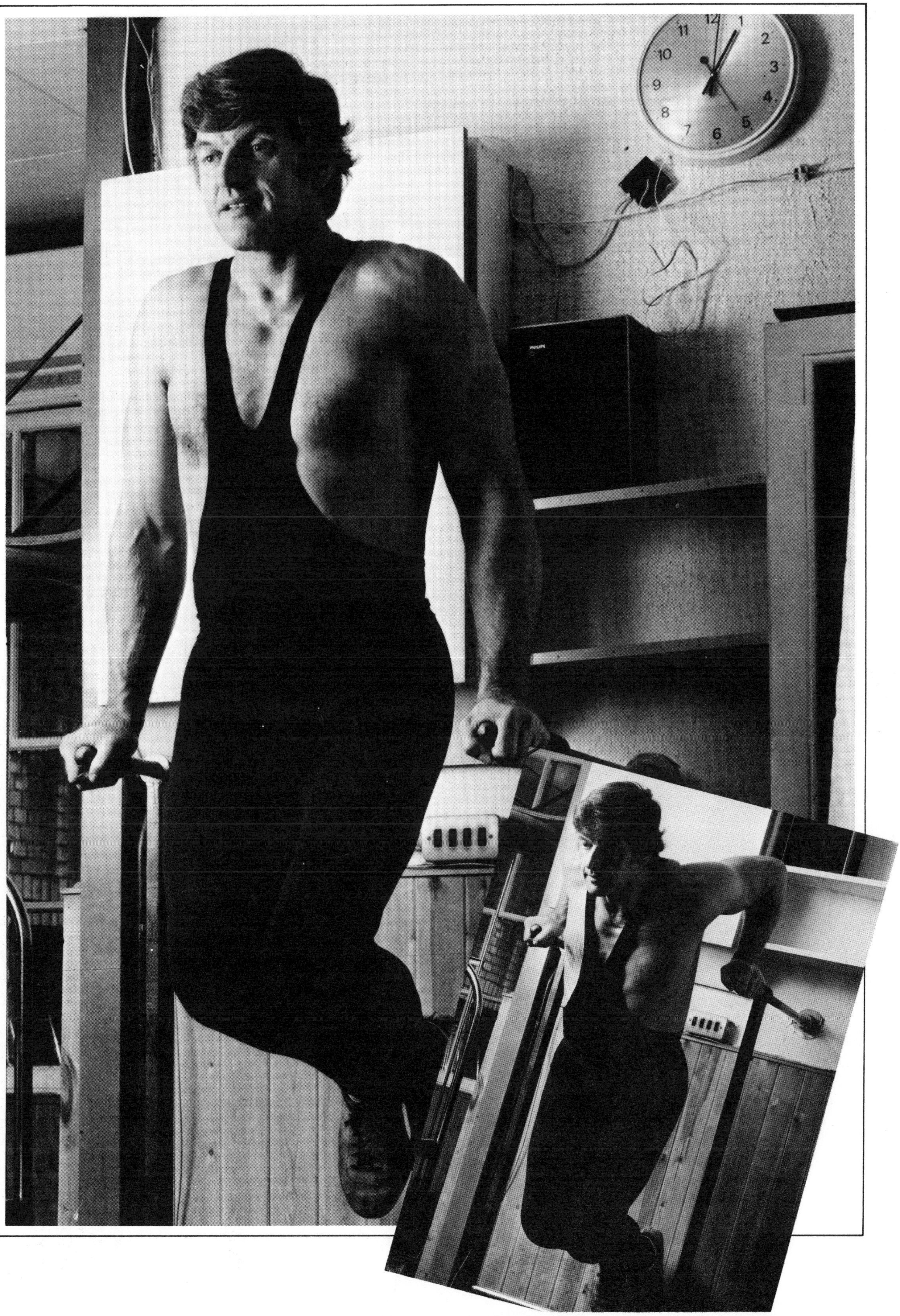

Triceps Press

1. Grasp the barbell centrally as in the upright rowing exercise.
2. Bring the bar up to your shoulders in the clean position.
3. Place the bar over your head onto your shoulders behind the neck.
4. Force your elbows backwards and as close to your ears as possible.
5. From this position straighten your upper arms until the weight rises above your head. This is the start of the exercise. So breathe *in* on way down, *out* on way back up.
6. Lower to the behind-neck position, trying to keep the arms as still as possible.
7. Repeat 10 times (up to 3 sets).

This can also be done as a single-handed dumbell exercise when the arm is straightened against the resistance of the dumbell. It will probably help to hold your upper arm in position by placing your other hand on your biceps.

The next triceps exercise has been the favourite of several famous body-builders and musclemen, including John Citrone from Chester-Le-Street, a former winner of the Mr Universe competition.

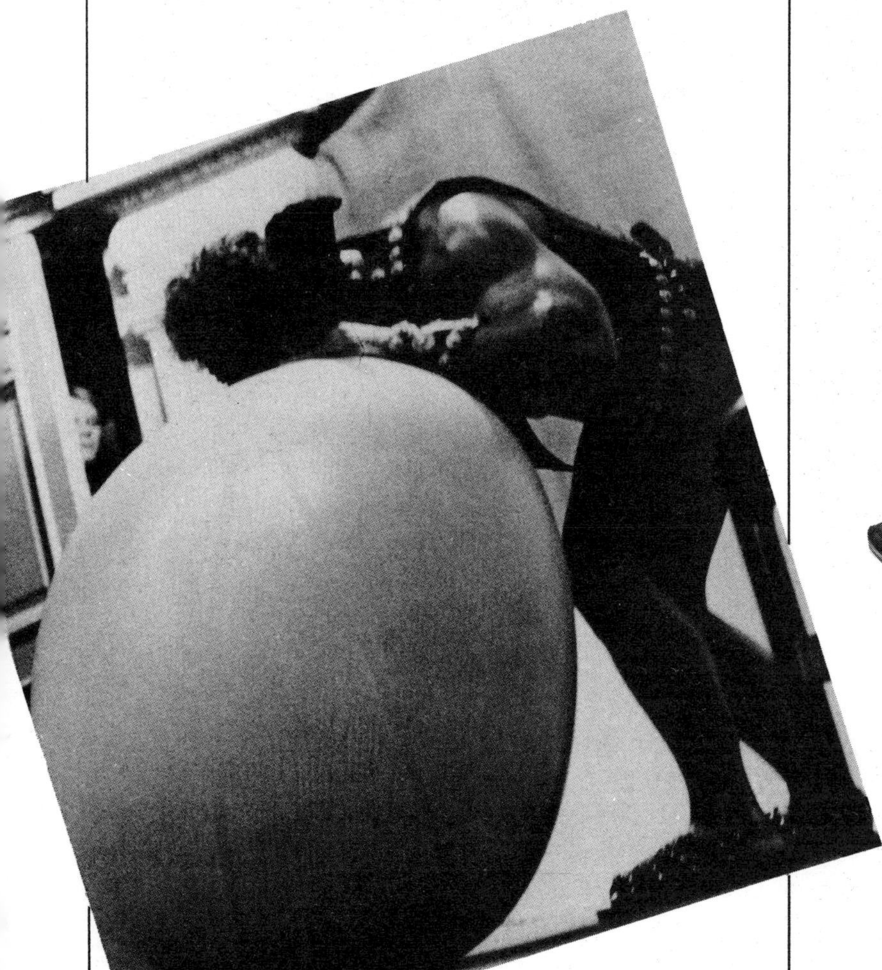

ABOVE: LUNG POWER – JOHN CITRONE BLOWS UP A HOT-WATER BOTTLE.

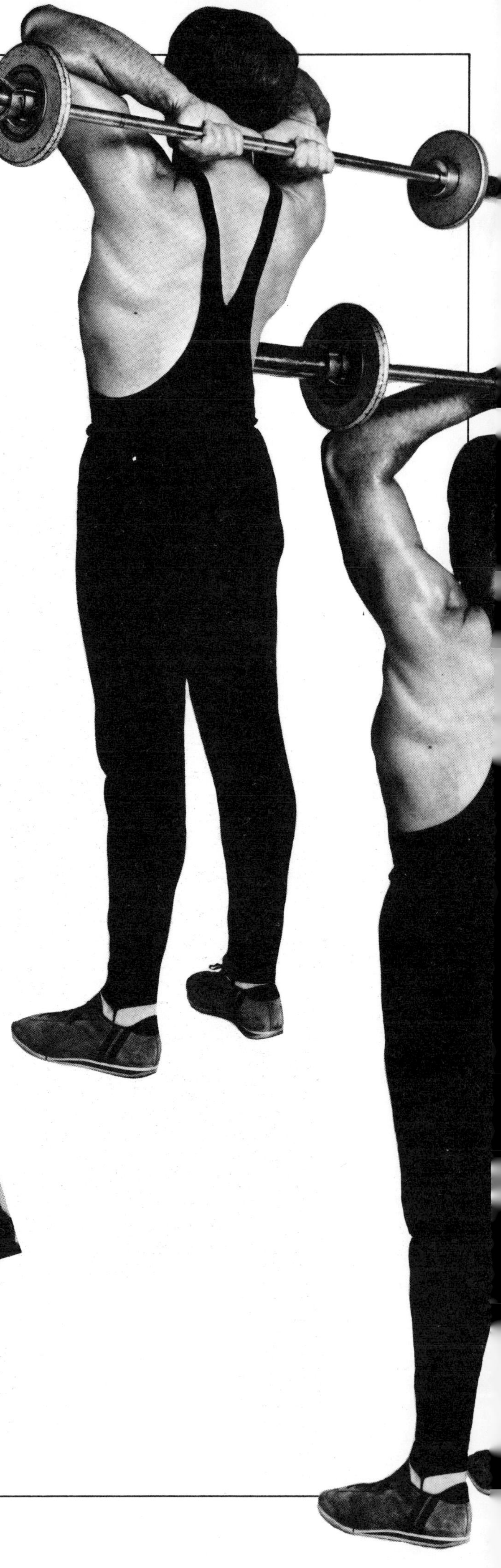

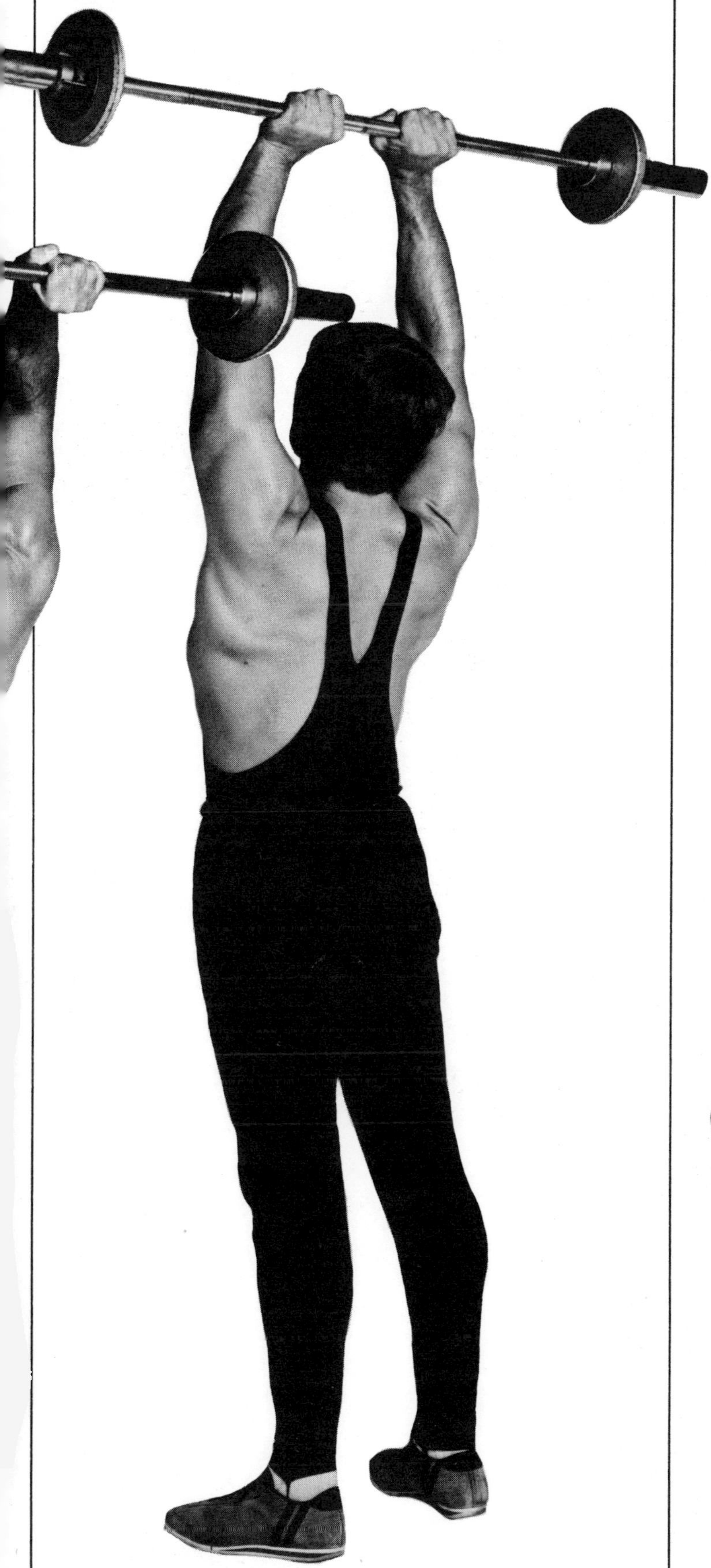

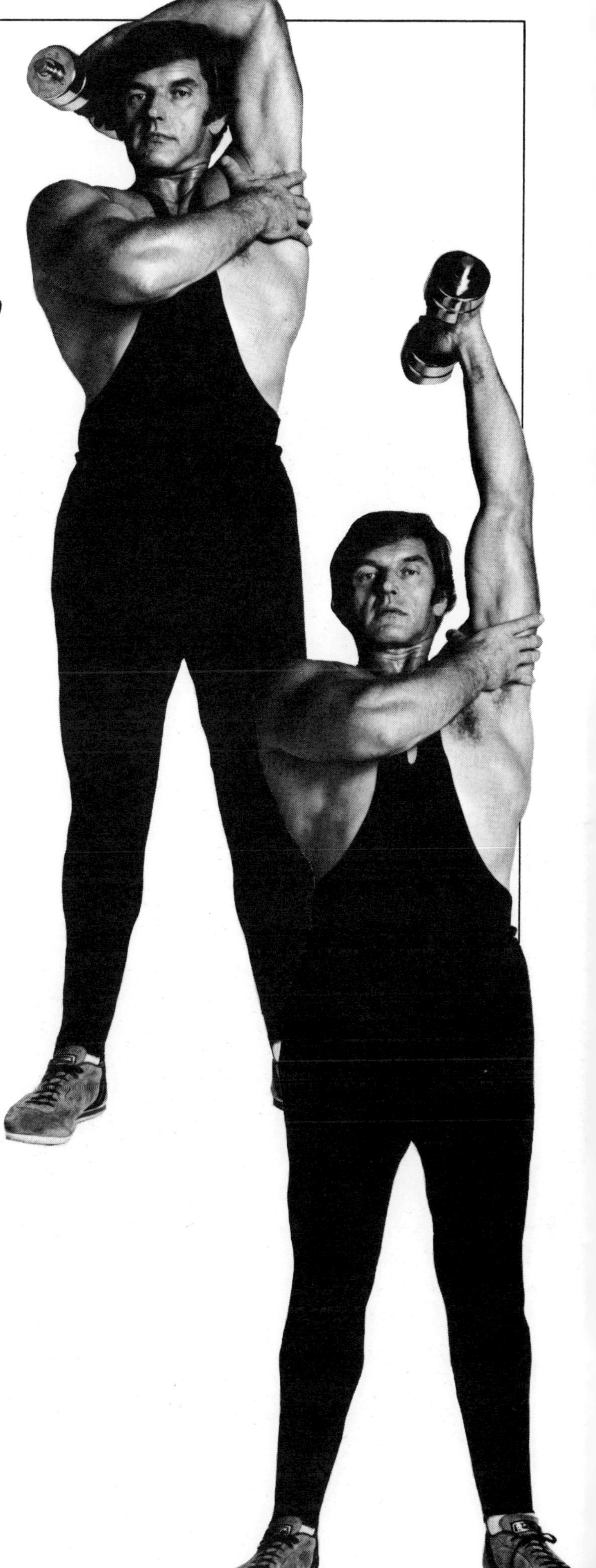

Triceps Travel

You'll need a bench to lie on for this one. And a barbell.

1. Sit on the end of the bench. Pick the barbell up with the closehand spacing again, and with overhand grip.

2. Lie back on the bench and bring the barbell up to the clean position. You'll be lying on your back with the barbell across your chest under your chin, palms facing upwards.

3. Describe an arc with the barbell, starting at your chest, going past your nose and then raising it upwards. Do not lock the arms at all. This keeps the pressure on the triceps the whole way through.

4. The end position of the barbell is out past the head.

5. Describe an arc back to starting position.

6. Watch your nose. Repeat 10 times (up to 3 sets).

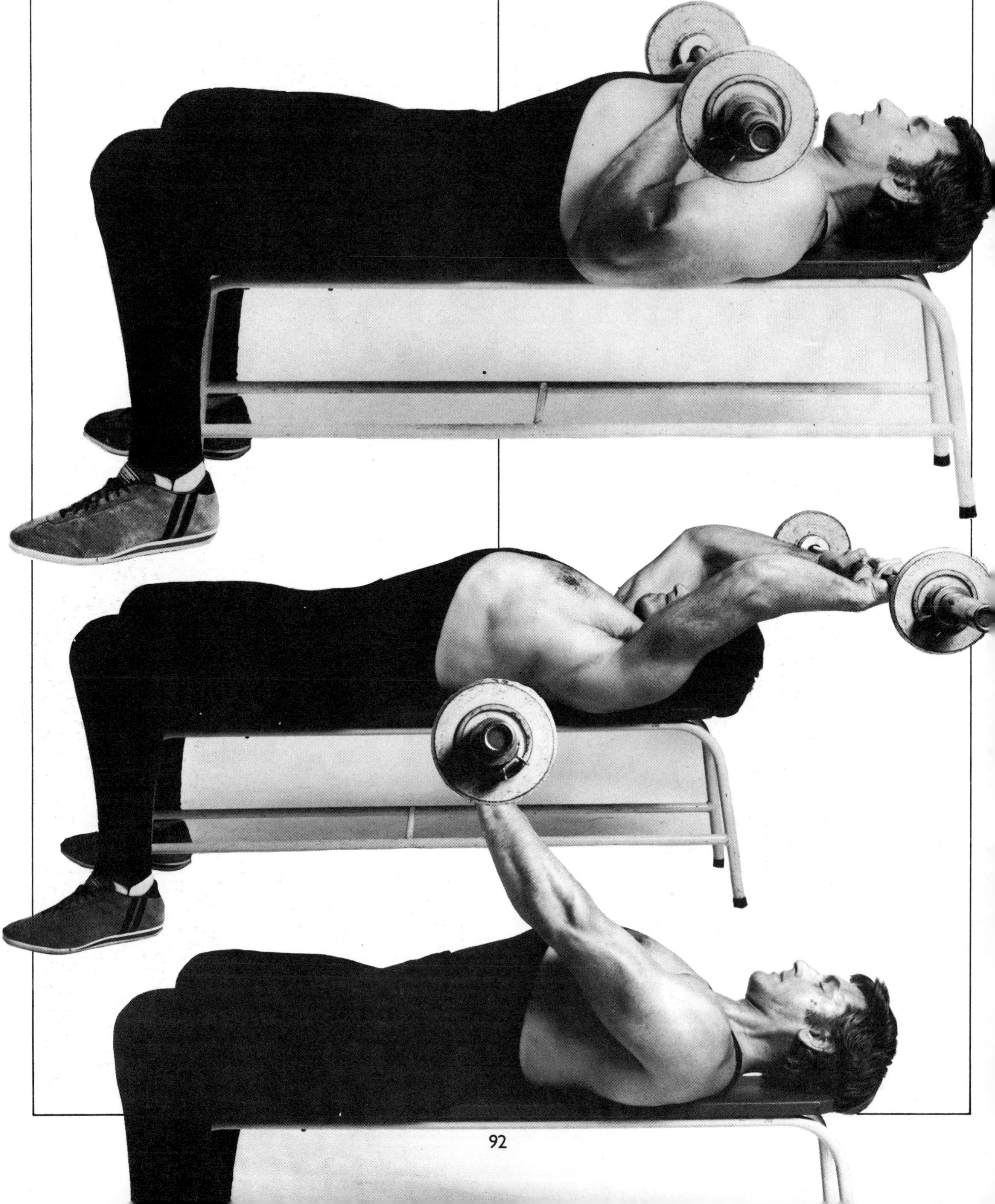

Press-up

And lastly, an excellent exercise for the triceps, if you have no equipment, is the common-or-garden press-up, but doing it with the hands close together.

1. Get into the normal press-up position on the floor.
2. Bring your hands together until your thumbs touch.
3. Try to ensure that your elbows are kept in all the time and that your upper arms end up alongside your chest.
4. Press up ten times (up to 3 sets).

NB This is a super exercise for girls who are a bit overweight and want to take the weight off their upper arms.

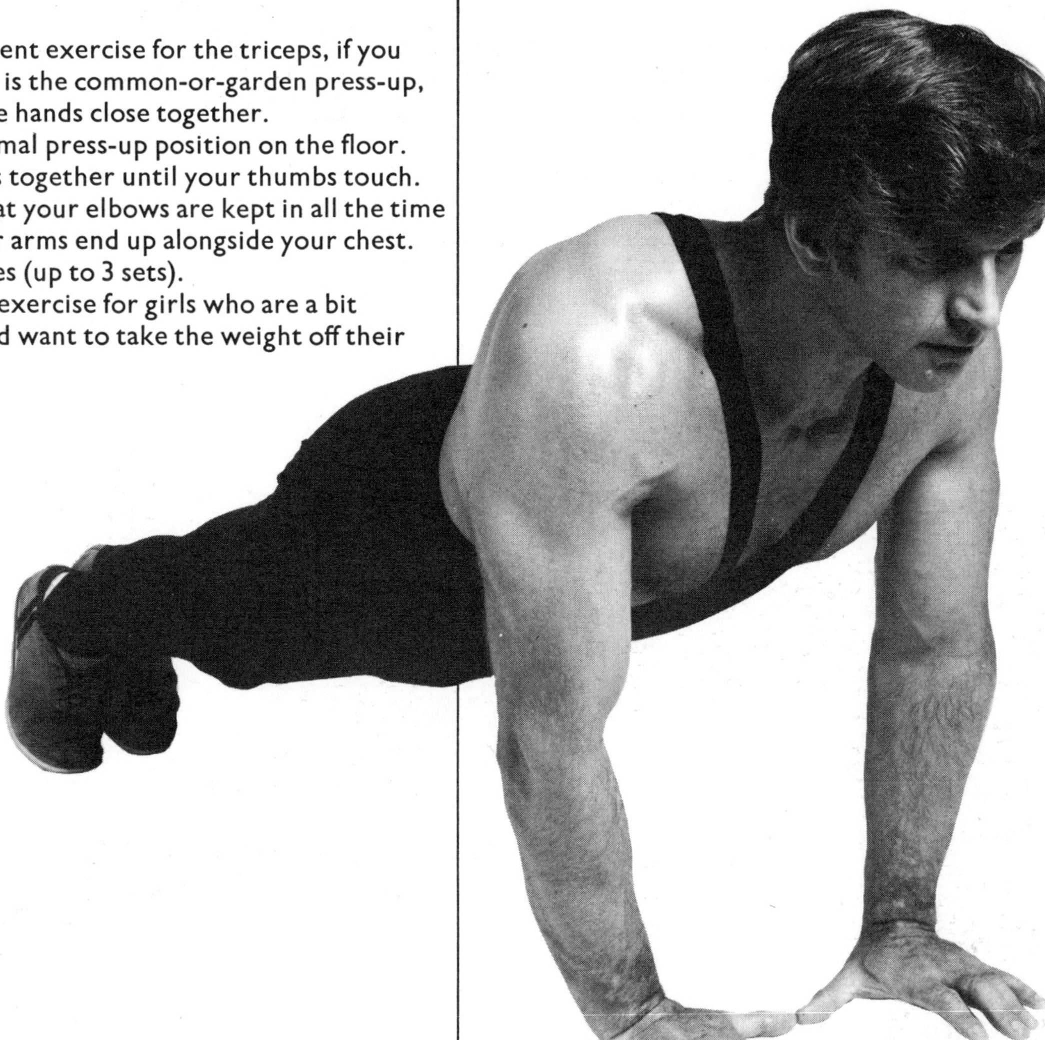

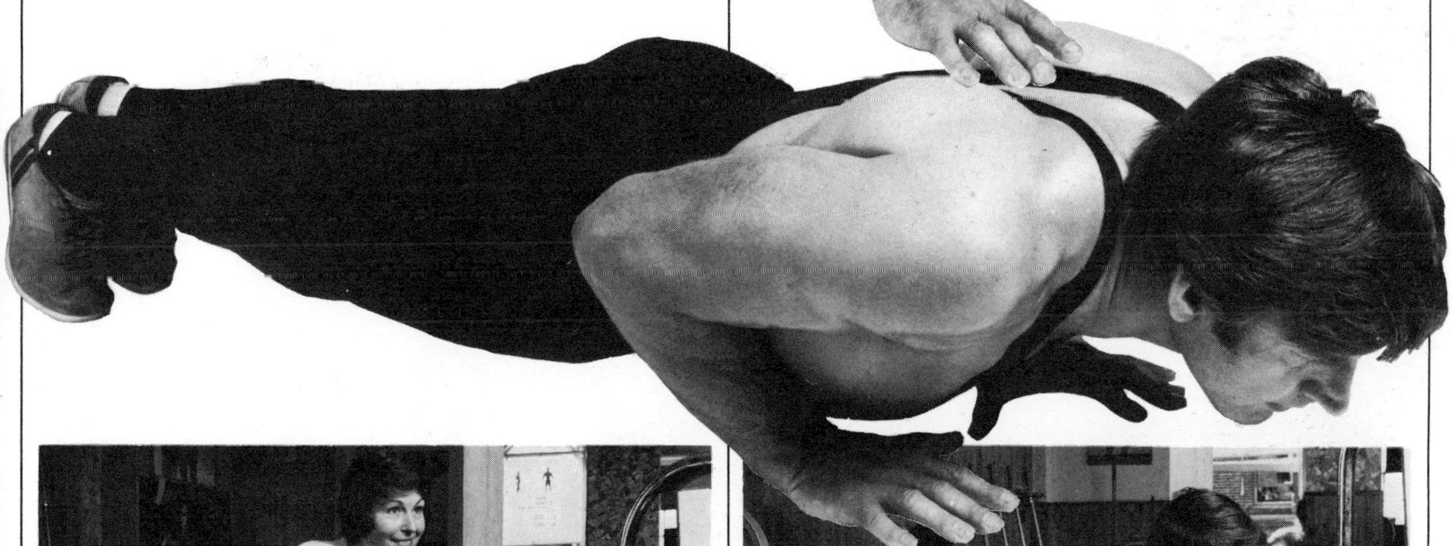

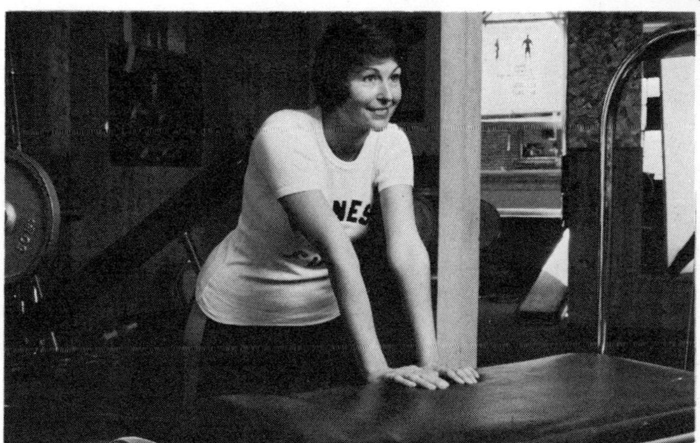

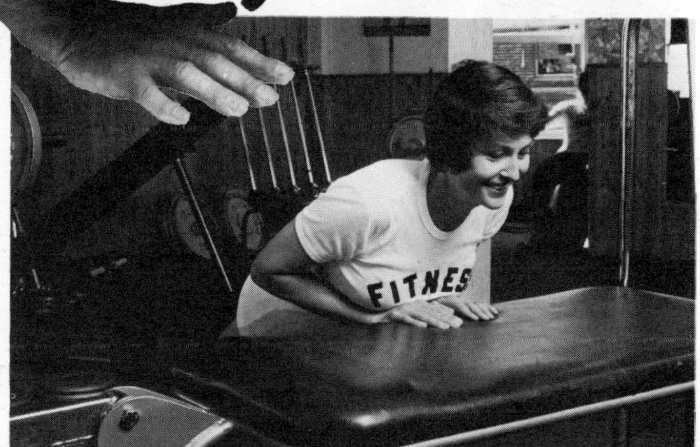

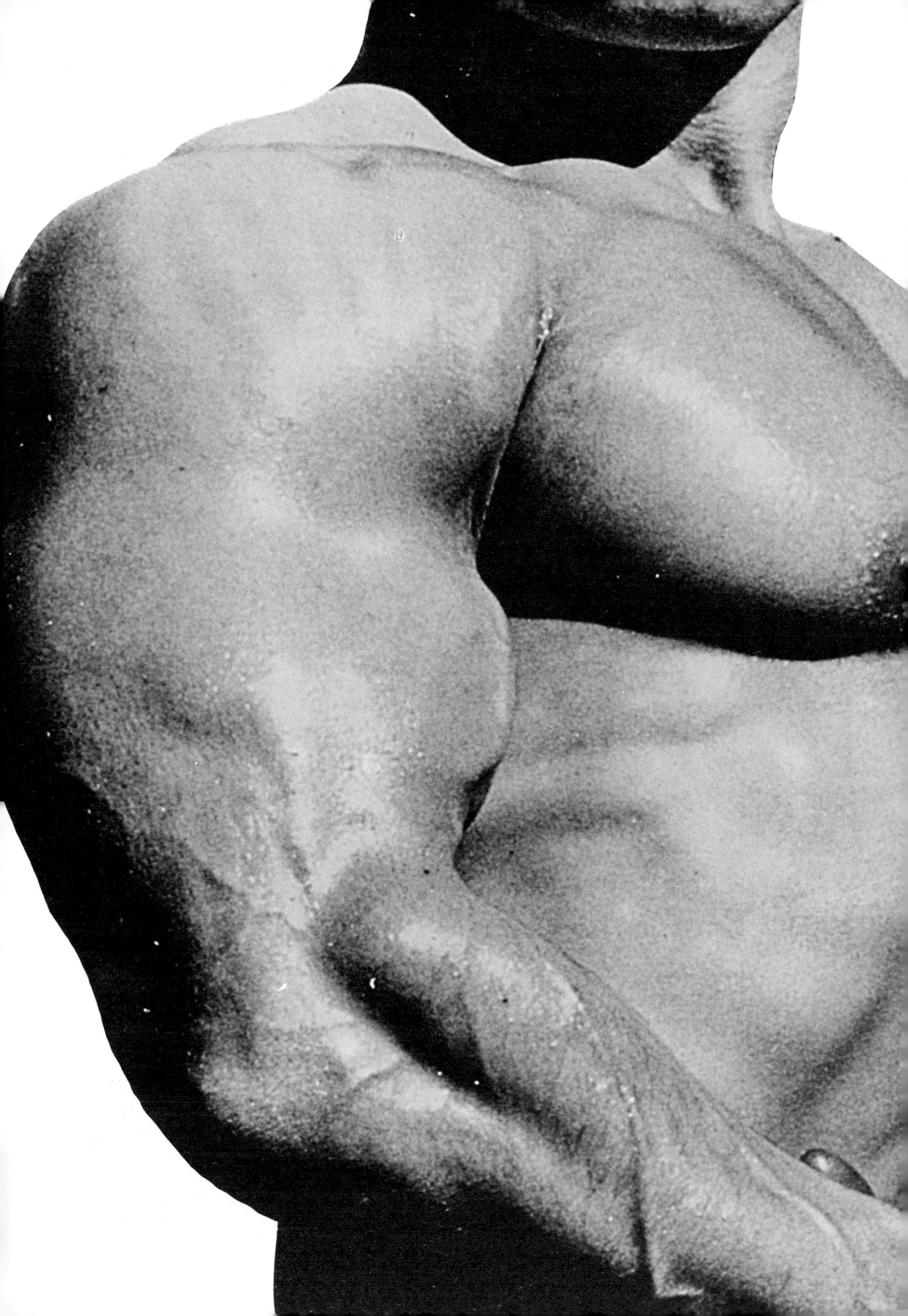

Chapter 12

KEEPING ABREAST OF FITNESS

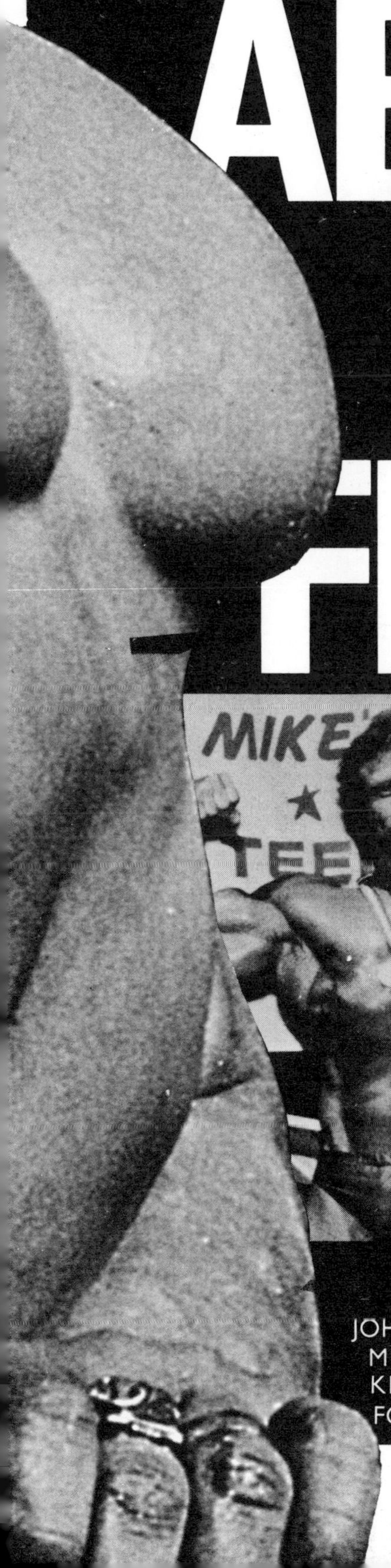

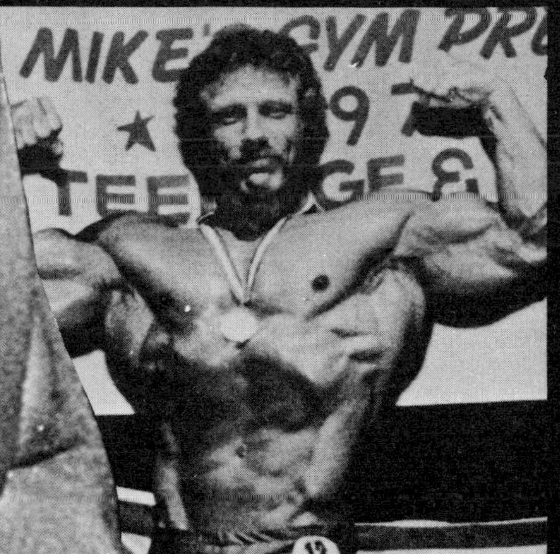

JOHN CITRONE, FORMER MR UNIVERSE. **INSET:** KENT KUEHEN, OVER FORTY MR UNIVERSE.

The chest muscles consist of the pectoralis major, the pectoralis minor sub-clavius and the serratus anterior, better known as the serratus magnus. These are the muscles on the side of the chest, that look very much like ribs. The pectoralis muscles are the main ones that interest us, for they are the big showy chest muscles, and they consist of the clavicular, or upper portion, and the sternal or lower portion which are attached to the collar bone, the whole length of the sternum and the cartilage of the ribs.

The largest mass of the pectorals starts at the upper arm bone where it fastens just under and above where the deltoids attach to the humerus. The serratus fans out to cover the rib cage and appear very much like an additional rib. The action of the pectoralis muscle is to pull the arm across the front of the body and this is why the bench press and all forms of lying, pressing movements are good for this particular muscle group. The pectorals are also brought into play in activities like swimming and even throwing a ball.

First and most popular of all chest exercises is the bench press, and for this you're going to need a bench 18 ins high and about ten ins wide. It helps if the bench is padded for comfort and it also helps if you have weight supporting stands at one end.

Bench Press

1. Lie back on the bench with the weight held at arm's length above you. Hand spacing is optional. Feet should be flat on the floor.

2. Breathe *in*. Lower weight slowly to your chest and then push it back slowly to the arm's length position. Breathe *out* when you get past the hard bit.

3. Repeat 10 times (up to 3 sets).

NB Although I've said hand spacing is optional, remember that the closer your hands are together the less the exercise works the pectoralis muscle and the more it becomes a triceps exercise. Placing your hands closer together will also limit the weight you can handle.

This exercise can be expanded into an incline press where the bench is adjusted to various angles. The purpose of using an incline bench is to affect the inter-relationship of the pectoralis and the deltoids. The steeper the angle of the bench the more effect the exercise has on the upper chest and deltoid muscles.

You can in fact use the bench in reverse, as it were, with your feet higher than your head. By doing this you'll find you work your pectoralis muscles slightly

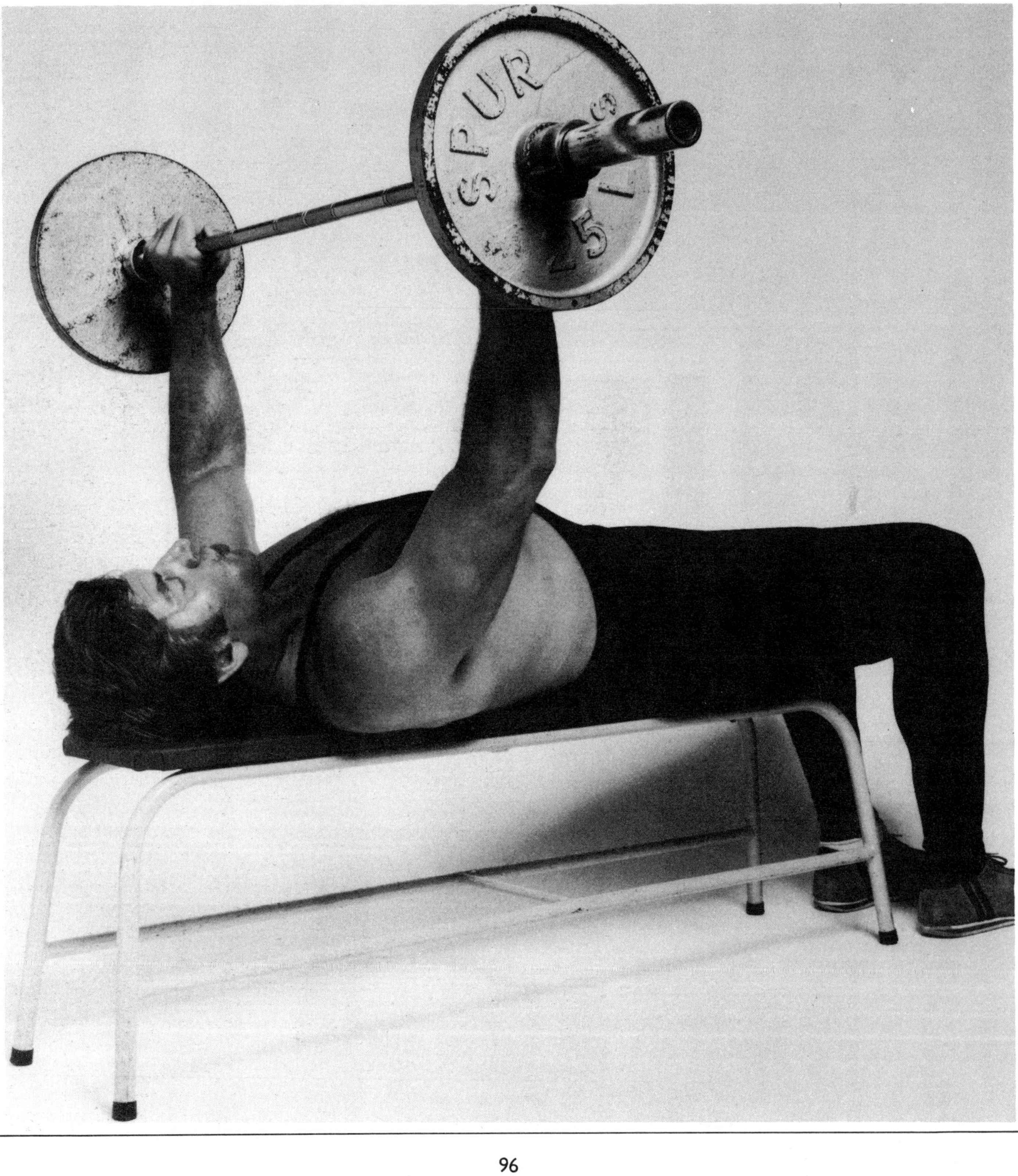

differently, and you'll find it a stronger lift, pushing slightly away from yourself as well as upwards. Not only can you handle more weight, but the exercise works the lower part of the pectoralis. I myself am not a great lover of this particular exercise. I feel that it tends to over-develop the lower part of the pectoralis which can give a man a 'tittified' appearance.

Parallel bar dips, described in the section on arm exercises, is also a marvellous chest exercise, and one usually finds that it affects the centre of the pectoralis, i.e. your cleavage. For this you will either need a set of parallel bars or a similar, smaller piece of apparatus usually attached to a wall and found in most gymnasia. You can also do the exercise between the backs of two chairs, provided they're properly anchored. It's a great combination movement for the pectoralis and the biceps. The trainee should aim to do *as many repetitions as possible*. You'll probably begin with 10 to 15, but there's no reason why you shouldn't work up to doing 25 to 30 at a set. If you begin to go above the 30 mark, then you can increase the resistance by tying weights around your waist.

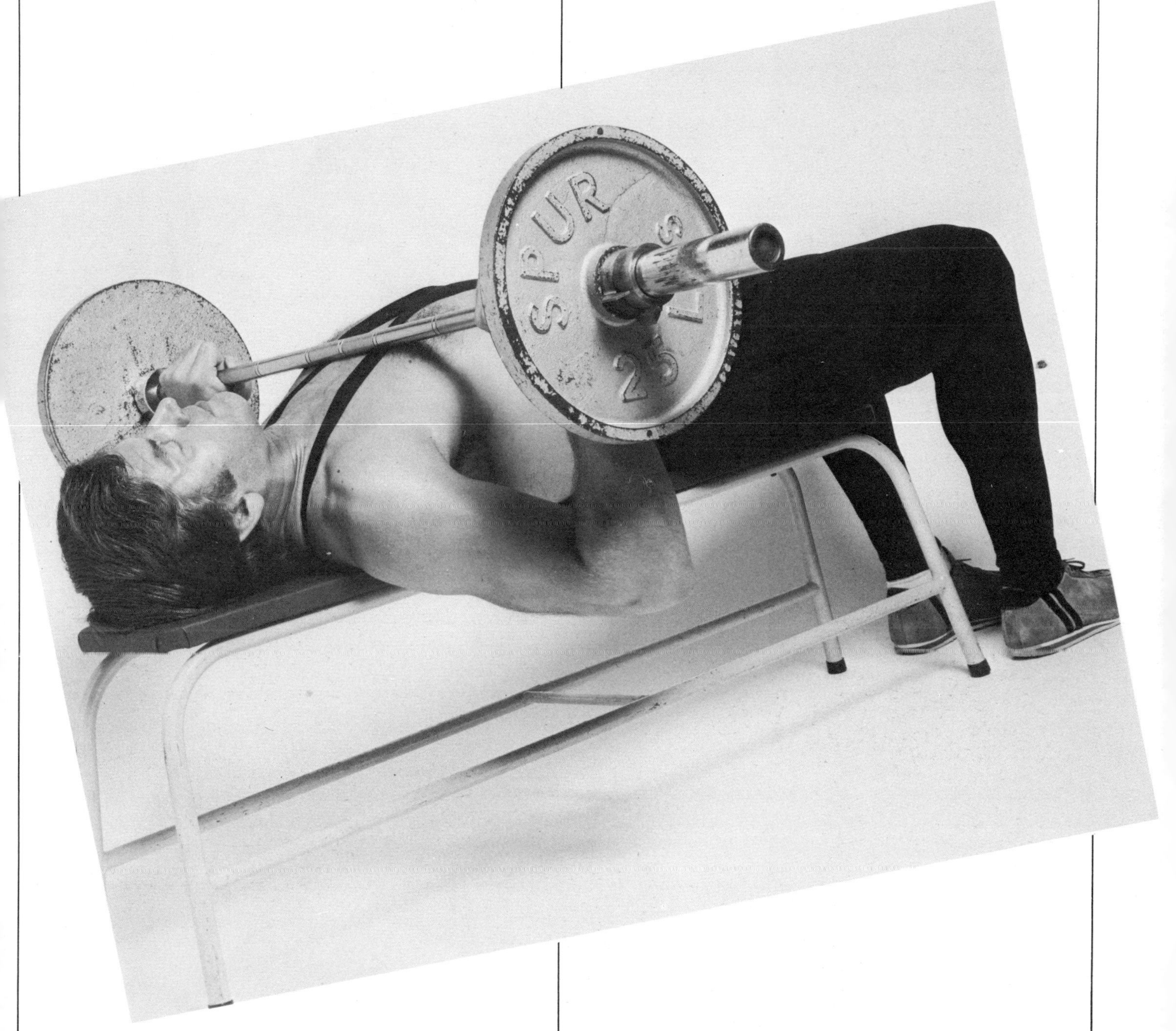

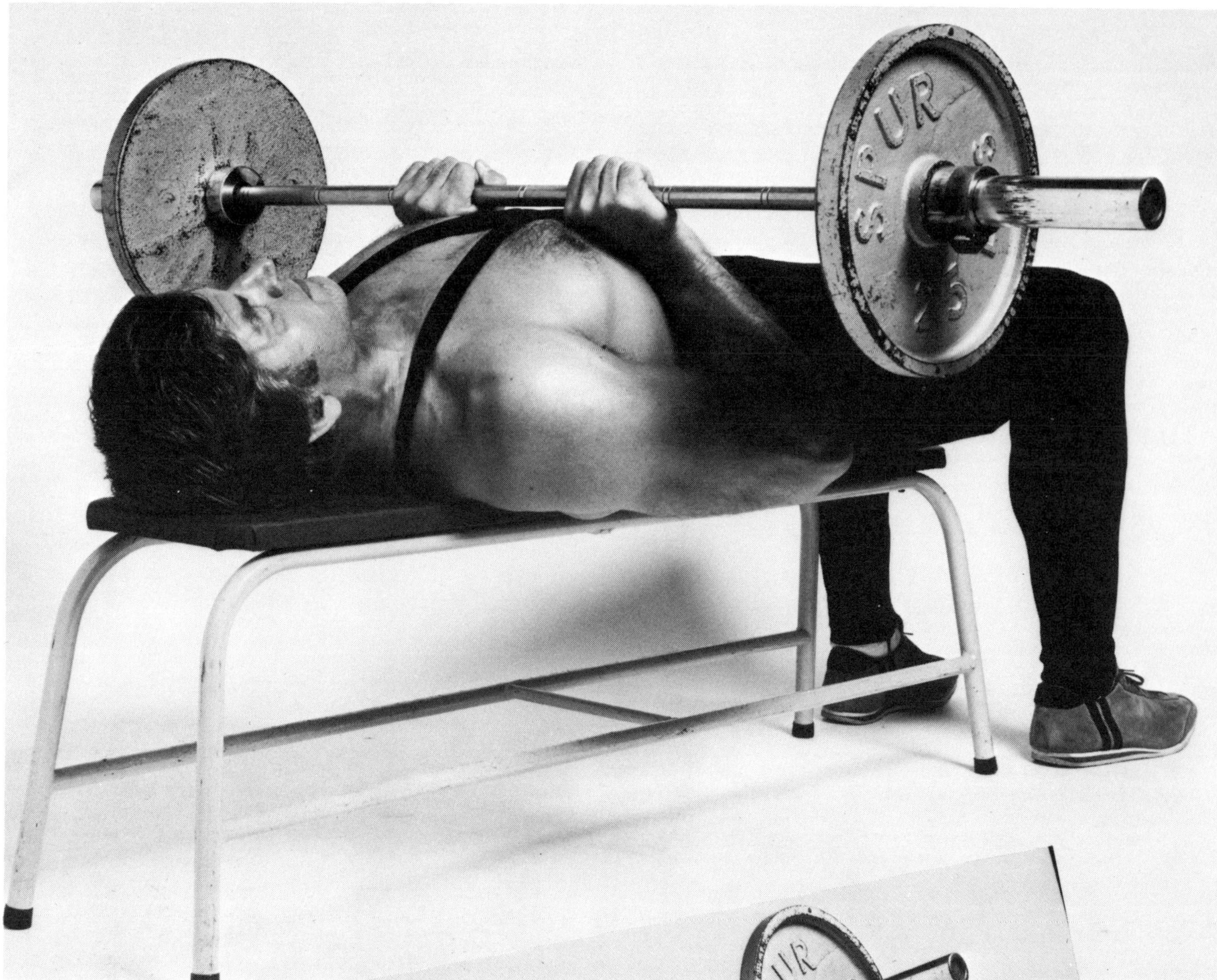
SPUR

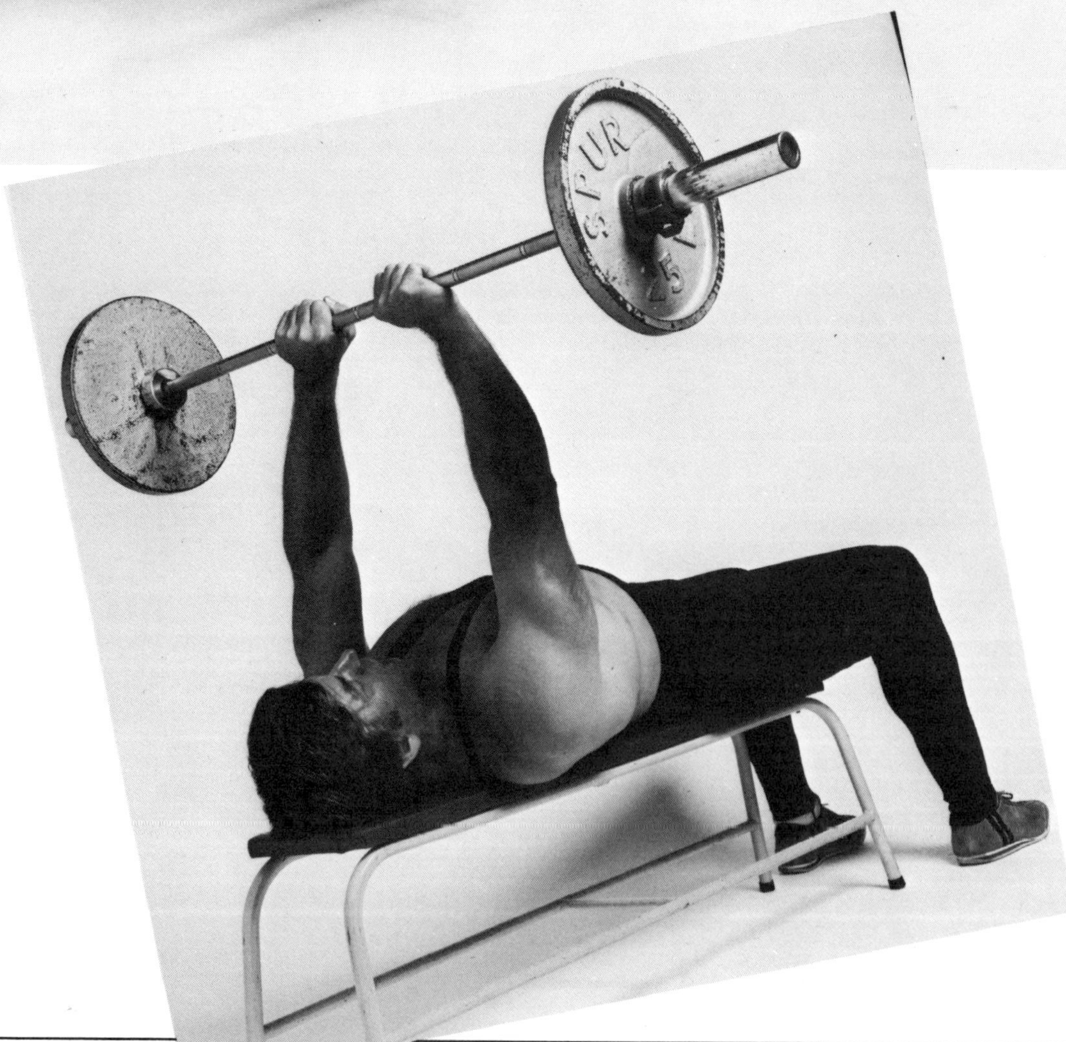
SPUR

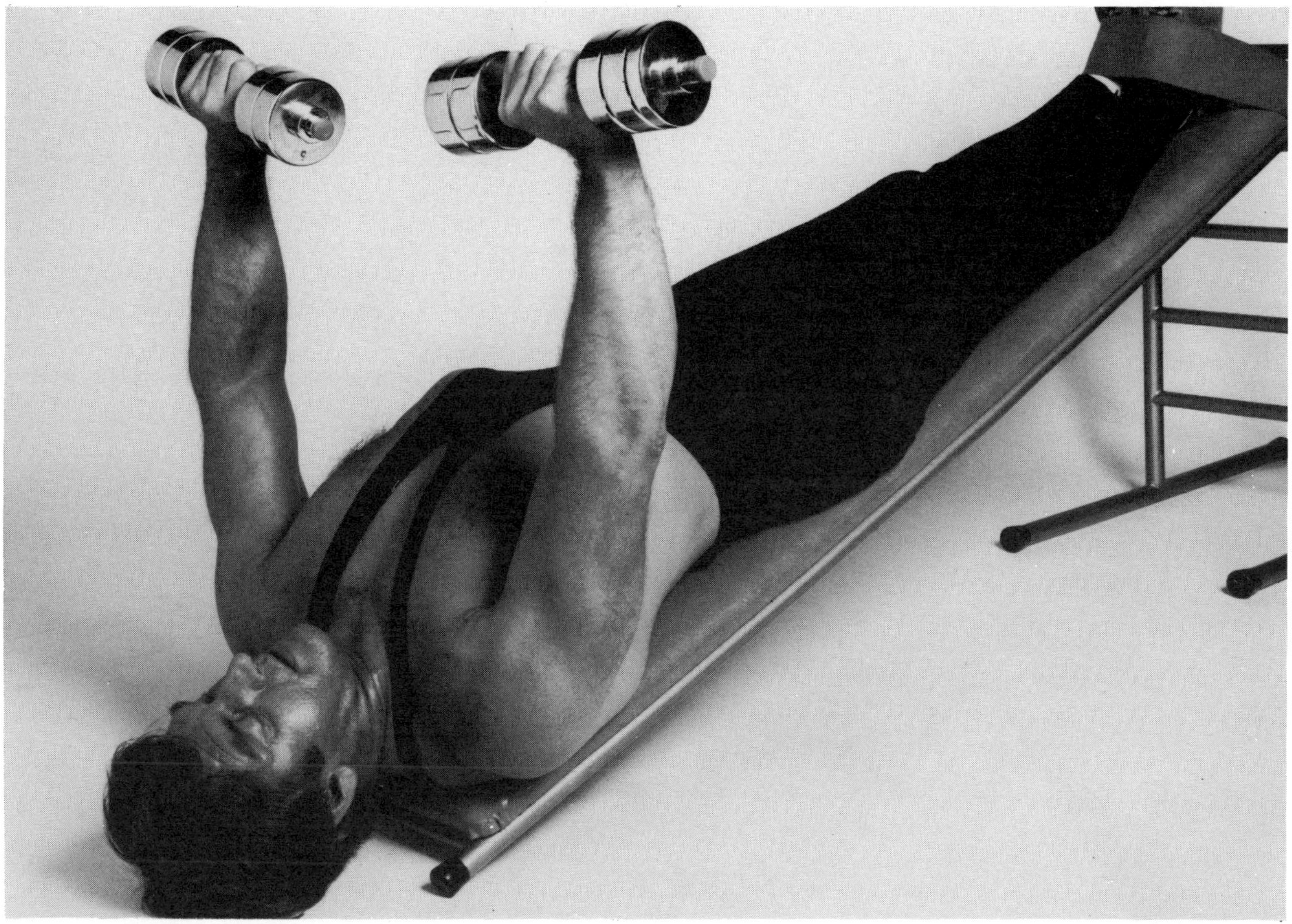

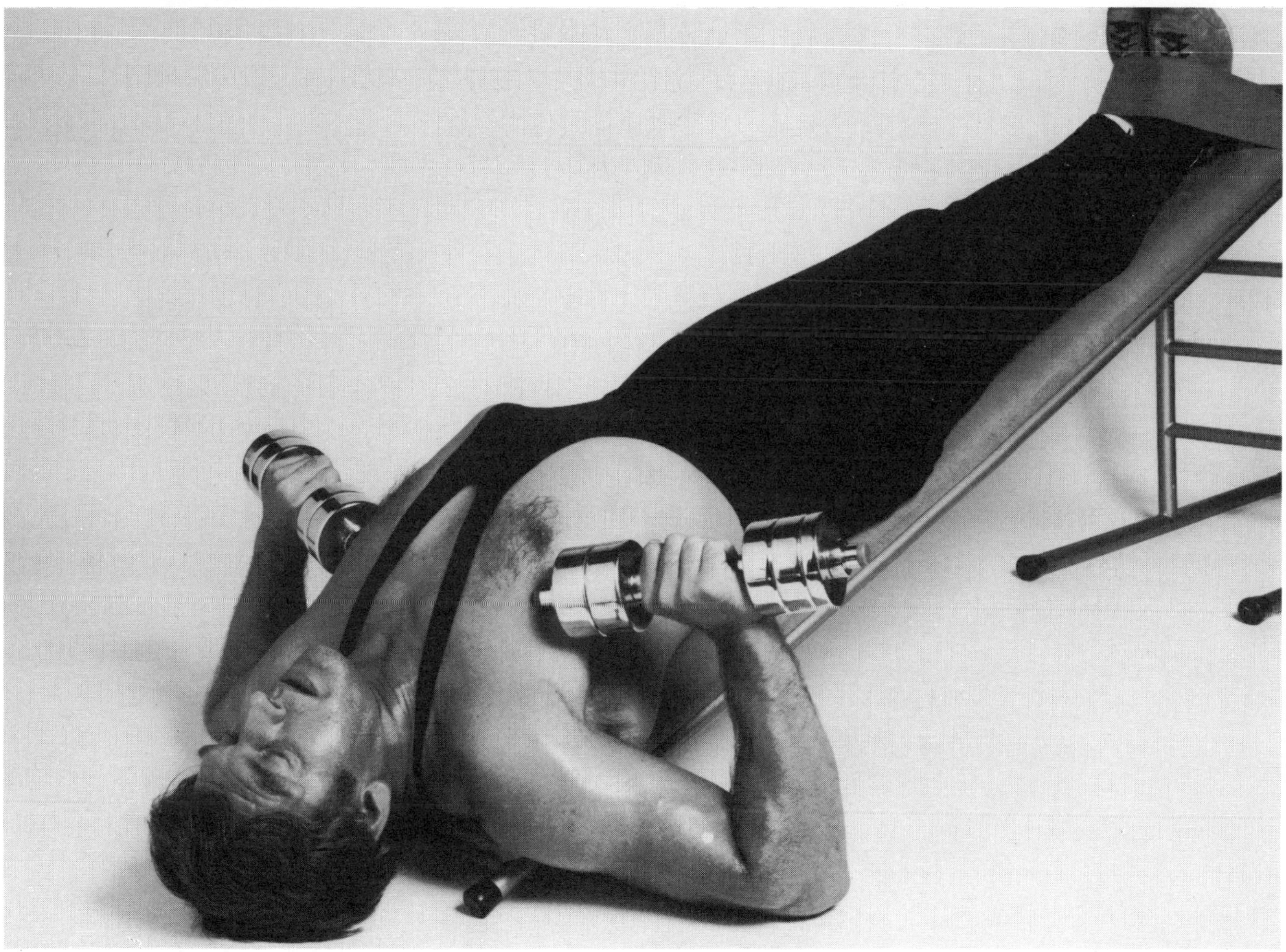

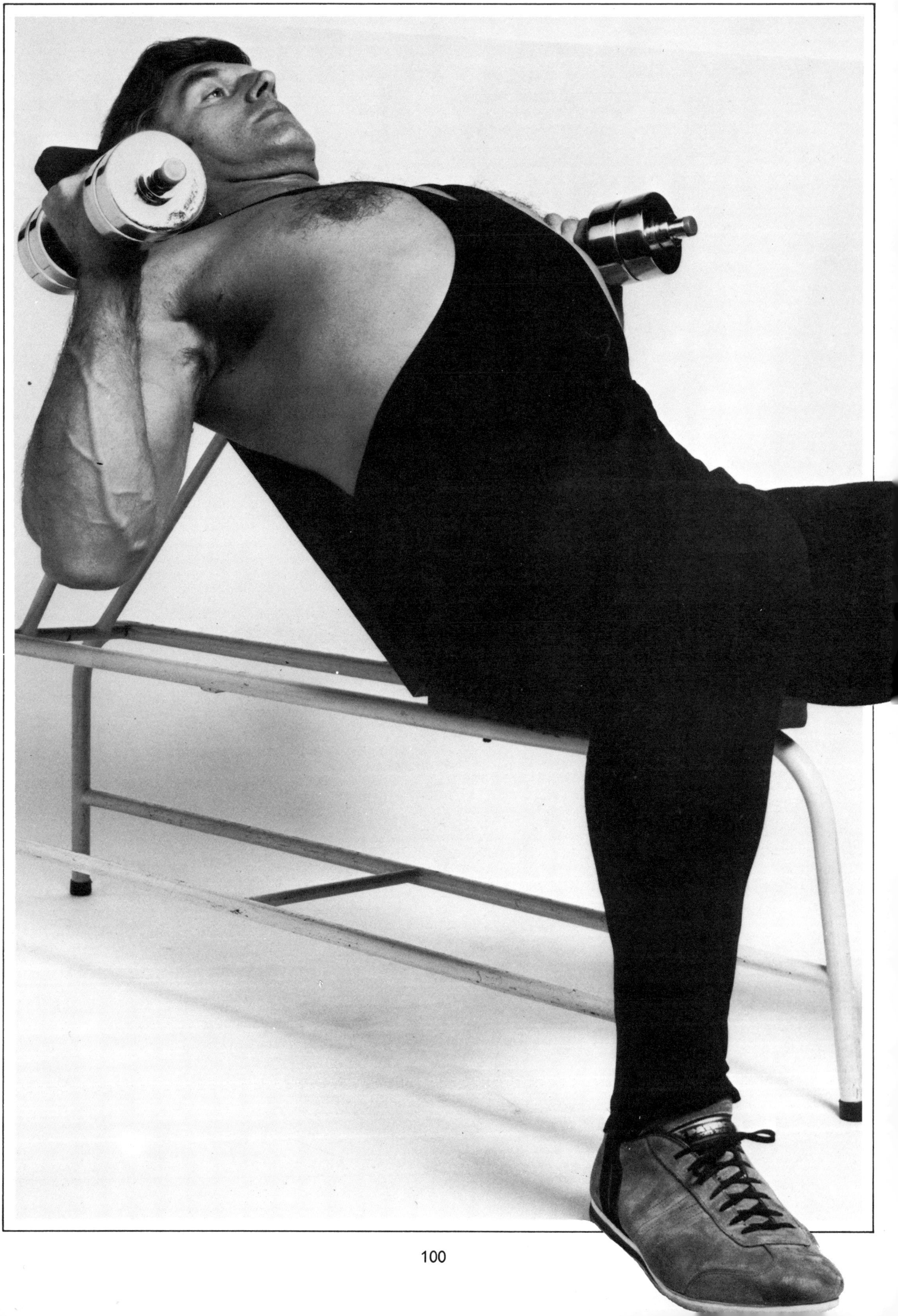

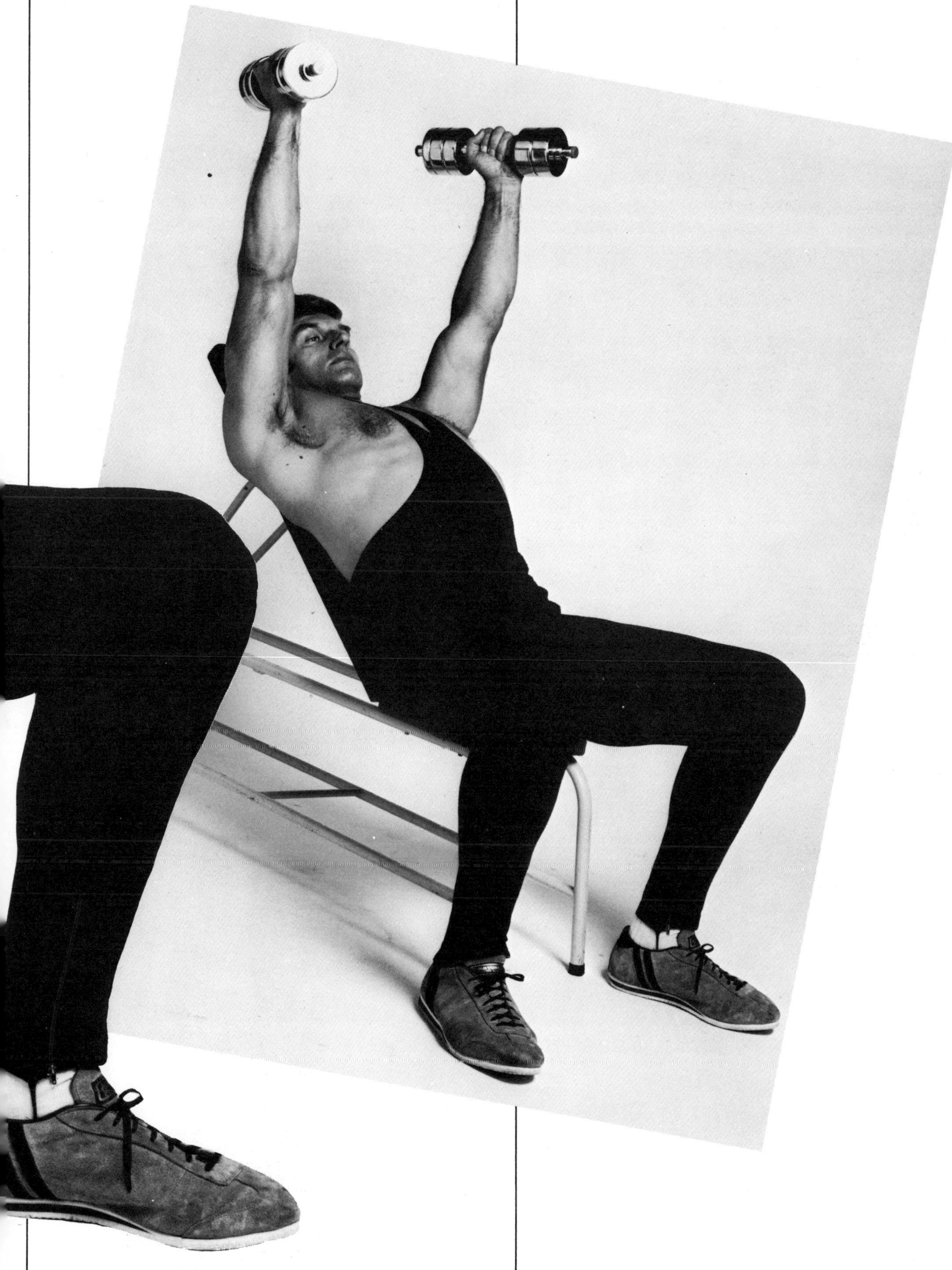

Flying Exercise (flat or incline bench) for Men

1. Select reasonably weighted dumbells (10–15 lbs).
2. Lie on bench. Lift the dumbells until they are directly above chest level and at arm's length.
3. Keeping the arms fairly straight, bring the weights down as low as they'll go on either side.
4. Breathe in. Return weights to starting position above you.
5. Repeat 20 times (up to 3 sets, as a shaping exercise). But if you want to use it as a development exercise, increase the weight, decrease the repetitions and increase the number of sets i.e. four to five sets of eight to ten repetitions.

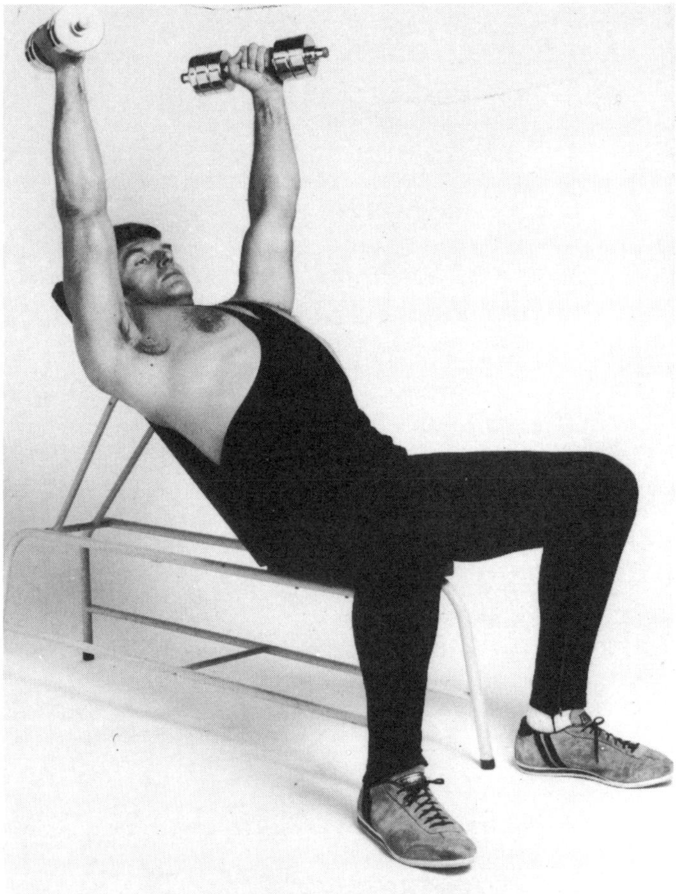

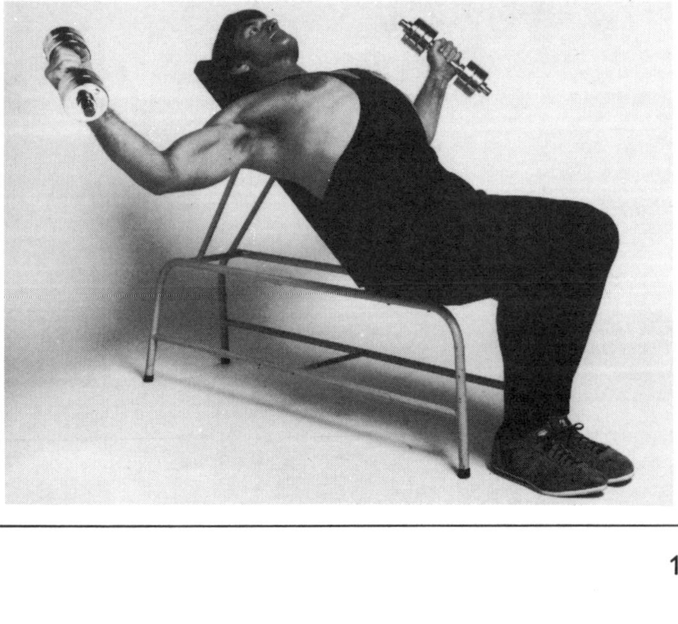

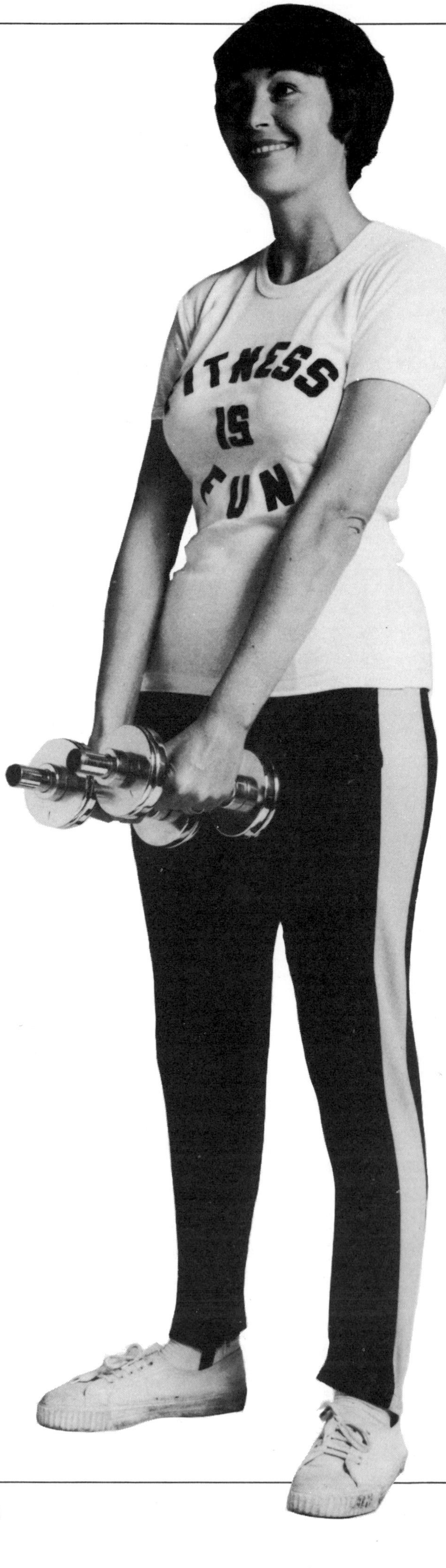

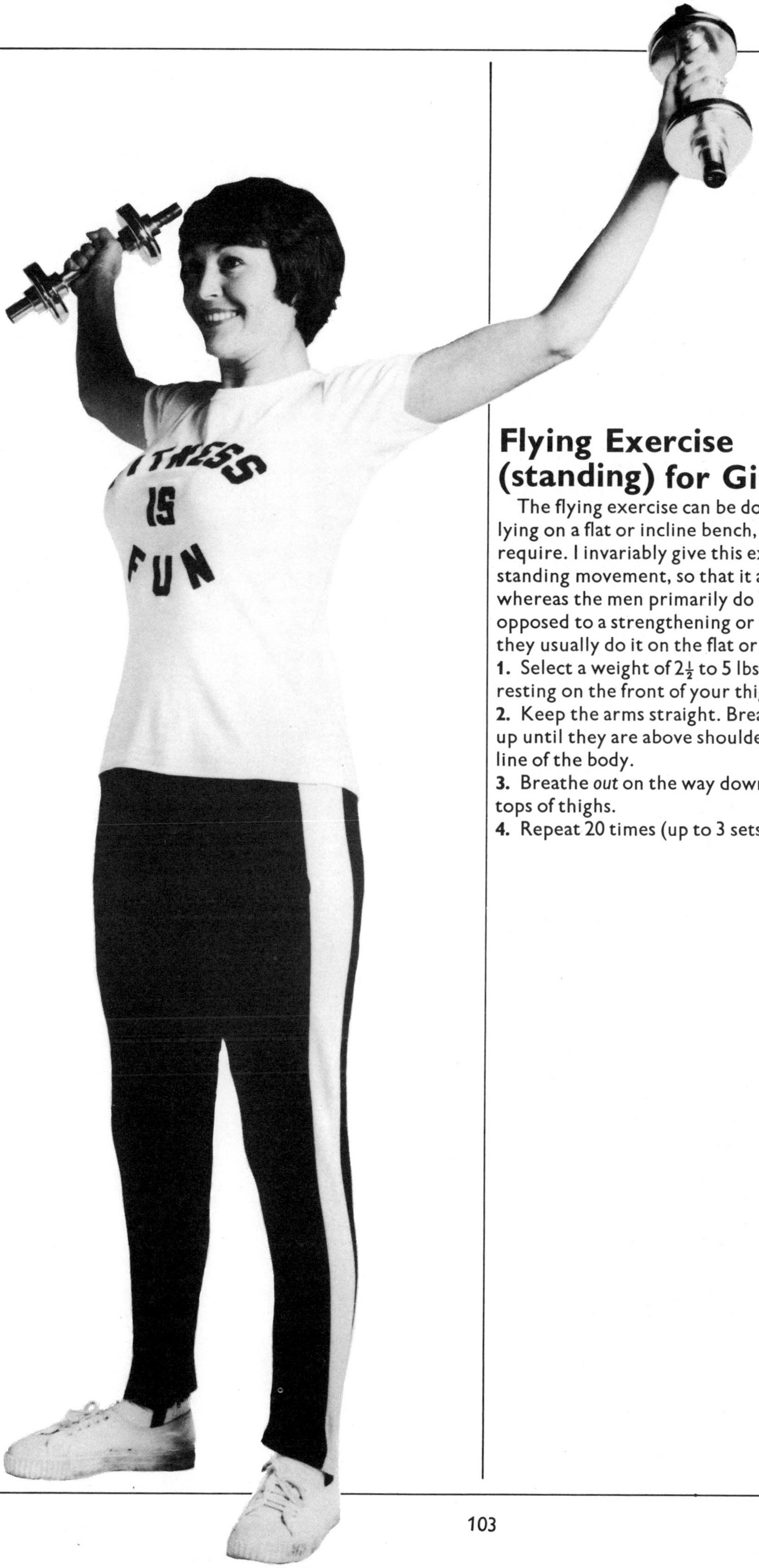

Flying Exercise (standing) for Girls

The flying exercise can be done either standing up or lying on a flat or incline bench, depending on what you require. I invariably give this exercise to girls as a standing movement, so that it affects the breast muscles, whereas the men primarily do it as a shaping exercise as opposed to a strengthening or developing one and so they usually do it on the flat or the incline bench.

1. Select a weight of $2\frac{1}{2}$ to 5 lbs held at arm's length resting on the front of your thighs.

2. Keep the arms straight. Breathe in. Bring the weights up until they are above shoulder level and behind the line of the body.

3. Breathe *out* on the way down, returning weights to tops of thighs.

4. Repeat 20 times (up to 3 sets).

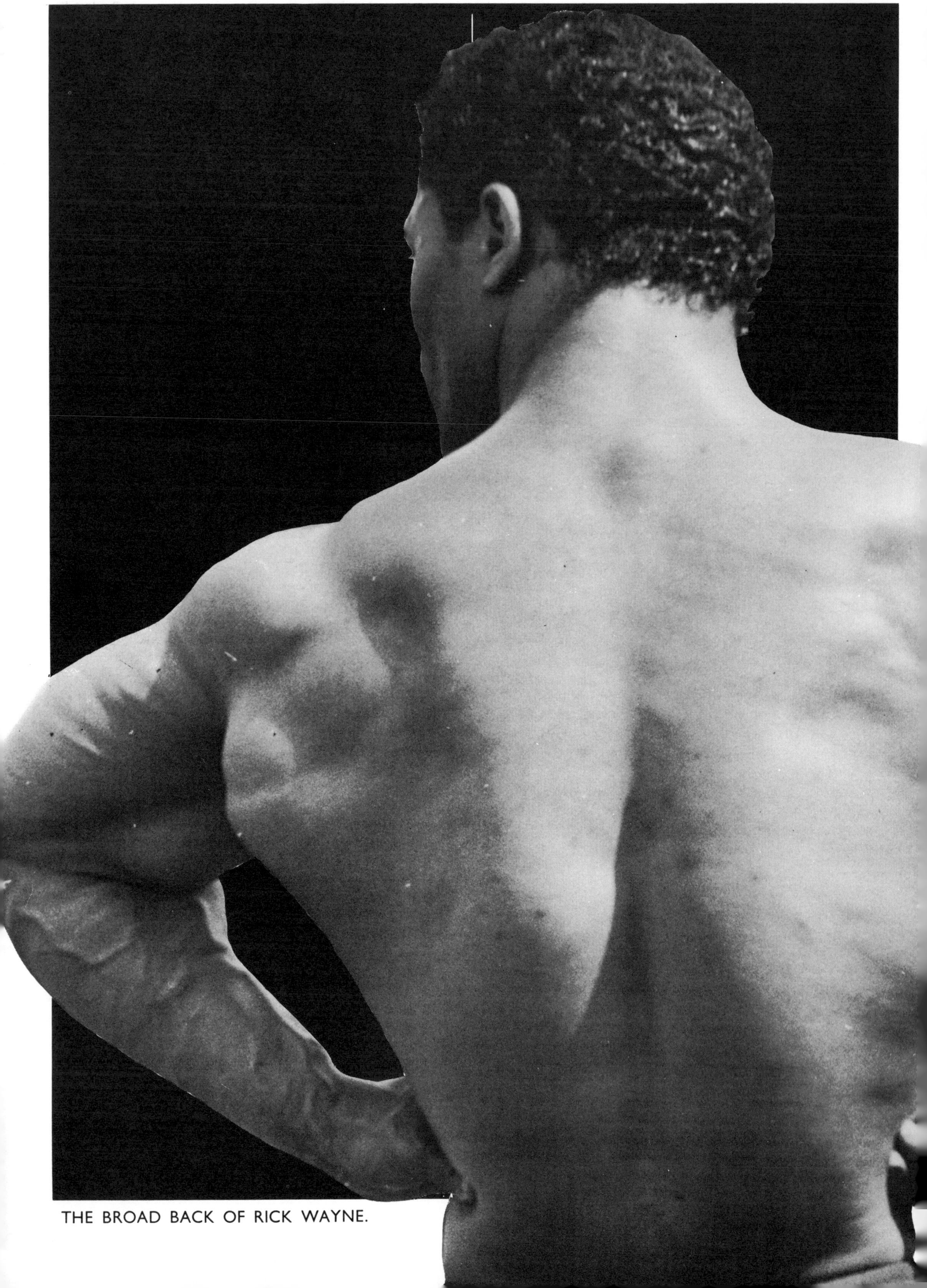

THE BROAD BACK OF RICK WAYNE.

Chapter 13

THE POWER LIFTS

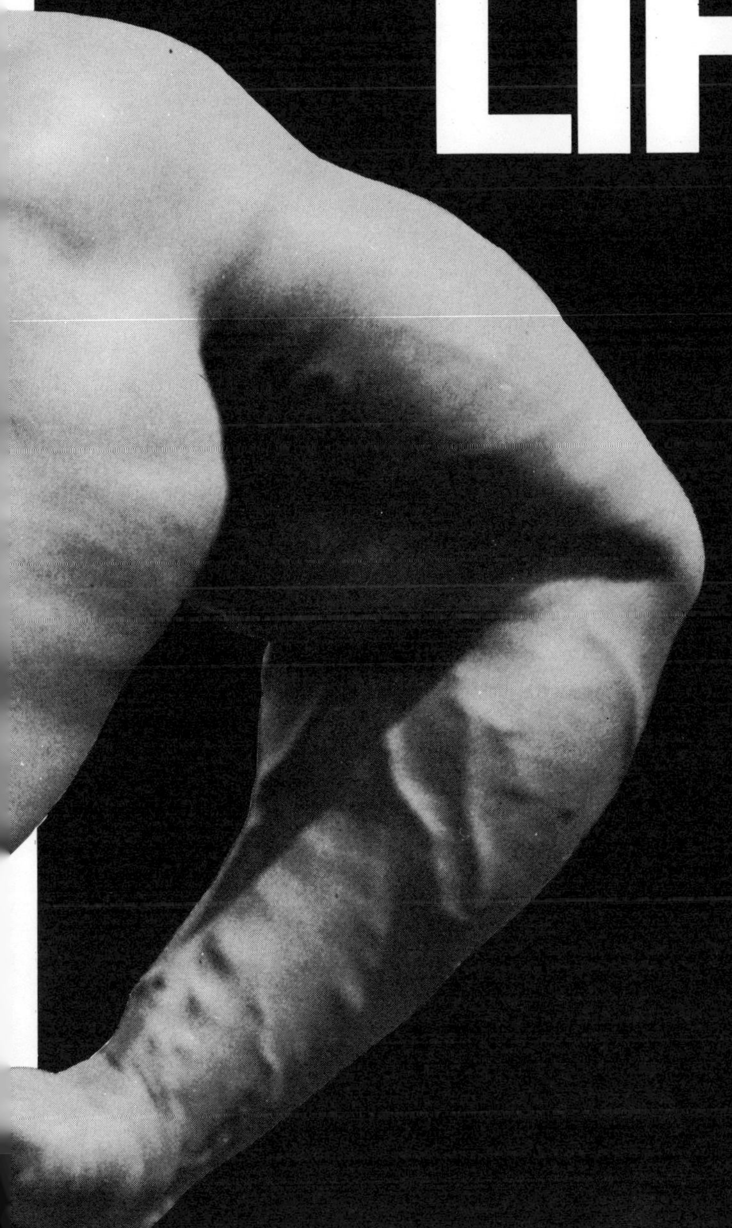

The major muscles of your back are the trapezius, the latissimus dorsi, and the spinae erector muscles which help to keep the spine upright.

The trapezius is a diamond-shaped muscle that covers parts of the neck, shoulders and upper back. It arises from the base of the skull, reaches out to the deltoids, and runs down to approximately the middle of the spine. Its function is to raise and lower the shoulder blade and help lift the shoulders from the front.

The latissimus dorsi, affectionately termed by body-builders the 'lats' is a large triangular muscle that starts in the lumbar region of the back and then fans out wide at the top near the shoulders. Its function is to bring the arms to the centre of the body. It also draws the shoulders downwards and backwards.

The erectors are the antagonists of the abdominal muscles. Your abdominal muscles help you flex the spine and sit up. The erectors control the straightening of the spine.

The back exercises can be specifically divided into latissimus dorsi exercises and erector spinae exercises.

Bent-over Rowing

This is by far the most popular latissimus dorsi exercise. Select a barbell of a reasonable weight (for a beginner say 60 to 70 pounds).

1. Stand at the bar with your feet about two feet apart (slightly wider than normal).
2. Grasp bar with much wider than normal hand spacing.
3. Bend the knees slightly. Breathe in. Raise the bar off the floor until your back is parallel with the floor.
4. The bar is now hanging directly beneath you, with your knees slightly bent, back flat, head up.
5. Breathe in. Bring bar up to touch your throat, keeping the elbows up all the time.
6. Lower weight back to starting position.
7. Repeat 8–10 times (3 sets).

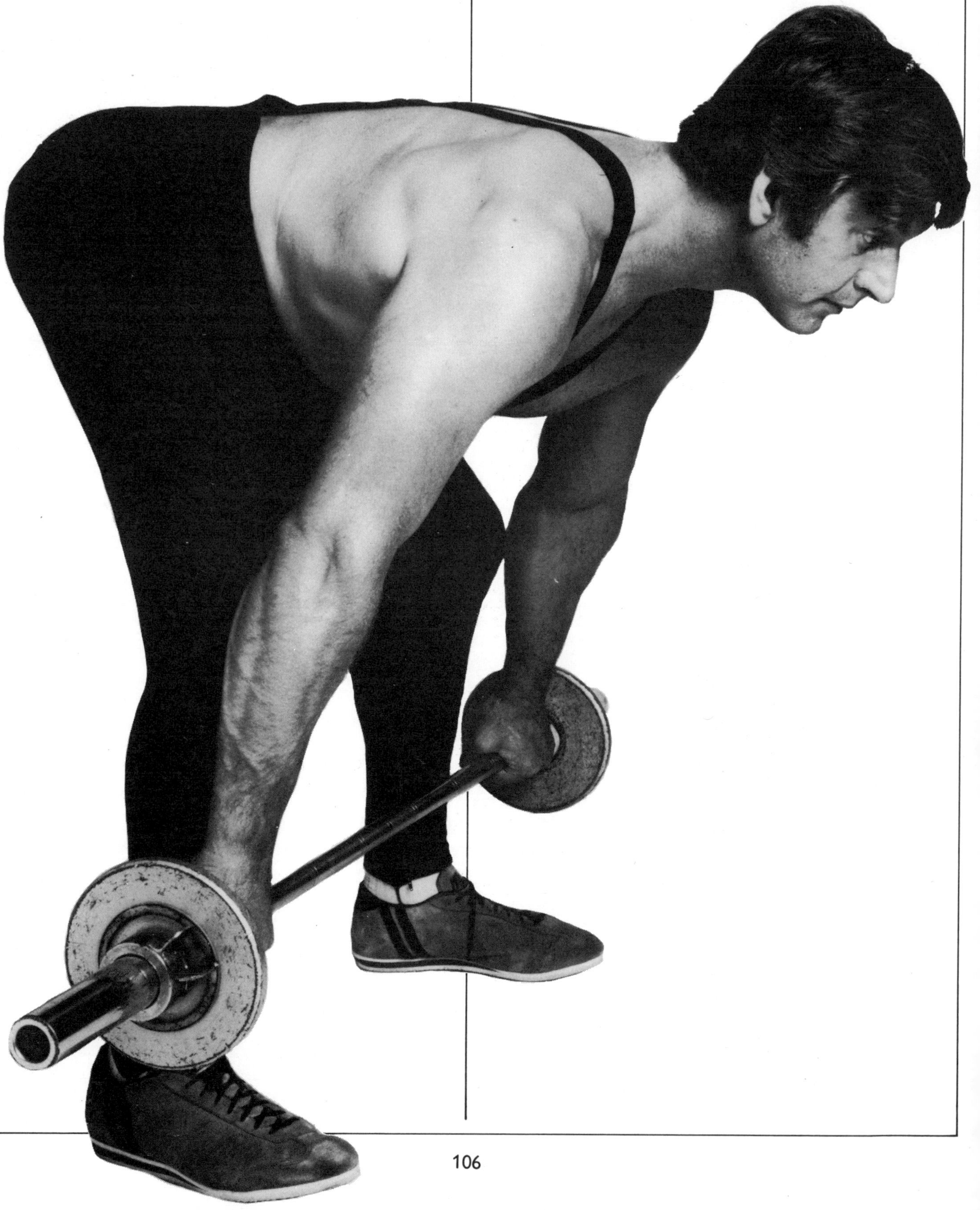

NB It's all-important to keep the exercise position. It will probably feel quite awkward at first, but you'll soon find the exercise position becomes quite natural.

You can also do this particular exercise with dumbells rather than a barbell. It then becomes the single arm bent-over row. Use a fairly heavy dumbell.

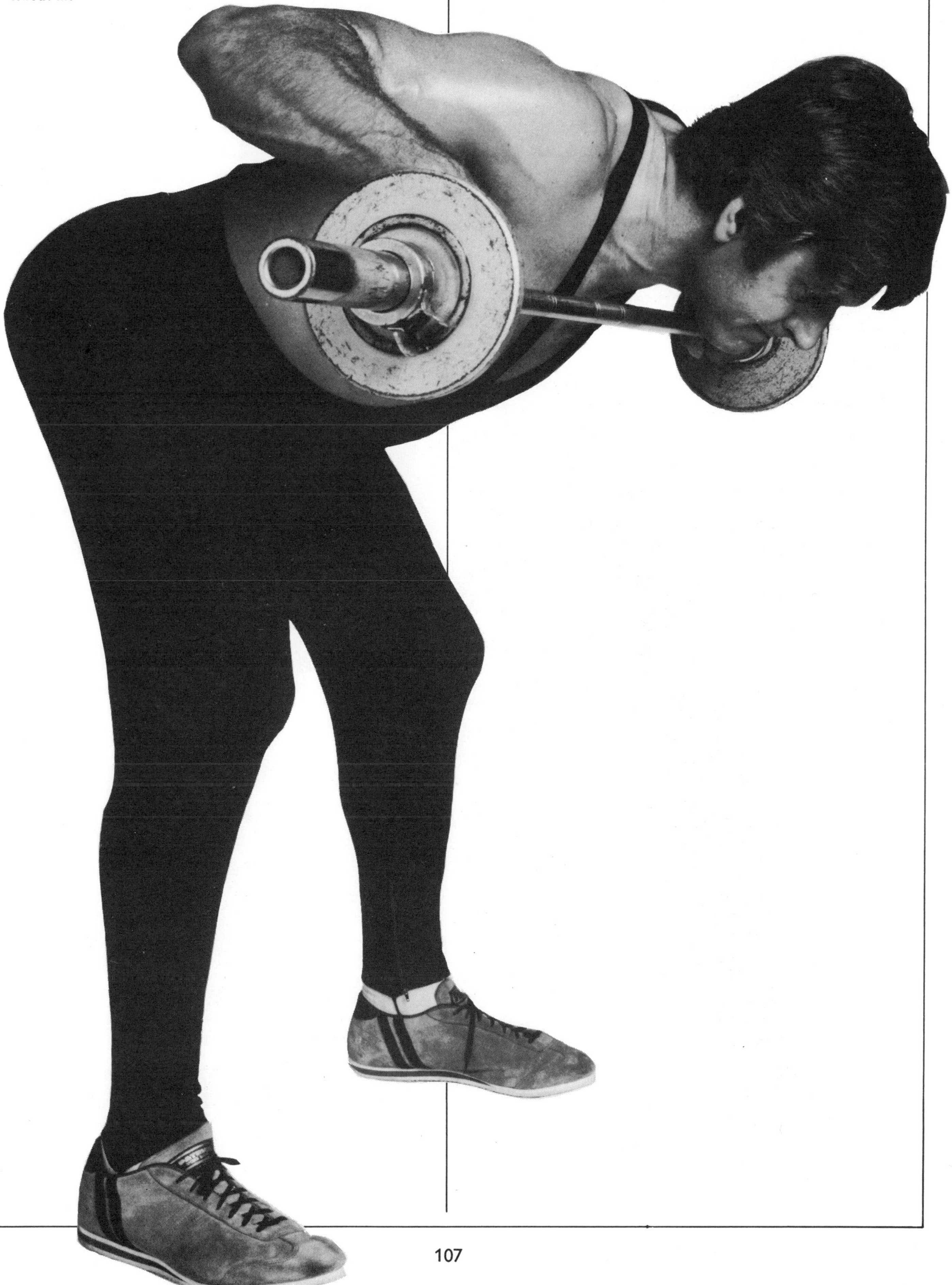

Single Arm Bent-over Row

1. Get into a similar position as that described above, but this time support yourself by your free arm, using a bench or the wall.
2. Place the dumbell by the foot opposite to the side you're going to work. You aim to get as big a stretch to the body as possible when reaching for the dumbell and when bringing it up to the limit of your pull.
3. Breathe in. Pull the dumbell up to the full extent of your arm and above your shoulder level.
NB If it goes too high, then the weight's too light. Increase it.
4. Do 10 repetitions, then change hands (3 sets in all).

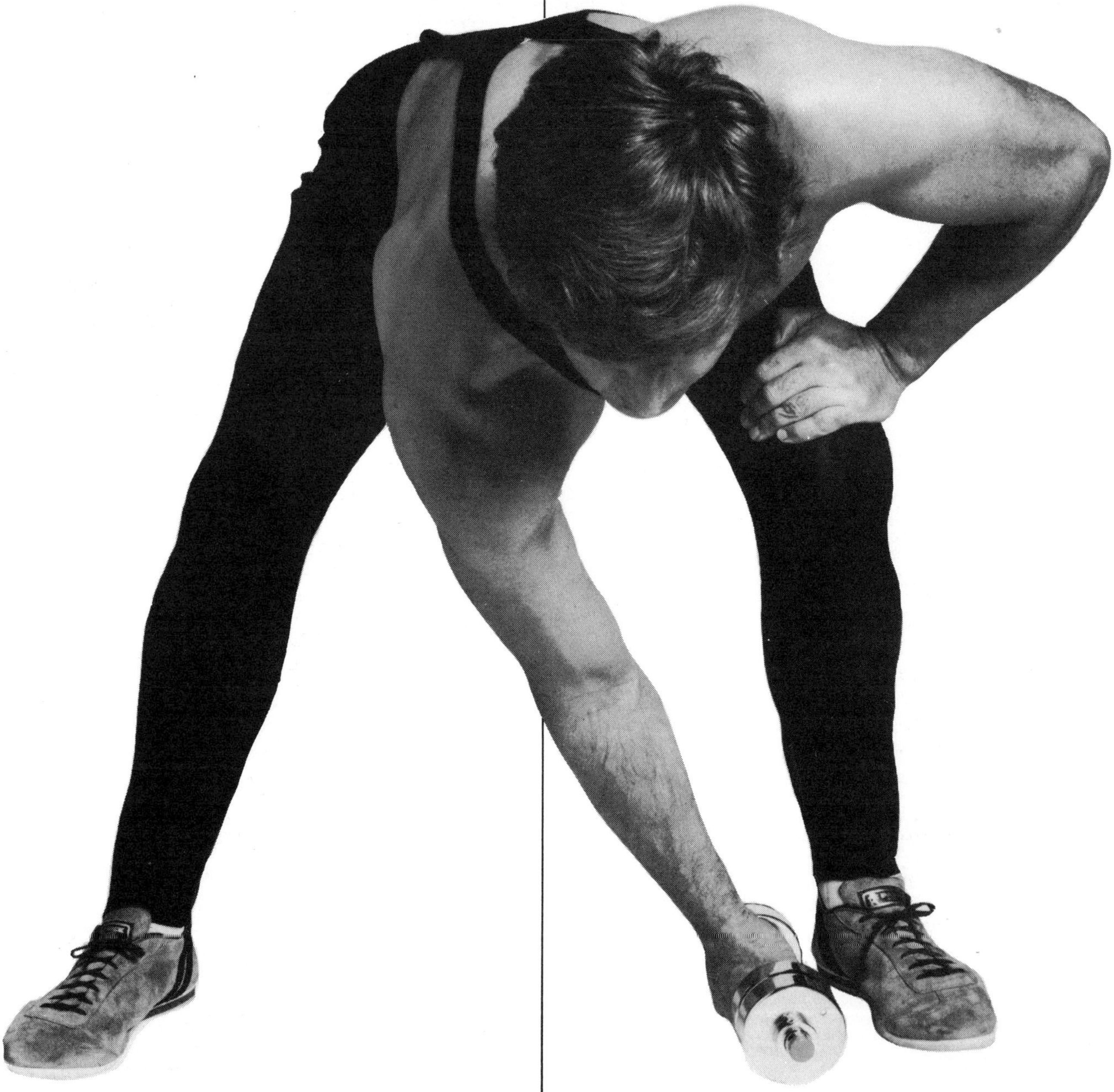

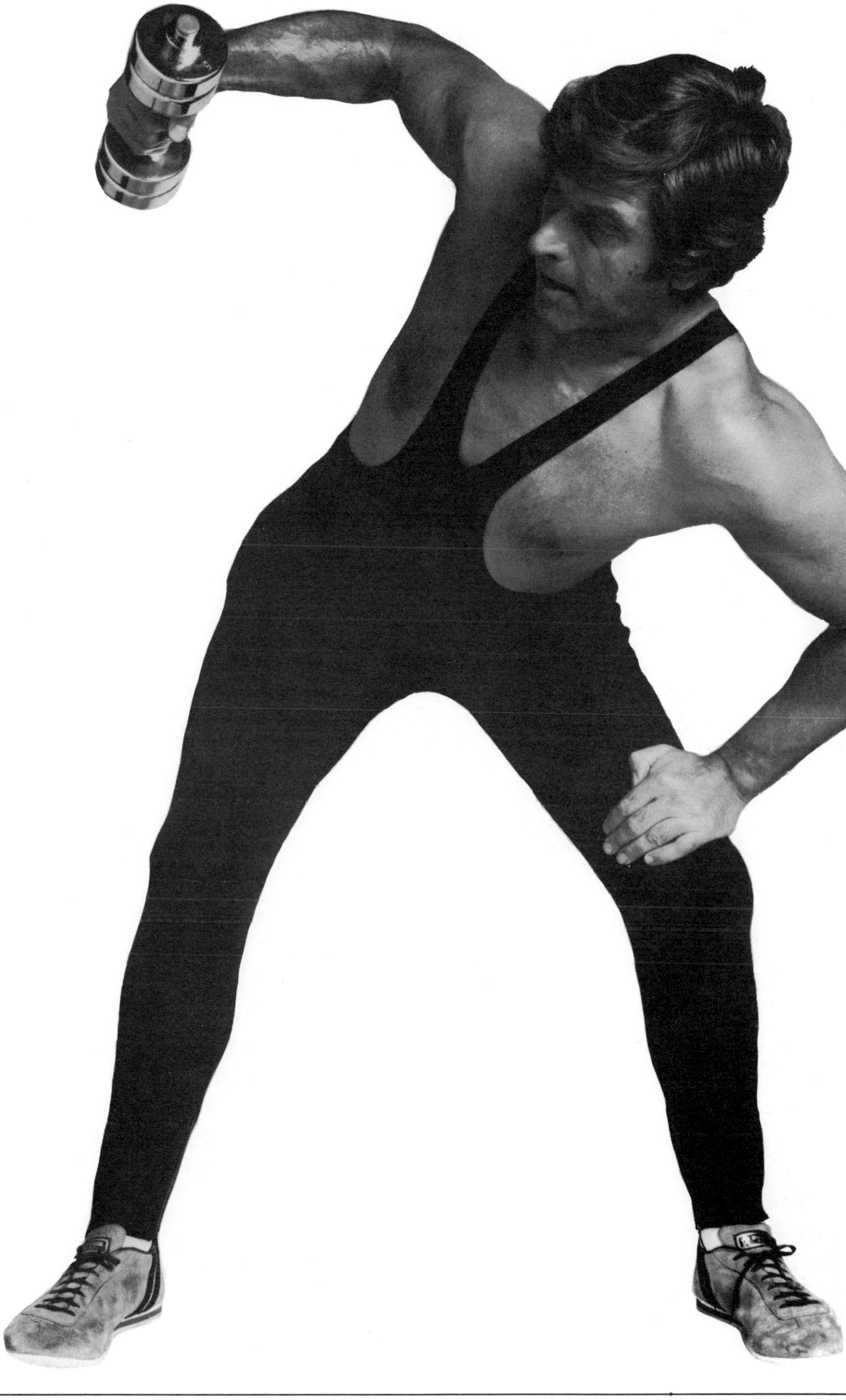

Two Hands Dead Lift

1. Stand with your feet 10–12 ins apart, ankles touching the bar.
2. Crouch down until hands are at the barbell, shoulder width apart, one hand over and one hand under the bar. Keep back straight, head and shoulders up, arms straight.
3. Breathe *in*. Straighten legs, and back and stand up.

Since my day, the record for the dead lift has risen to over 800 pounds and some world lifters are nearing 900 pounds, so you can see how standards have risen.

Remember you're doing this exercise from a strength and development aspect, so it's important to use as heavy a weight as you can handle. I would suggest not more than six repetitions of this exercise, but aim to do five to eight sets. This is the heaviest exercise in the whole schedule, and it is quite normal for a relatively untrained person to lift over 200 pounds. You must always be trying to increase the amount of weight you can handle.

This is one of the most important basic all-round exercises in any schedule; it works the lower back, the hips, the thighs, the trapezius muscles, the wrists, forearms and hand strength for grips. If you do this exercise on a regular basis, you should never have any form of disc trouble. The erector muscles become so strong that they keep all the discs in place without any trouble.

At one period, in a competition held by TWW, the old Welsh commercial television station, I won a competition for the strongest man in Wales and the West when I lifted 678¾ lbs to establish a new British record, and I beat the Welsh champion, Terry Purdue, into the bargain. I subsequently tried 700 on the same night, but I couldn't get it above my knees. The deadlift is one of the three power lifts – the lifts which body-builders compete on as opposed to the three Olympic lifts. The power lifts then used to consist of the two hands curl, the dead lift and the squat, but they are now the squat, the dead lift and the bench press which has now superseded the two hands curl.

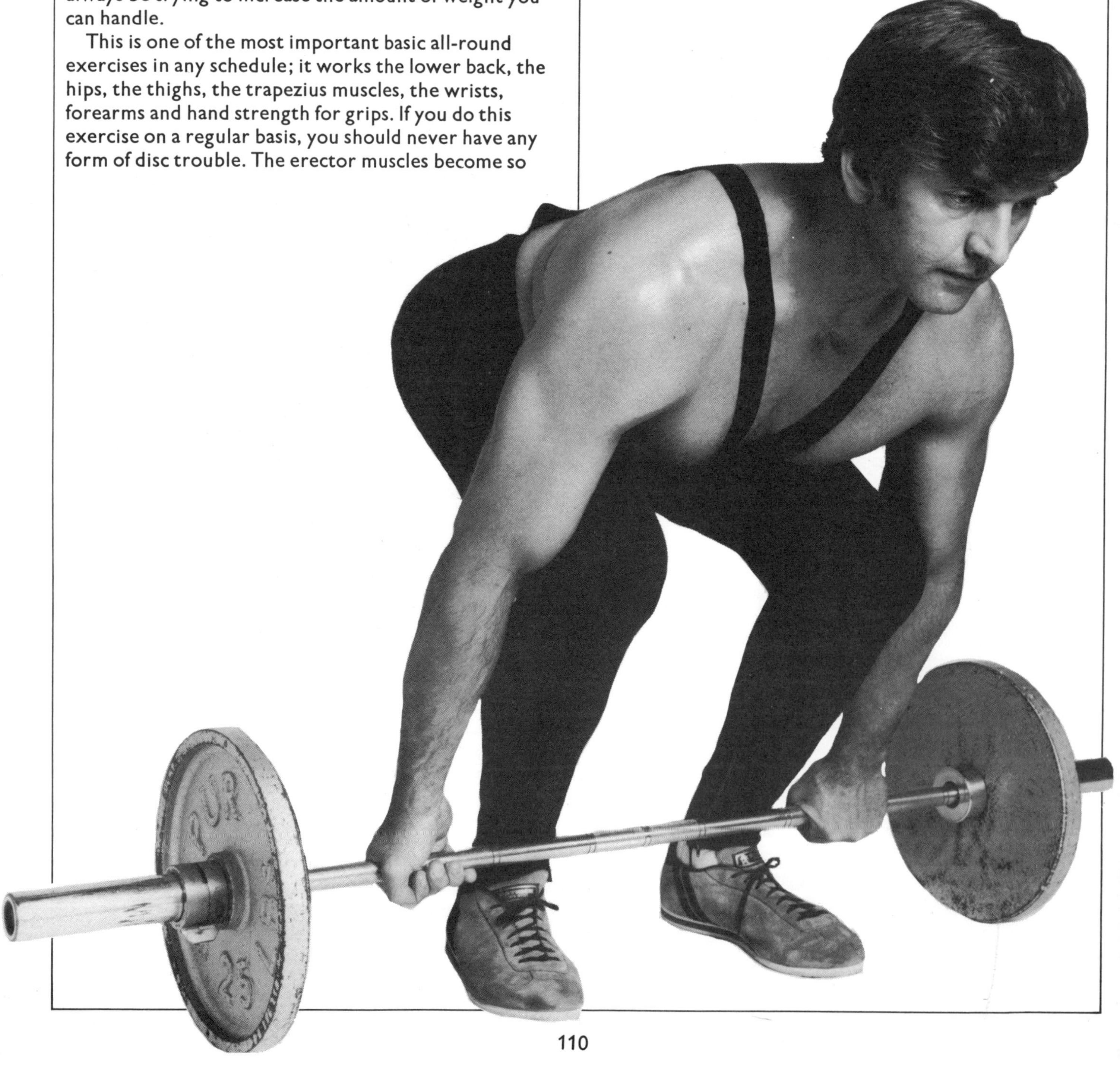

The two hands dead lift must be one of the most simple of all lifts to perform. The simple object is to stand up straight with as heavy a weight as possible. There are obviously rules which govern the lift, just as there are rules the lifter himself must apply to ensure he doesn't damage himself. For example, you bend your knees, and let the legs do most of the work; and a one hand under, one hand over grip will ensure the bar doesn't twist in your hands.

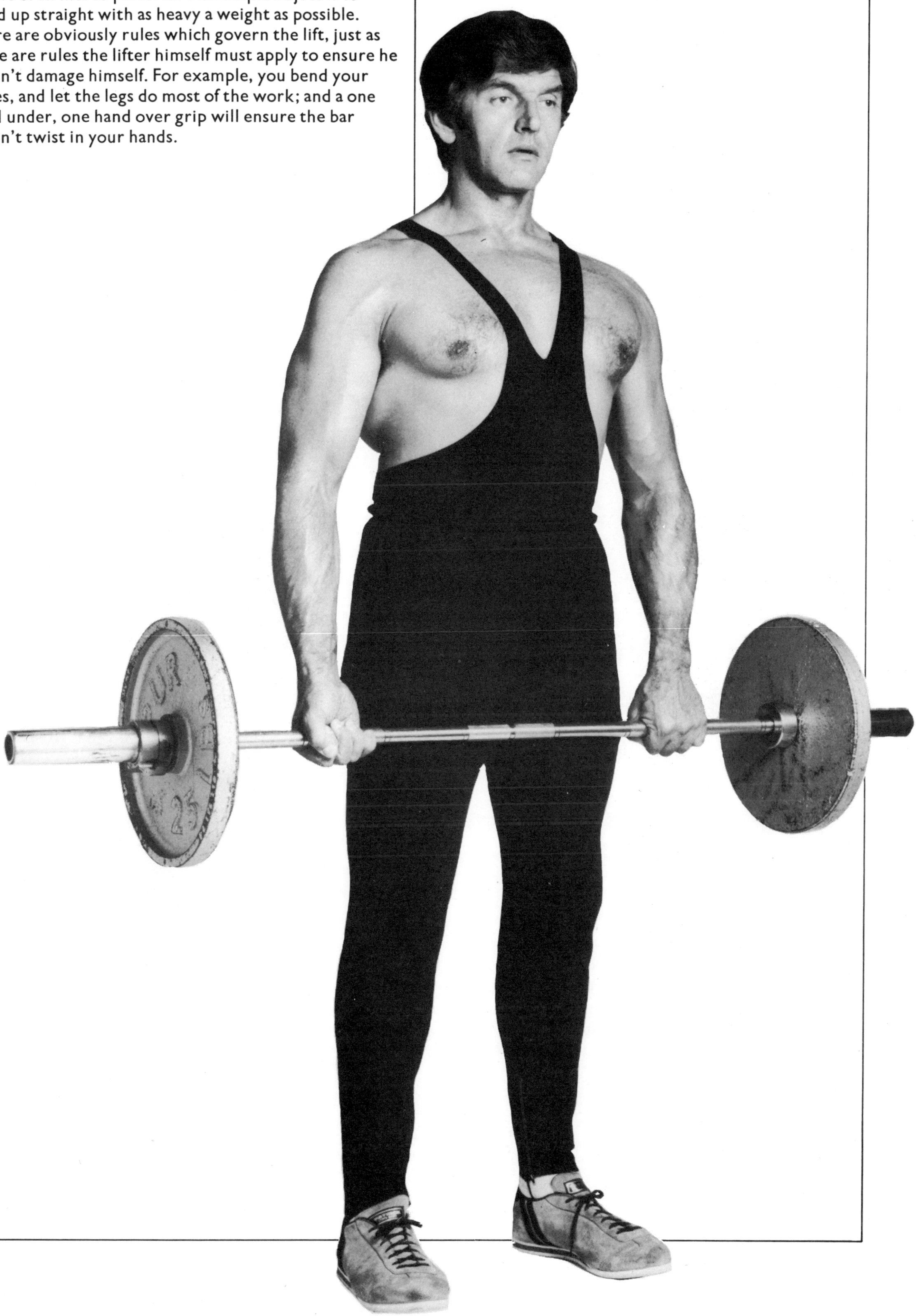

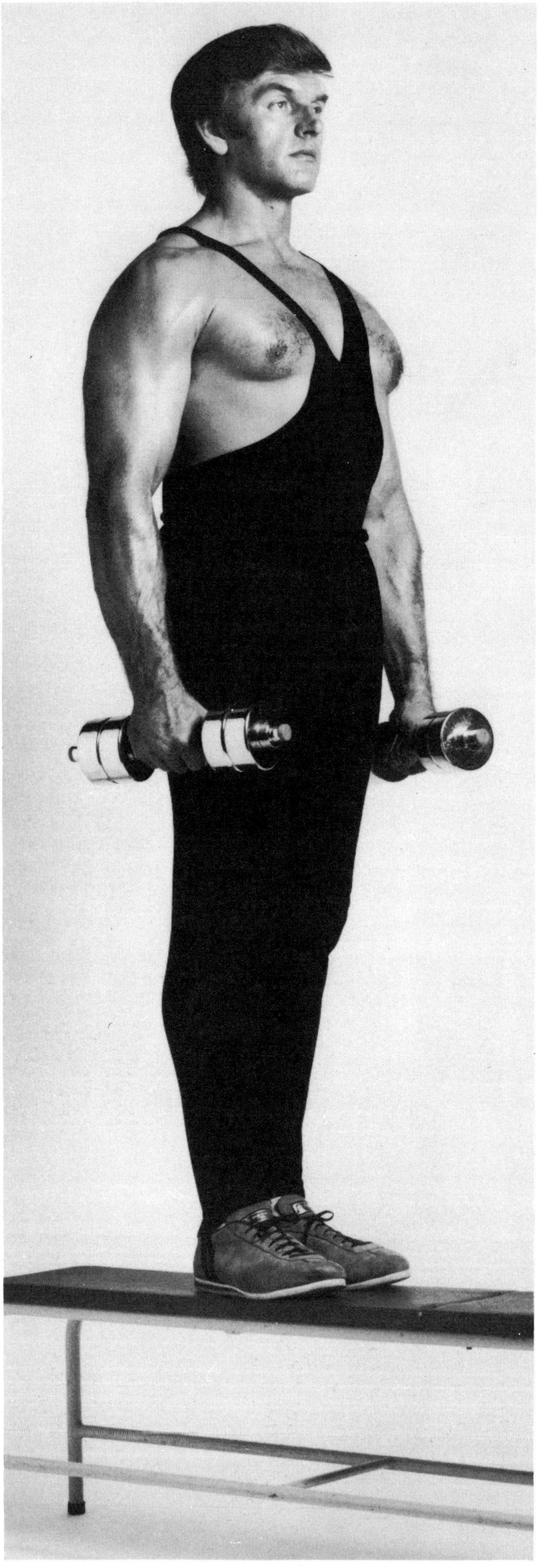

Two Hands Dead Lift with Dumbells

It's quite usual for the dead lift to be done as a suppleness and mobility exercise as well. This means the use of dumbells rather than a barbell, and also a bench.

1. Holding two dumbells stand up on the bench with your arms straight down at your sides.

2. Keep the legs as stiff as possible (just a slight knee bend). Bend forward and lower the dumbells below the level of the bench. Don't worry if you can't at first – some people are more supple than others – but you'll find with constant practice you'll be able to get lower and lower.

3. Straighten up.

4. Do 15 repetitions (3 sets).

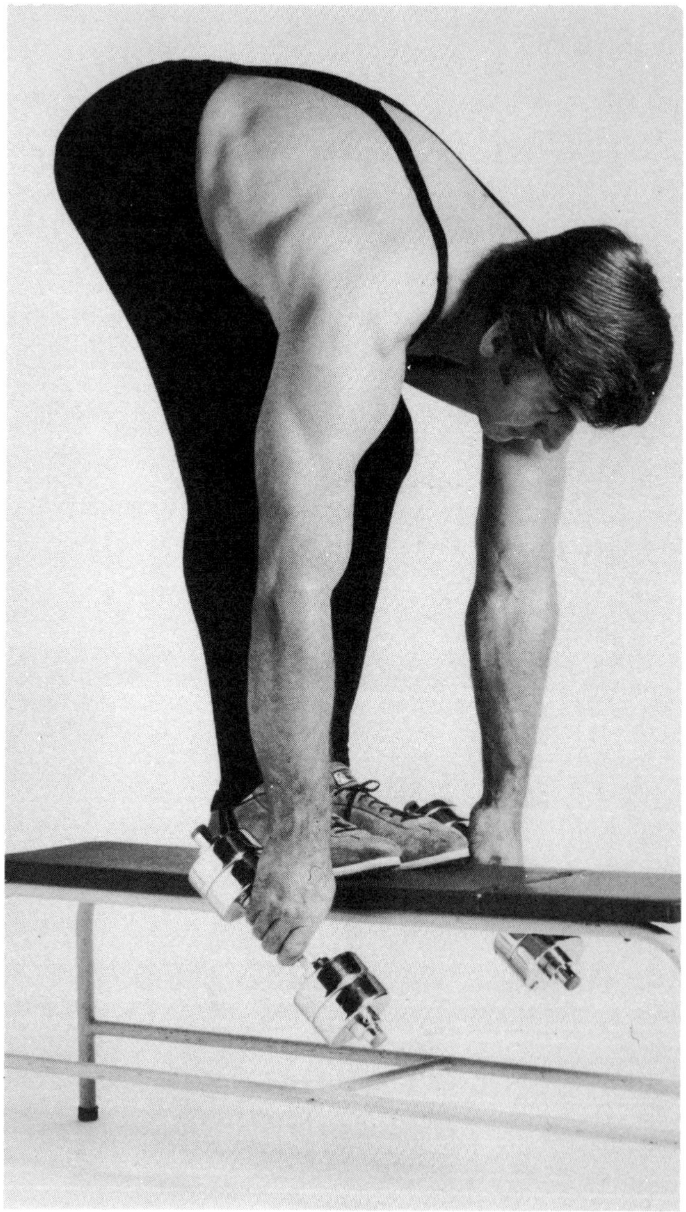

Hyper Extensions

These are a great exercise for the muscles of the lower back – the erector spinae. These really are the opposite of doing dead lifts – in which you bend forward to pick up the weights. In the hyper extensions you bend up backwards. You have to get into a position whereby the effort comes from arching the back, so basically you'll do the exercise lying face down on the floor with a companion anchoring your feet or hooking your ankles under a piece of furniture.

1. Lie face down on floor, hands behind your back, with your ankles anchored

2. Arch your back as high as possible.

3. Return to prone position.

4. Do 15 repetitions (3 sets).

To increase resistance, first fold your arms across your chest; then clasp your hands behind your neck. After that you can add further weights to the hands behind neck position, or increase the range of movement by doing it in different positions, say across a bench. You can work up to doing the hypers on a table, where you find you can get something like 130 degrees of movement.

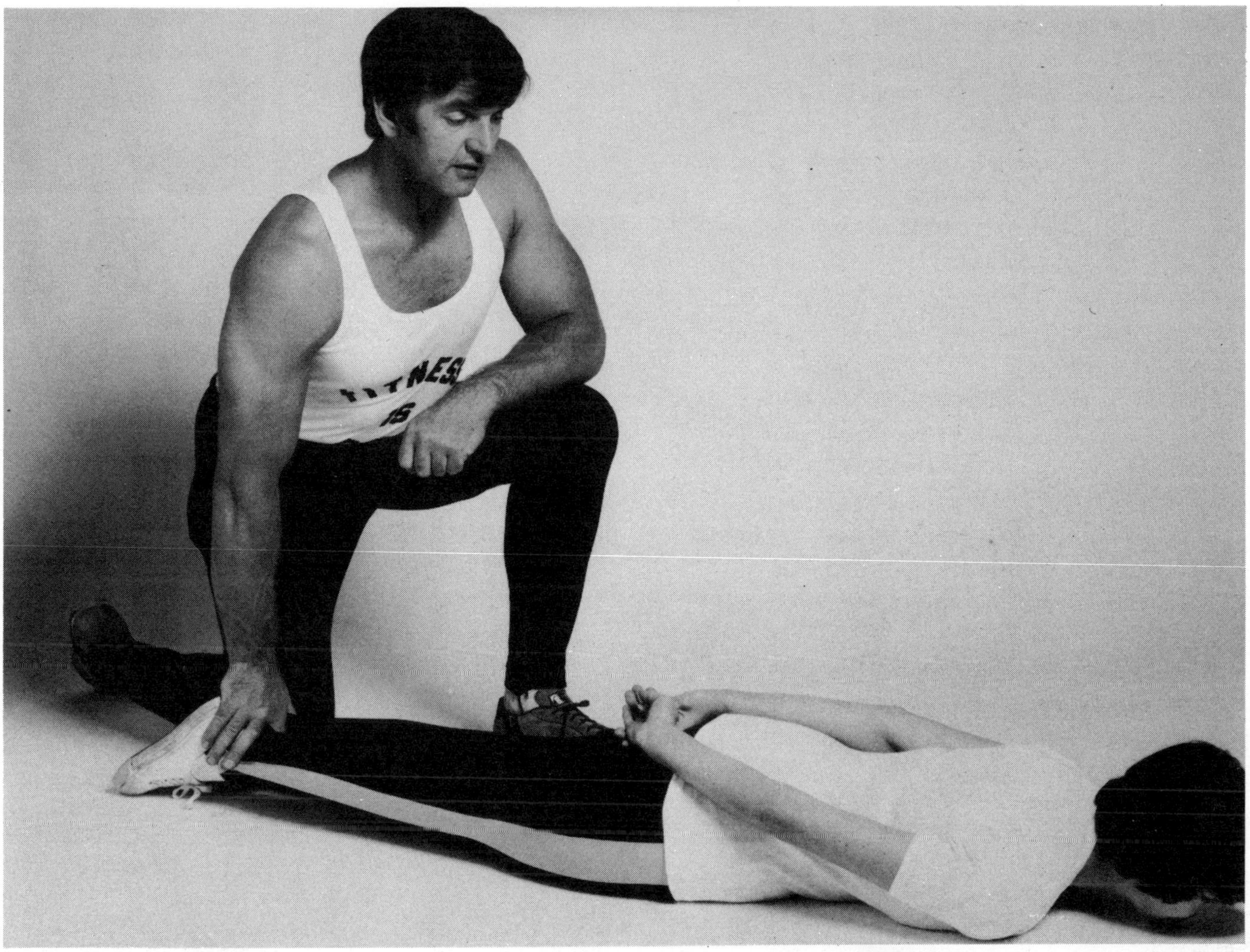

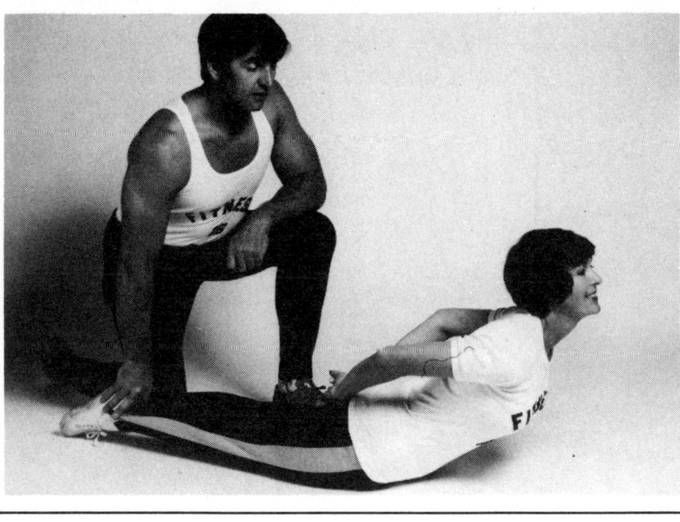

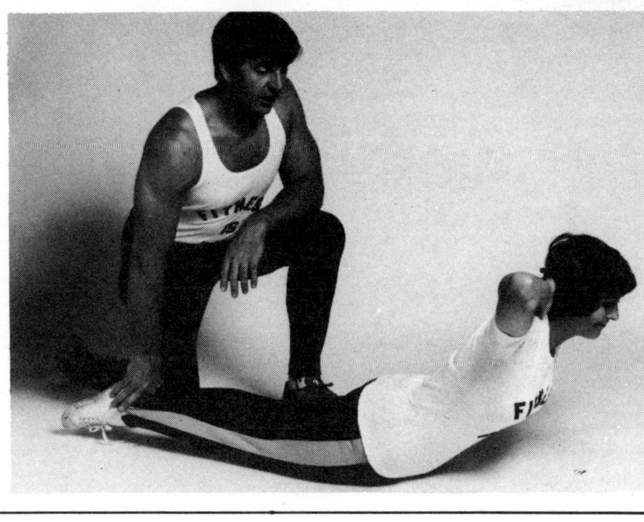

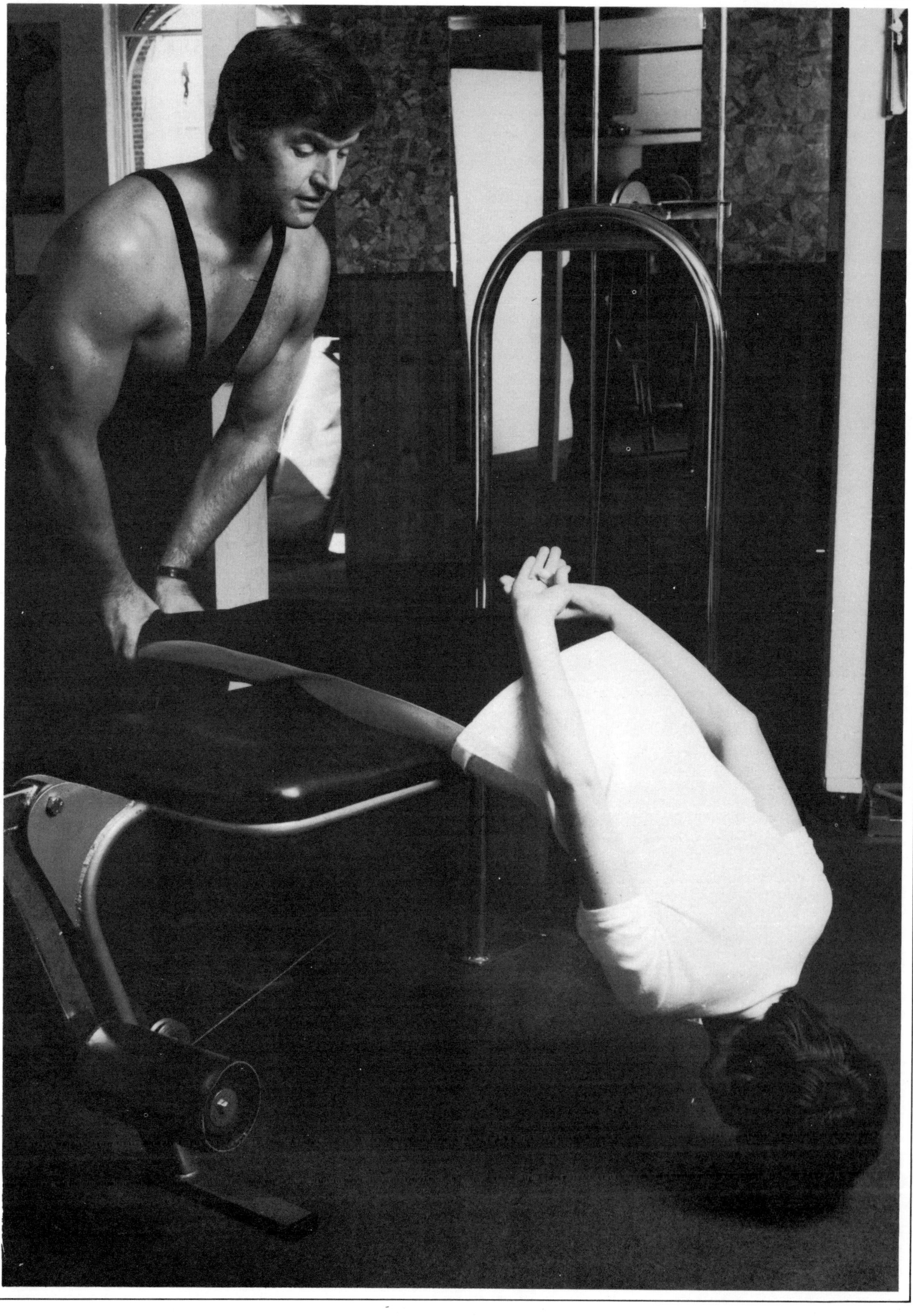

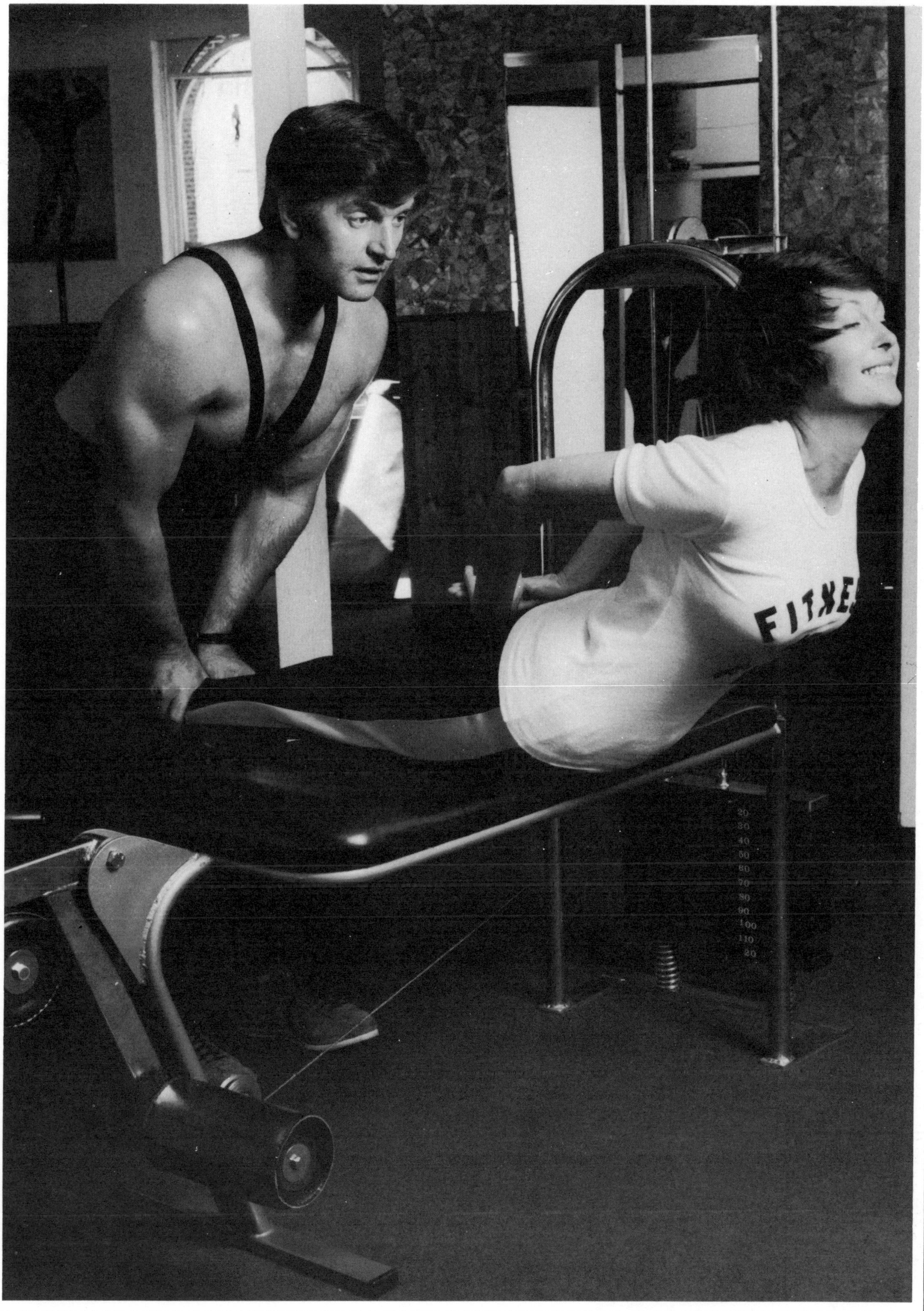
FITNES

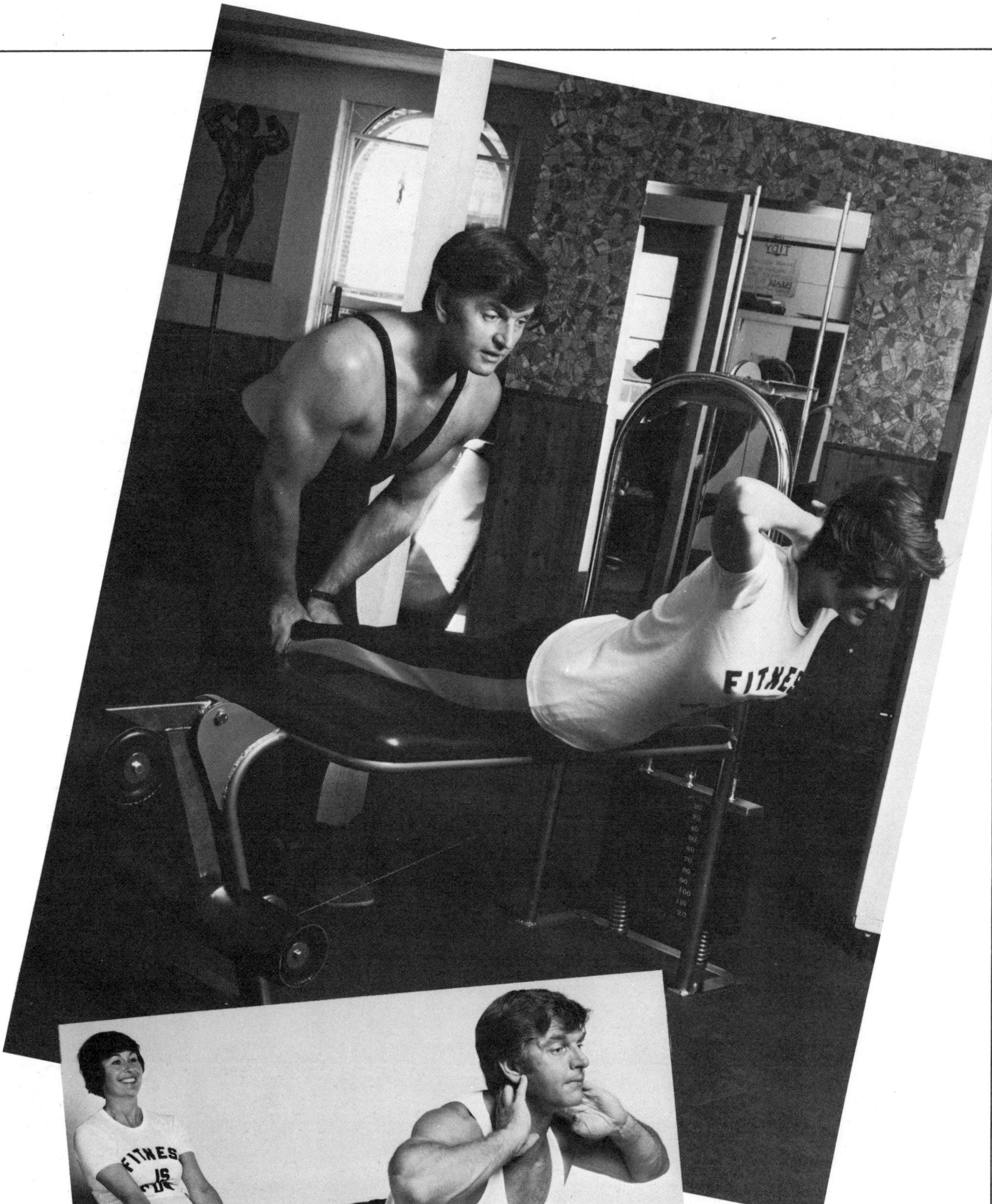
FITNES

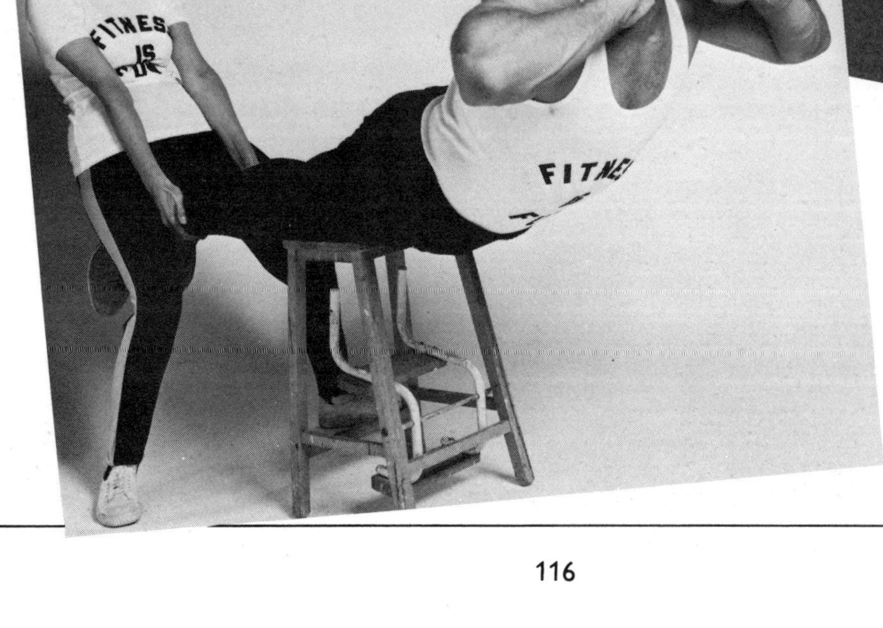
FITNES
IS
FITNES

The Chins or Pull-ups

This is a marvellous exercise for the upper back, and it entails the use of a pull-up or chinning bar. Basically it is a bar either in a doorway or between two walls that you have to jump up to reach.

1. Grasp the bar with an over grip, hands shoulder width apart.

2. Pull yourself up until your chin comes above the level of the bar.

3. Let yourself slowly back to full extent of arms.

4. Call the chin-up position the start; breathe *in* coming down and *out* after the hard bit going up.

You can vary the hand position of the exercise – over hand or under hand grip. If you use a narrow under hand grip this will also benefit your biceps muscles. Start off by trying to do as many repetitions as you can; do three sets. When you can do three sets of 15 repetitions, then is the time to increase the resistance by tying weights around your waist. But I've never yet found anyone who finds chinning easy.

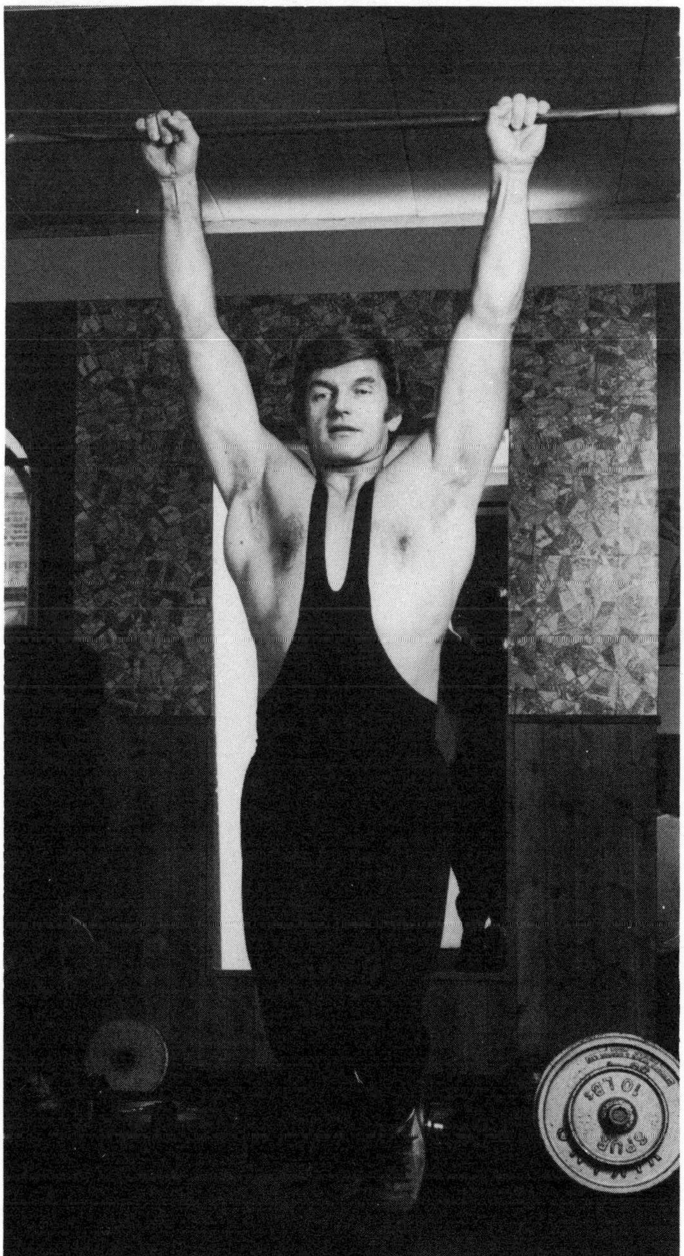

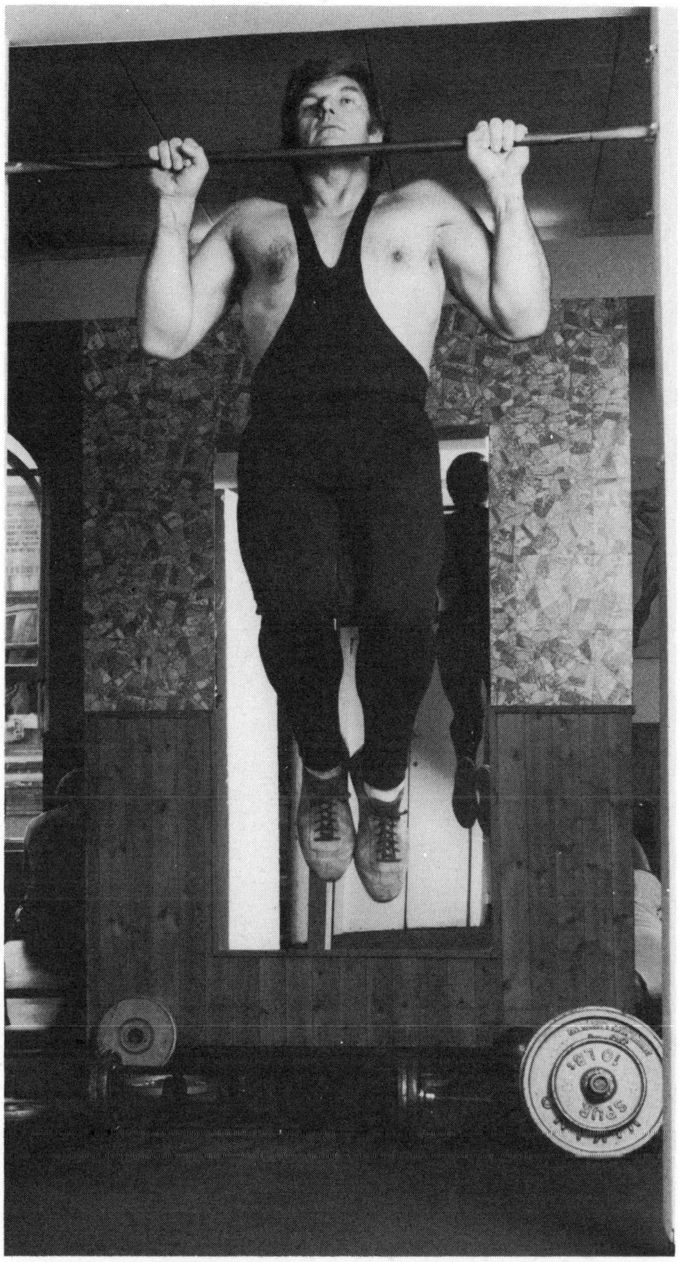

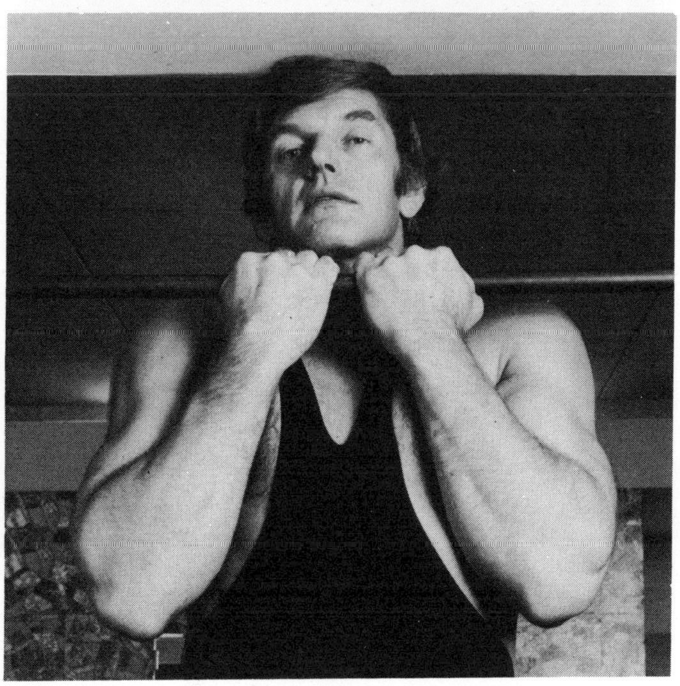

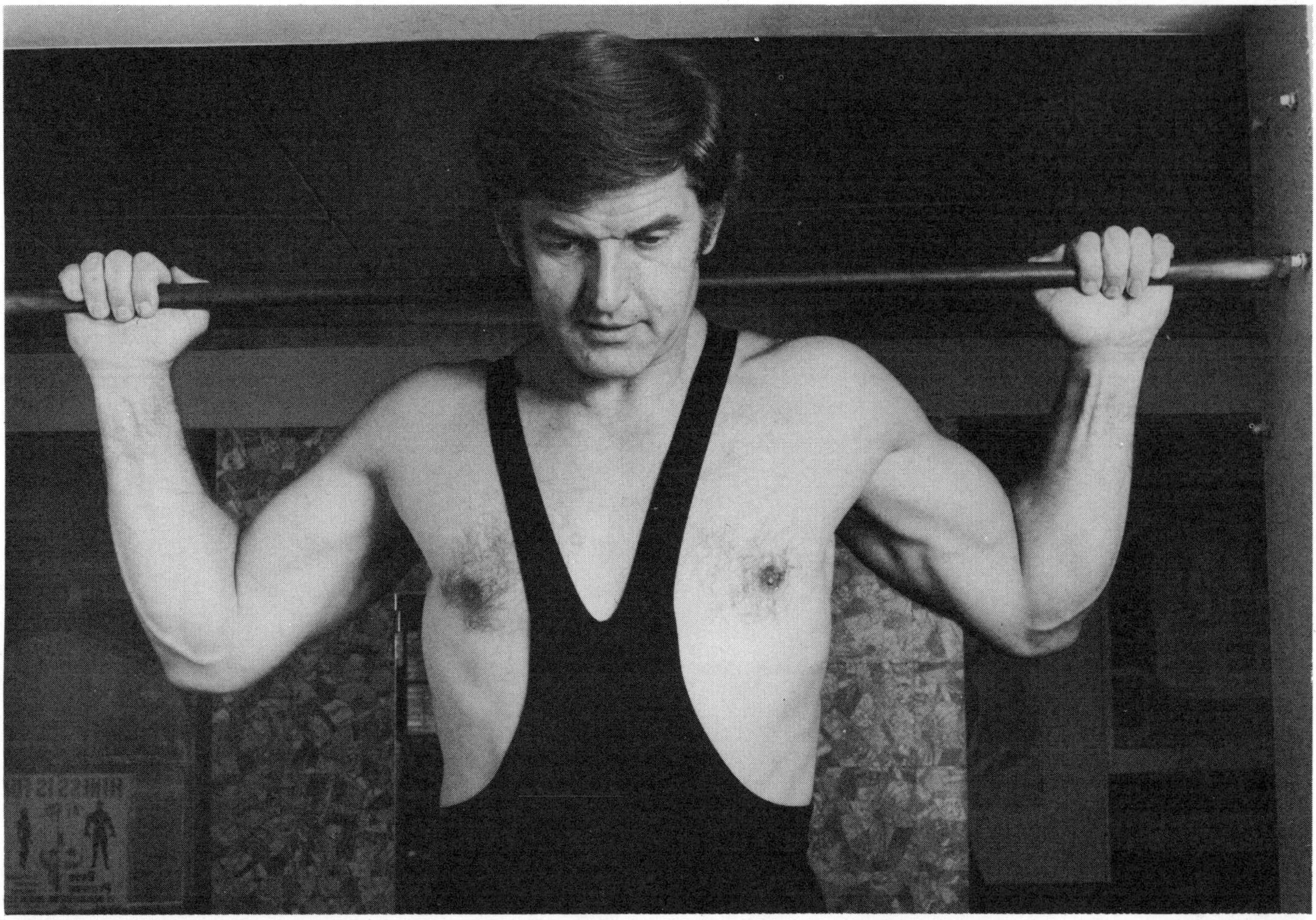

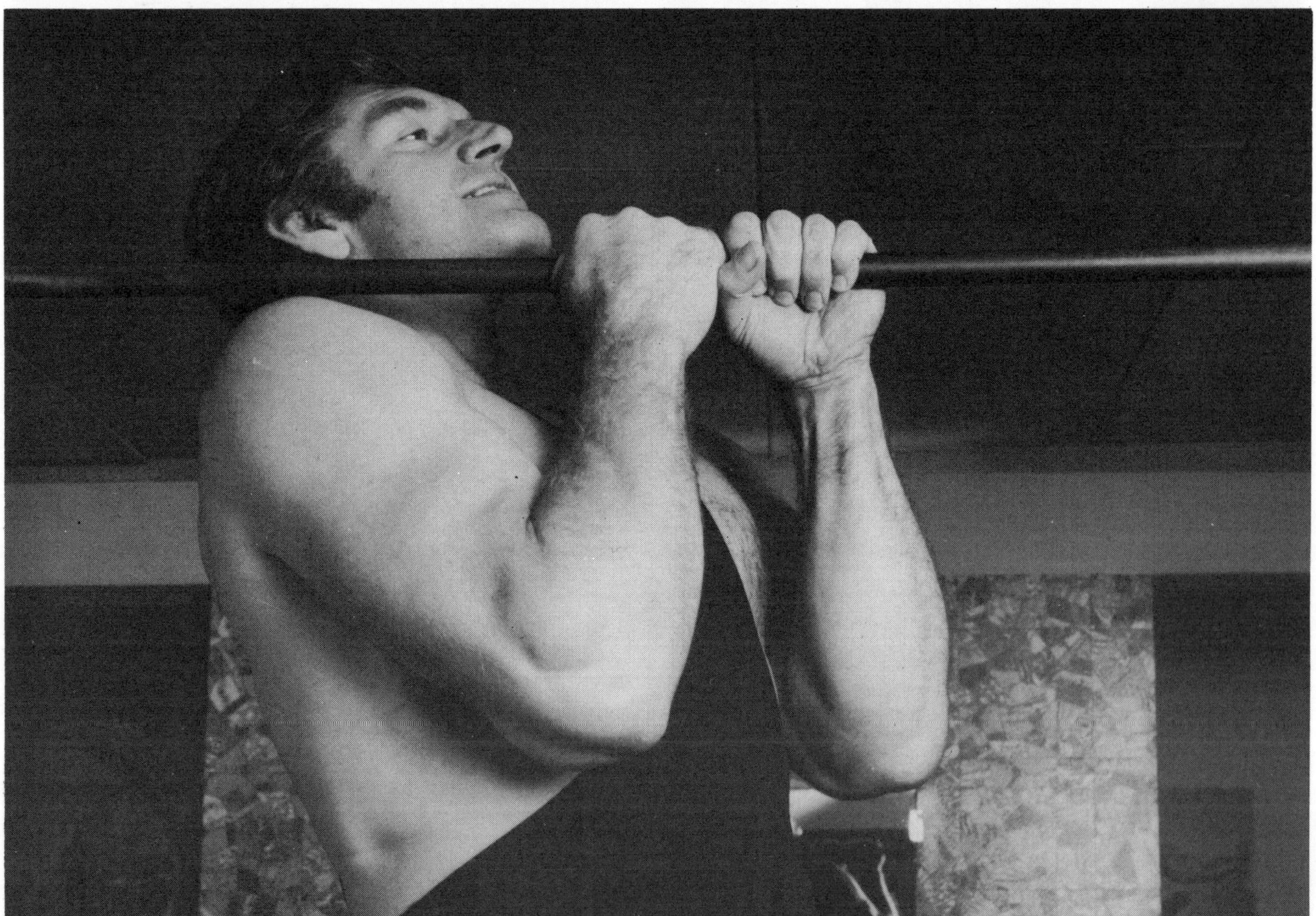

The Shoulder Shrug

Finally with the back exercises we come to the shoulder shrug, which is done either with barbells or dumbells. As the name implies, the shoulder shrug simply means raising the level of your shoulders as though you were shrugging, but of course you are doing it with the added resistance of a barbell or dumbell.

1. Pick up the weight and hold it at arm's length, resting against your thighs.
2. Try to make your shoulders touch your ears. Don't bend your arms.
3. You can if you like rotate your shoulders as you raise them.
4. Carry on until the shoulders and neck ache.

It's difficult to recommend a weight – as heavy as possible for this exercise – or a number of repetitions. Aim to do three sets of as many repetitions as are necessary to make your shoulders ache.

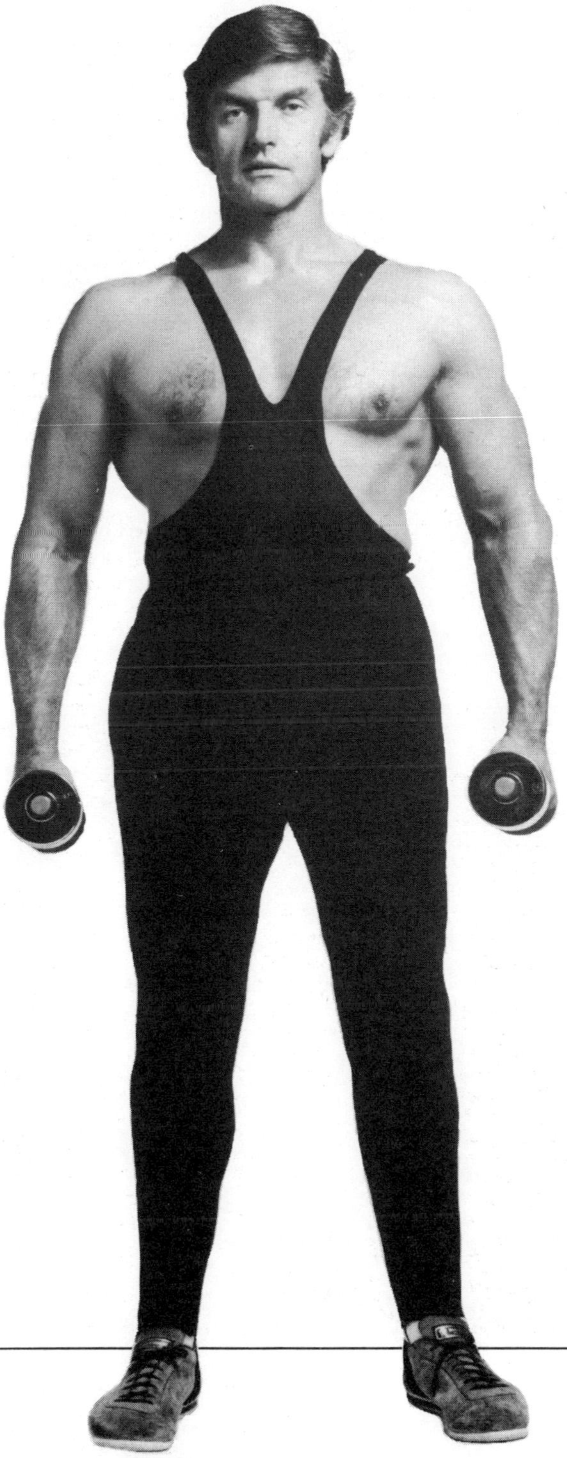

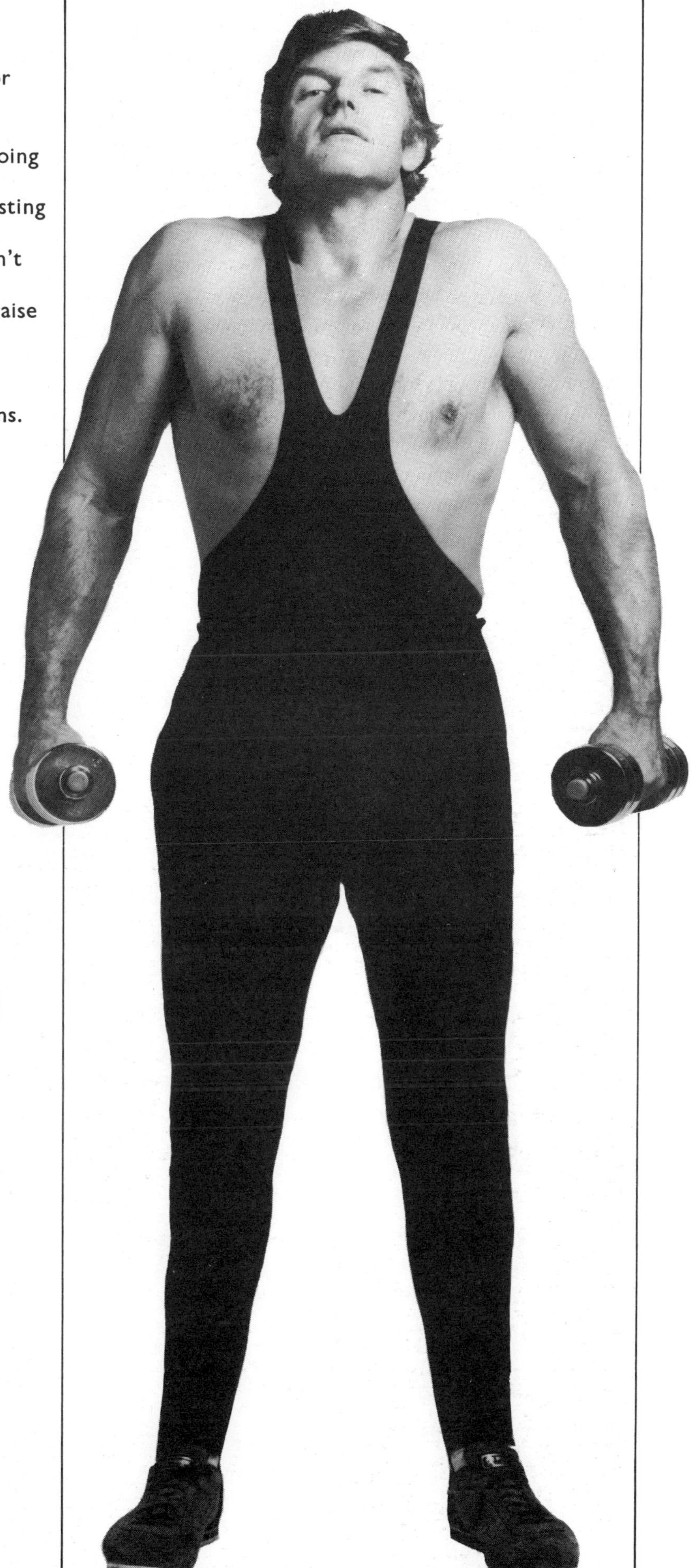

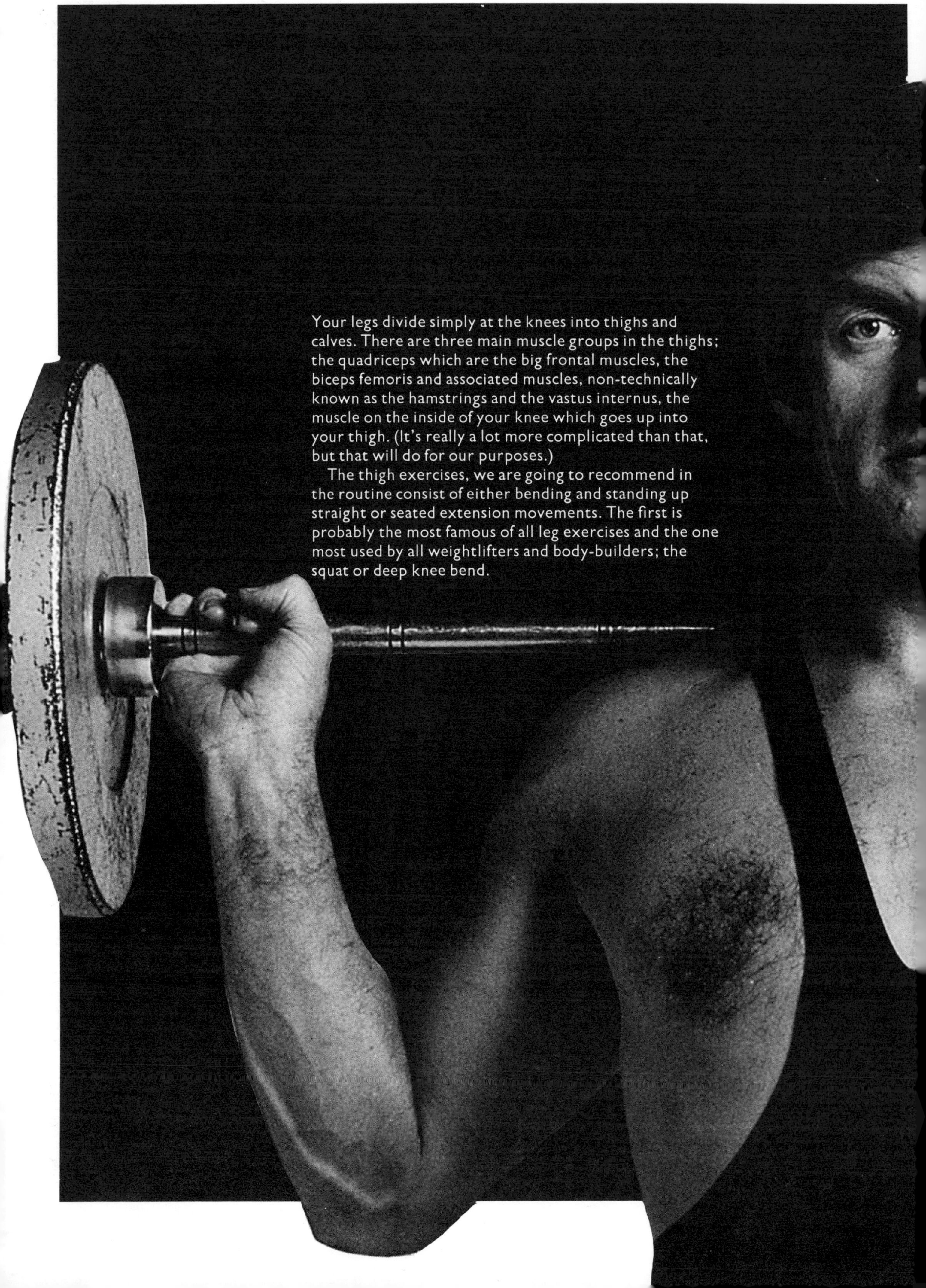

Your legs divide simply at the knees into thighs and calves. There are three main muscle groups in the thighs; the quadriceps which are the big frontal muscles, the biceps femoris and associated muscles, non-technically known as the hamstrings and the vastus internus, the muscle on the inside of your knee which goes up into your thigh. (It's really a lot more complicated than that, but that will do for our purposes.)

The thigh exercises, we are going to recommend in the routine consist of either bending and standing up straight or seated extension movements. The first is probably the most famous of all leg exercises and the one most used by all weightlifters and body-builders; the squat or deep knee bend.

Chapter 14

GETTING RIGHT DOWN TO IT

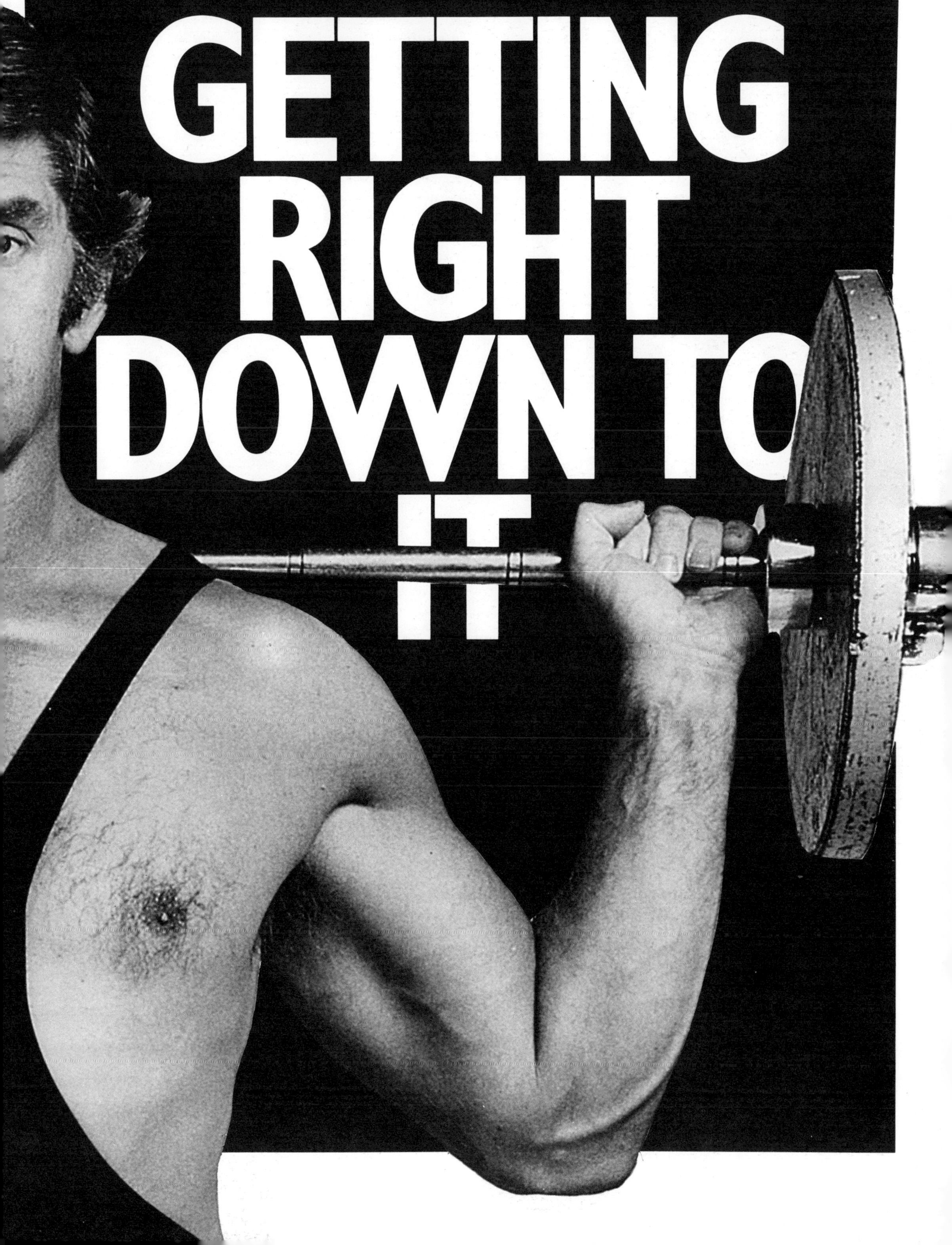

Deep Knee Bend

1. Place a weight (barbell) across your shoulders and stand with the feet 15 to 18 inches apart.
2. Sink down as low as you can go, or at least with your thighs below parallel. Stick your behind out, keeping your back as straight as possible. Head and shoulders should be upright.
3. Stand up straight again.
4. Do 20 repetitions (3 sets).

The exercise can be done in a variety of ways. You can squat to the parallel position, you can do quarter squats where you don't get as far as the parallel position, and full squats, which is going down as low as you can sink.

There is a lot of feeling, to which I don't subscribe, that very heavy full squatting is damaging to the knees. It derives from the discovery that the 'jumping squat' which was once very popular among athletes, could do more damage than good. I feel that, providing you squat within your limitations, there is no reason at all why you shouldn't do full squats.

There is another version of the squat called the breathing squat which is specifically for respiration and also for increasing the size of your thorax – rib cage. In this you squat in the normal way; but for the first ten repetitions you breathe once between each repetition. From 10 to 15 you take two breaths between each repetition; and from 15 to 20 you breathe three times between each repetition.

From my own experience, I have found that doing squats for basic power you will have to decrease the repetitions (come down to a maximum of six to eight repetitions) increase the number of sets to five or six and train with as heavy weights as possible. As with all exercises, if you do your twenty repetitions easily, then the time has come for you to increase the weight.

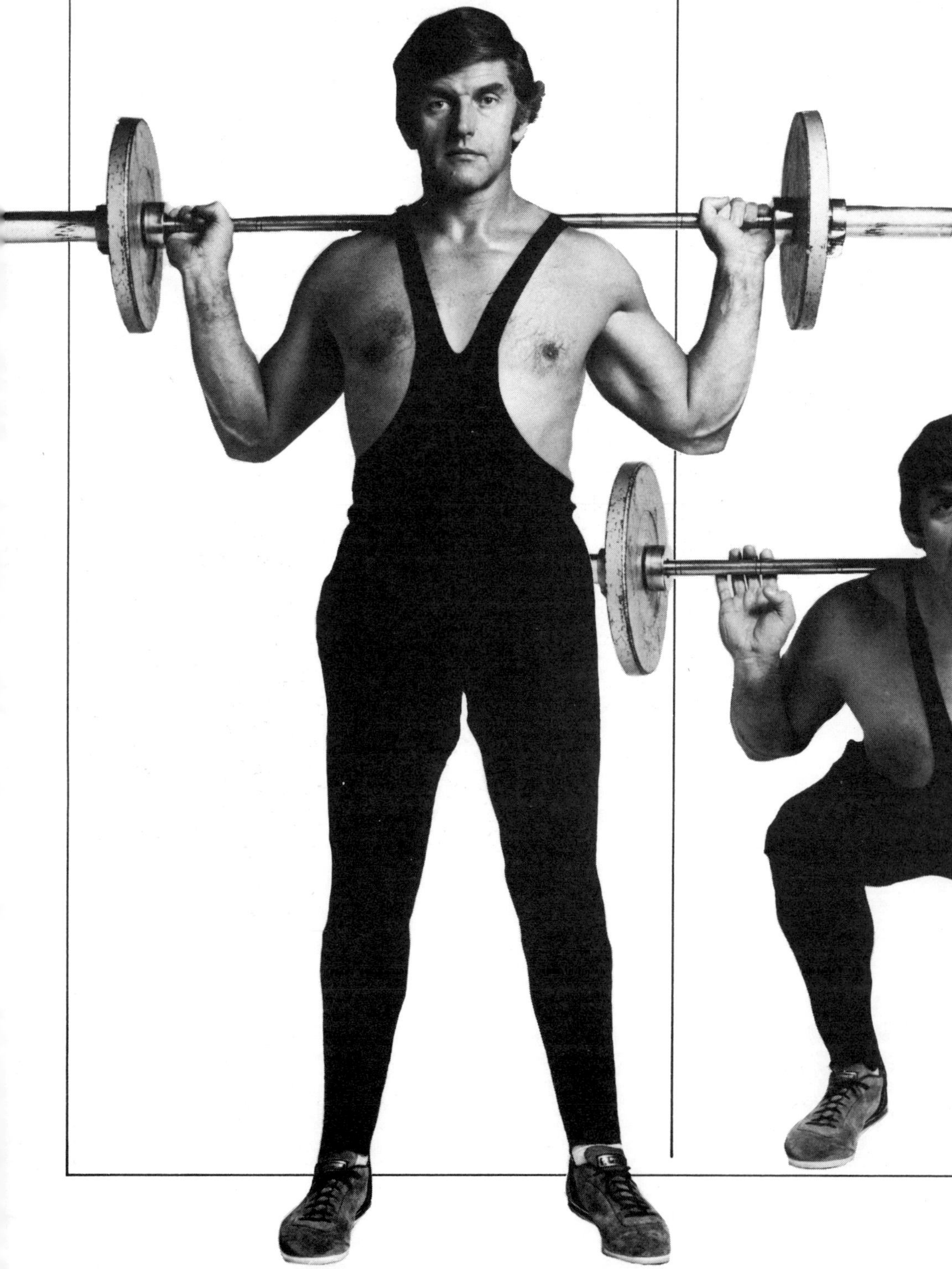

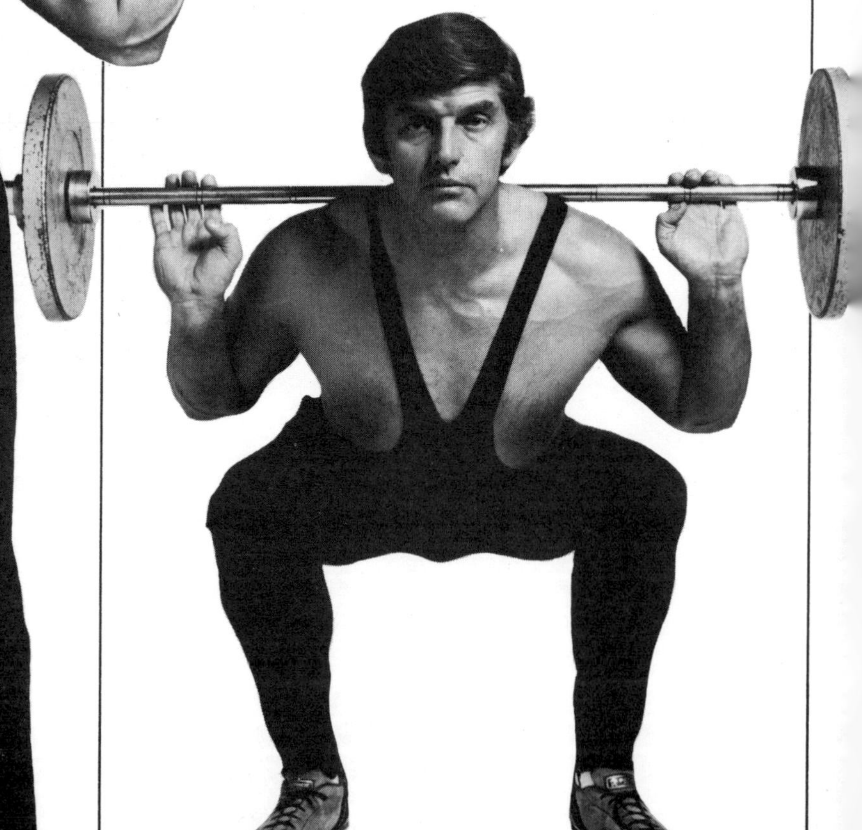

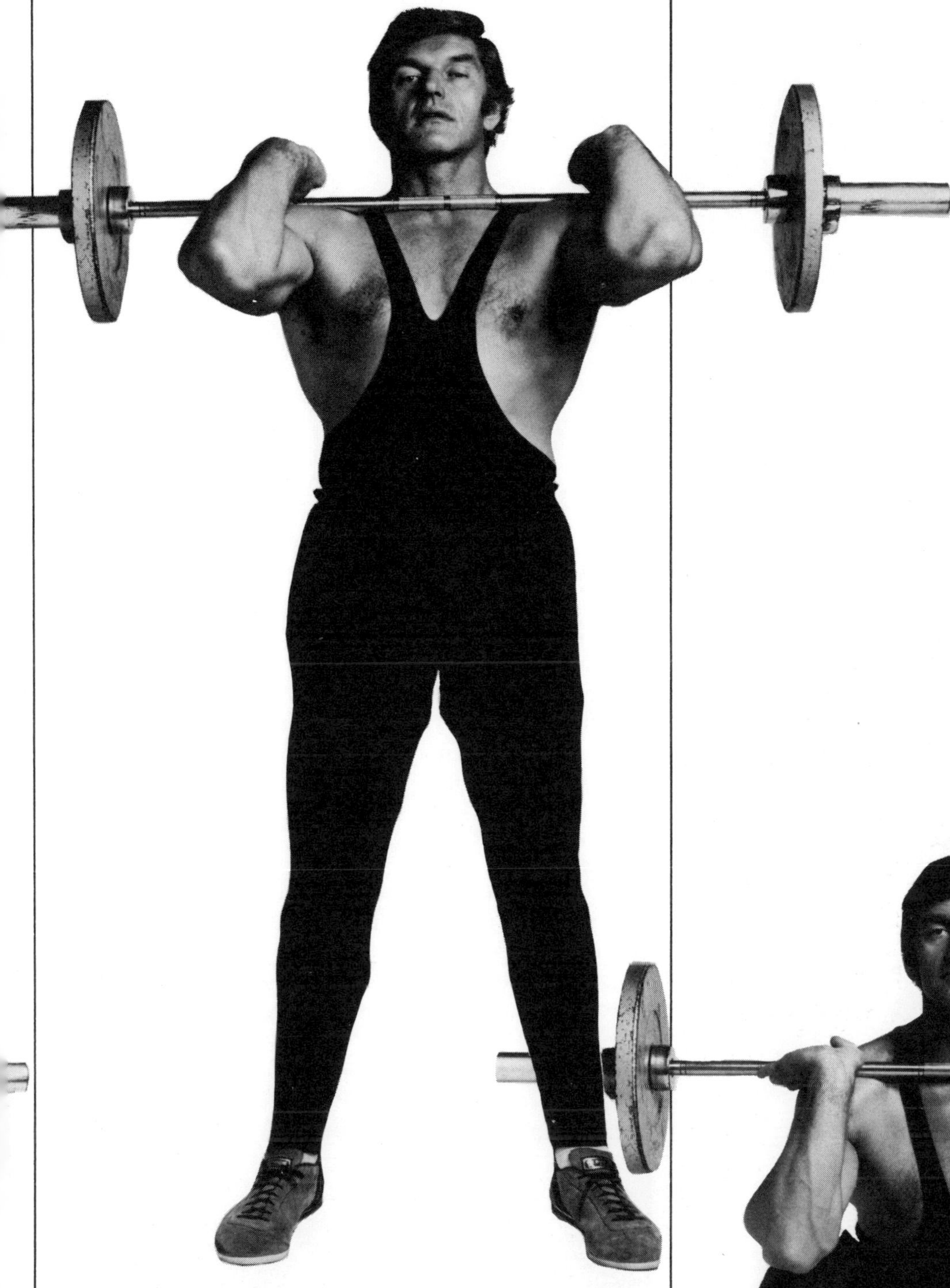

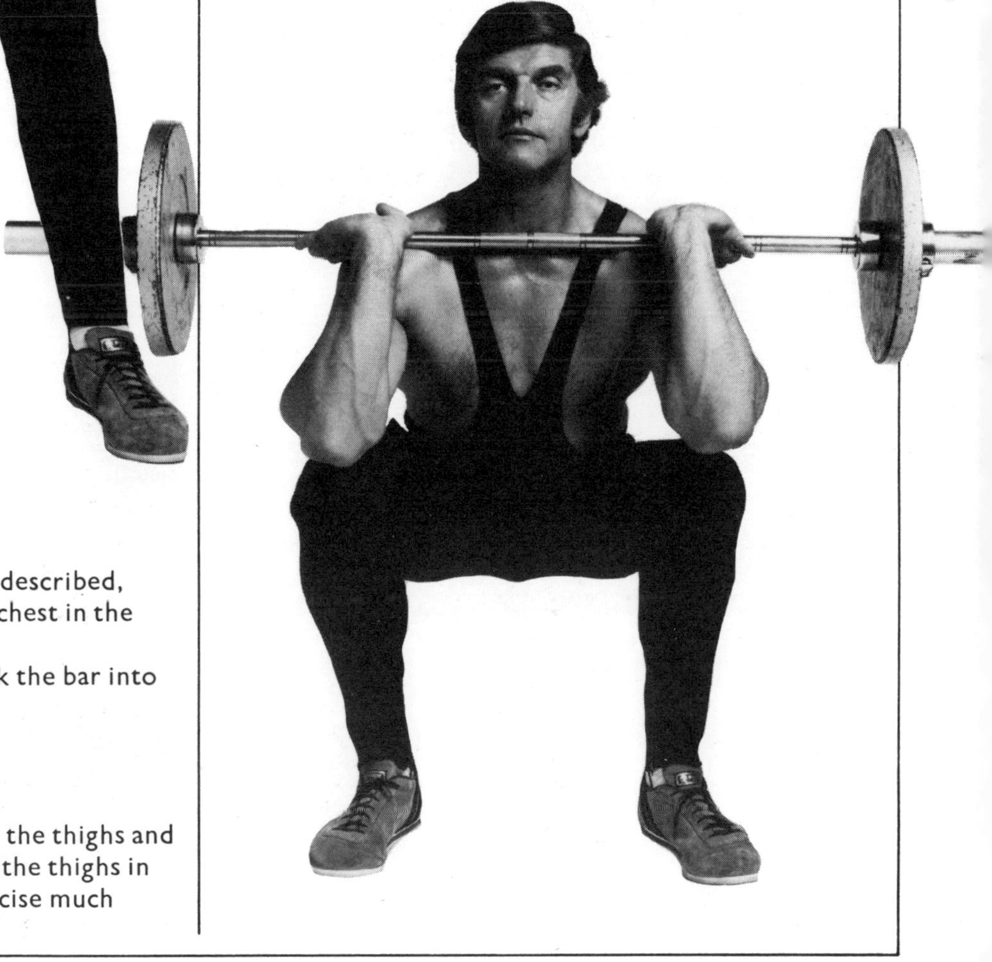

Front Squat

This is similar to the deep knee bend just described, except that the barbell is held across the chest in the clean position.

1. Breathe in. Force the elbows up to lock the bar into position.
2. Sink down to the squat position.
3. Recover to start position.
4. Repeat 20 times (3 sets).

This places a slightly different strain on the thighs and in fact tends to develop the lower part of the thighs in preference to the upper part. It's an exercise much favoured by weightlifters.

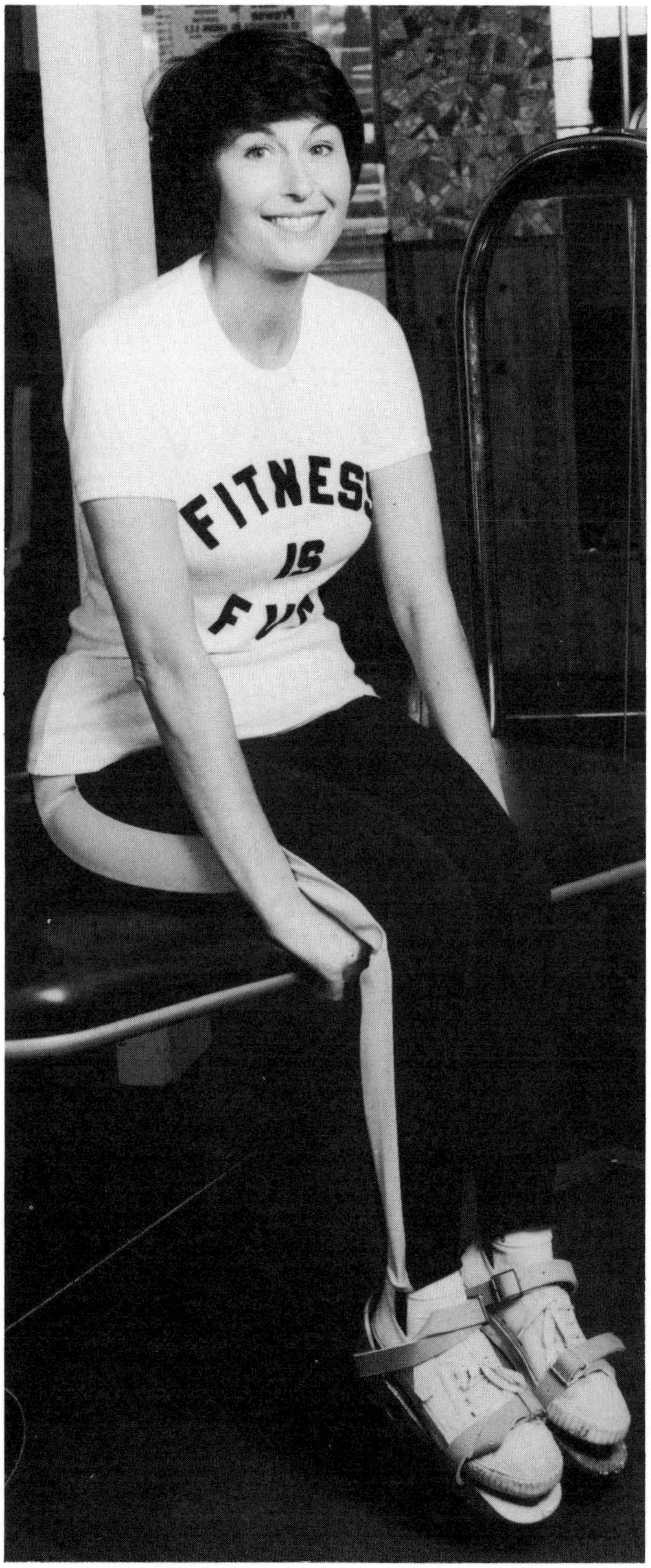

Leg Extensions

For these, you need the use of a leg extension machine; but if you haven't got one you can perform them easily by using an iron shoe on your foot.

1. Sit on the edge of a table.
2. With your upper leg flat on the table, straighten out your leg and bend it again.
3. Use alternate legs.
4. Repeat 10–15 times (3 sets).

This is specifically to strengthen the knee joint and the vastus internus muscle on the inside of the knee. Cartilage sufferers are always put on to leg extensions within a couple of weeks of the operation. It's amazing just how quickly some professional football players recover and are able to play within a few weeks of having the operation. If you're using an iron shoe, you can increase the weights to increase the resistance.

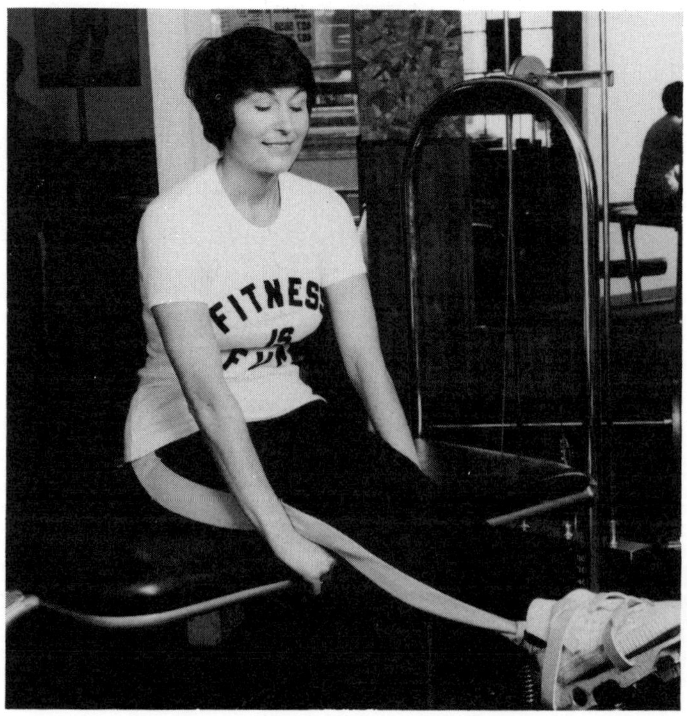

The Sissy Squat

This is very much favoured by body-builders, particularly because it does not enlarge your gluteous maximus (hip) muscles. You don't need any resistance for this exercise, but you will need something to hold on to to keep your balance.

1. Stand by a wall or post, up on your toes as high as possible, holding on for balance.

2. Do a deep knee bend but push your hips forward, so your knees come well forward, so all the strain is on the rest of the knee or thighs.

3. Repeat 20 times (3 sets).

NB Don't try this if you've any knee trouble at all.

The biceps femoris is very much the same as the biceps muscle in the upper arm in that its action is to draw the leg up to the hip, bending the knee. The action of the quadriceps is similar to that of the triceps – which is to straighten the limb.

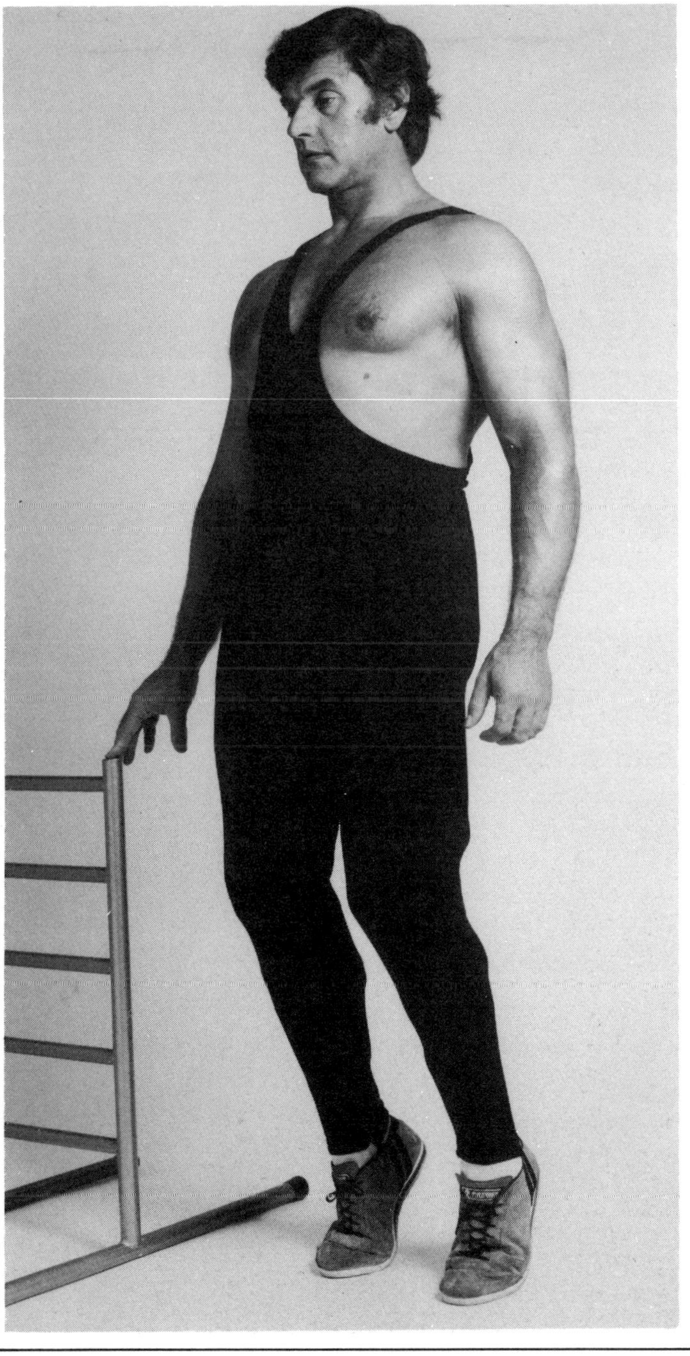

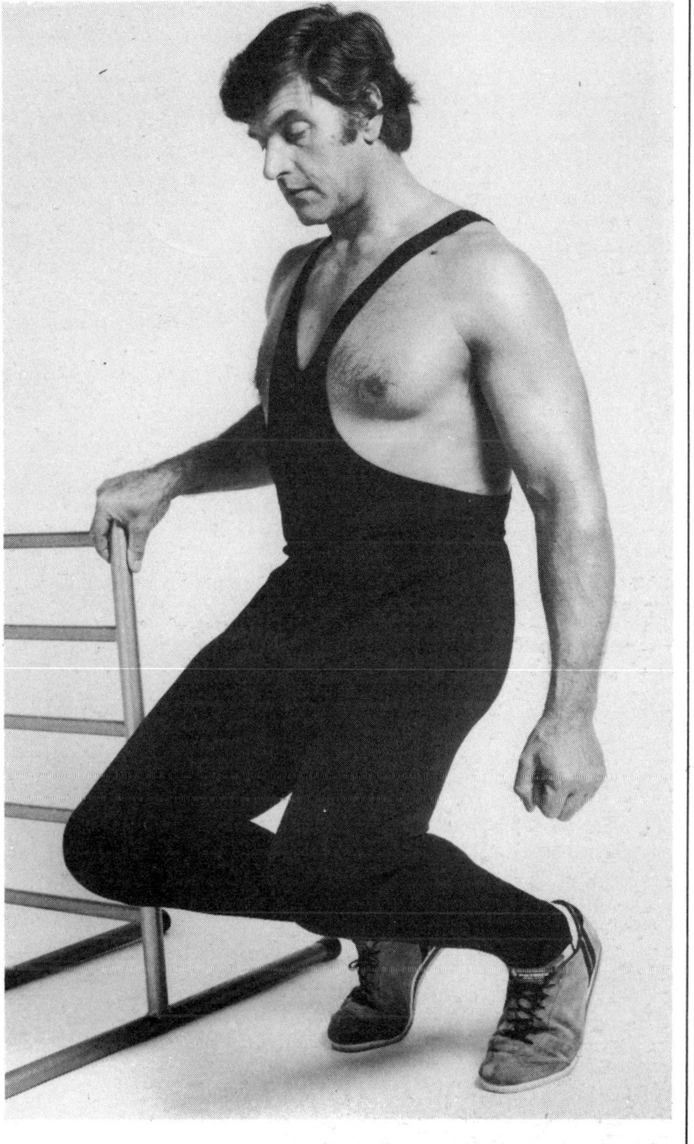

Leg Curl

1. Lie face downwards with a suitable weight on the iron shoe (about 20 or 30 lbs).
2. Bend the knees until your heels touch your behind.
3. Do 20 repetitions (3 sets).

You have to be careful about developing the biceps femoris, as it can have an inhibiting effect on speed. That's exactly why sprinters don't ride bicycles – all the wrong muscles are developed.

The calf muscles are a notoriously difficult area of the body to work. It has been established by a physiologist that every time you take a pace something like 500 lbs pressure goes onto the calf muscle. As a result, the calf muscles take an enormous amount of work during the day; and if you want to develop your calf muscles you have to place an even greater load on them. It's my opinion that unless you're going in for the Mr Universe competition the results of calf exercising hardly ever justify the effort involved. In the same way I hardly ever give specific exercises for neck or forearm muscles. You get plenty of exercise for those areas in the routine.

There are plenty of calf exercises if you wish, and lots of equipment on the market for developing the calves. There are two which are particularly effective.

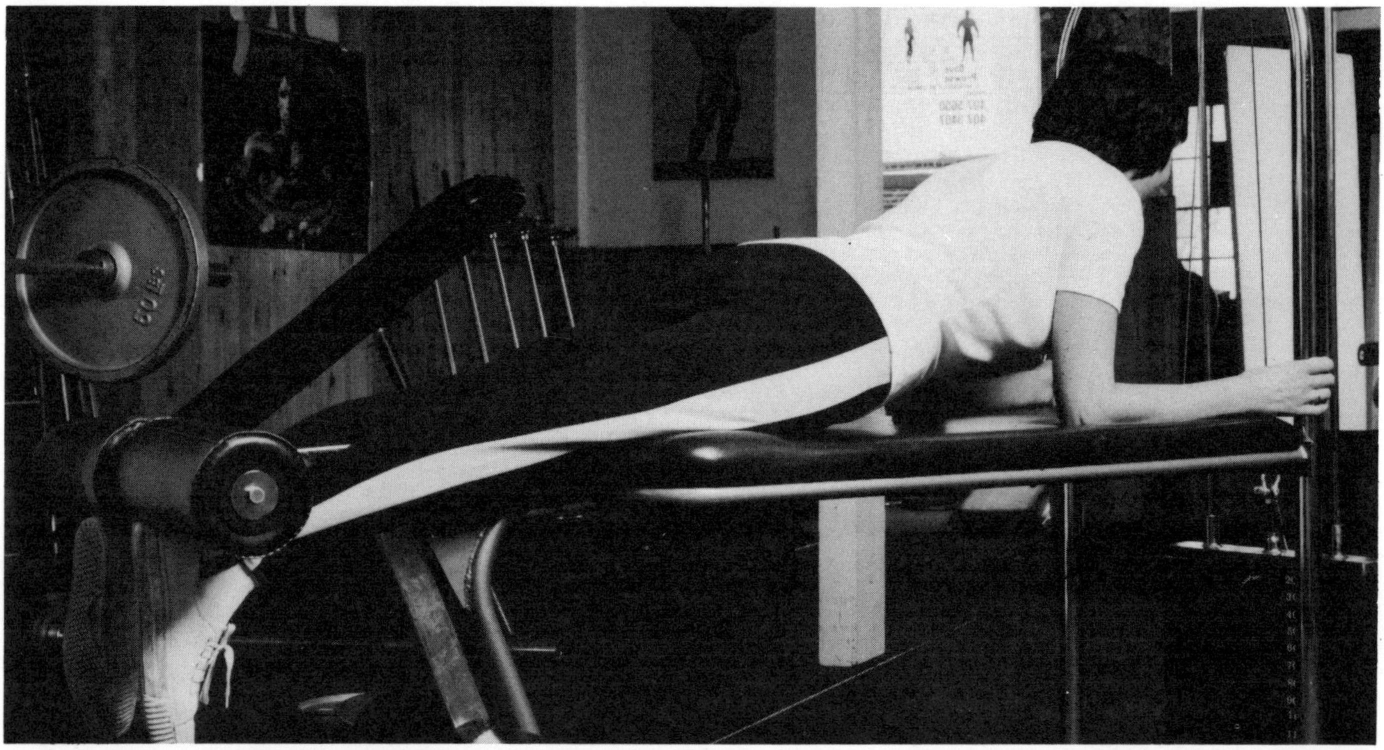

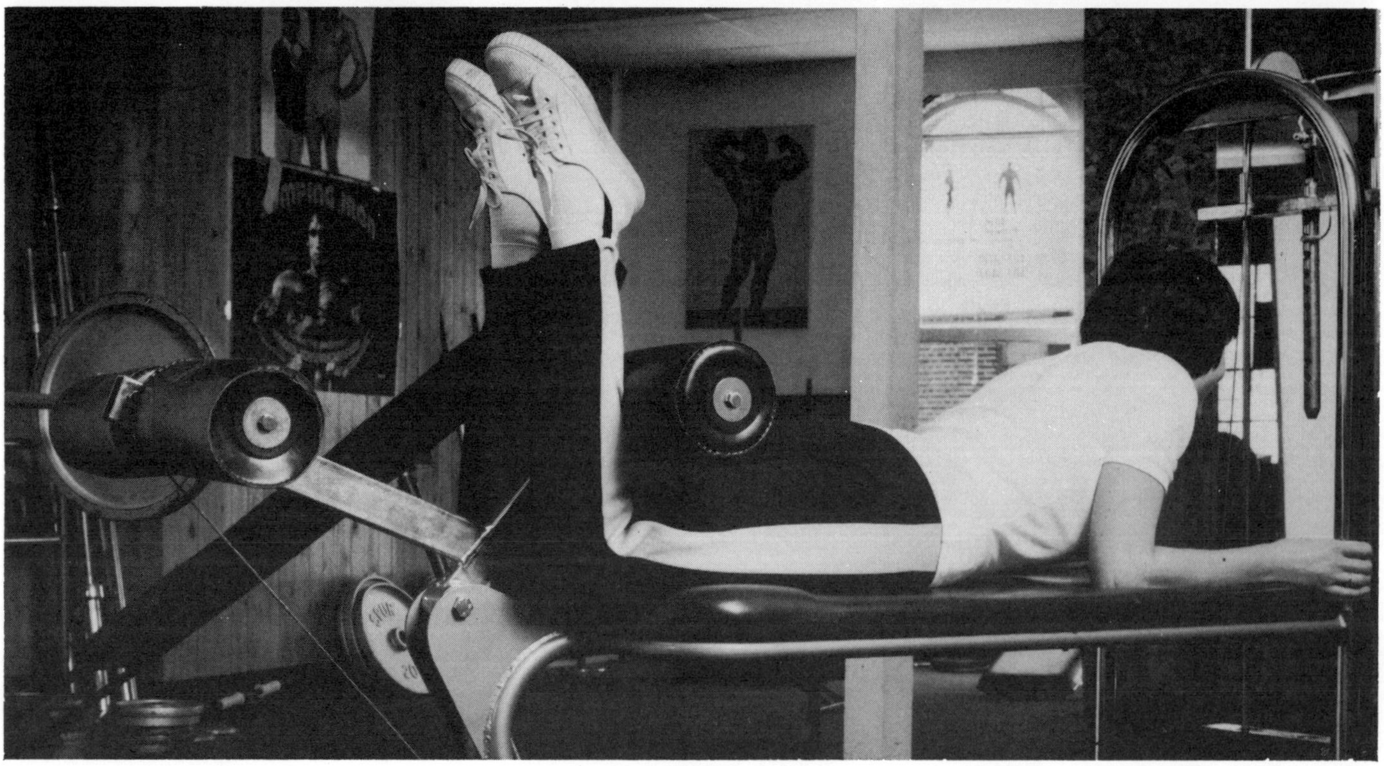

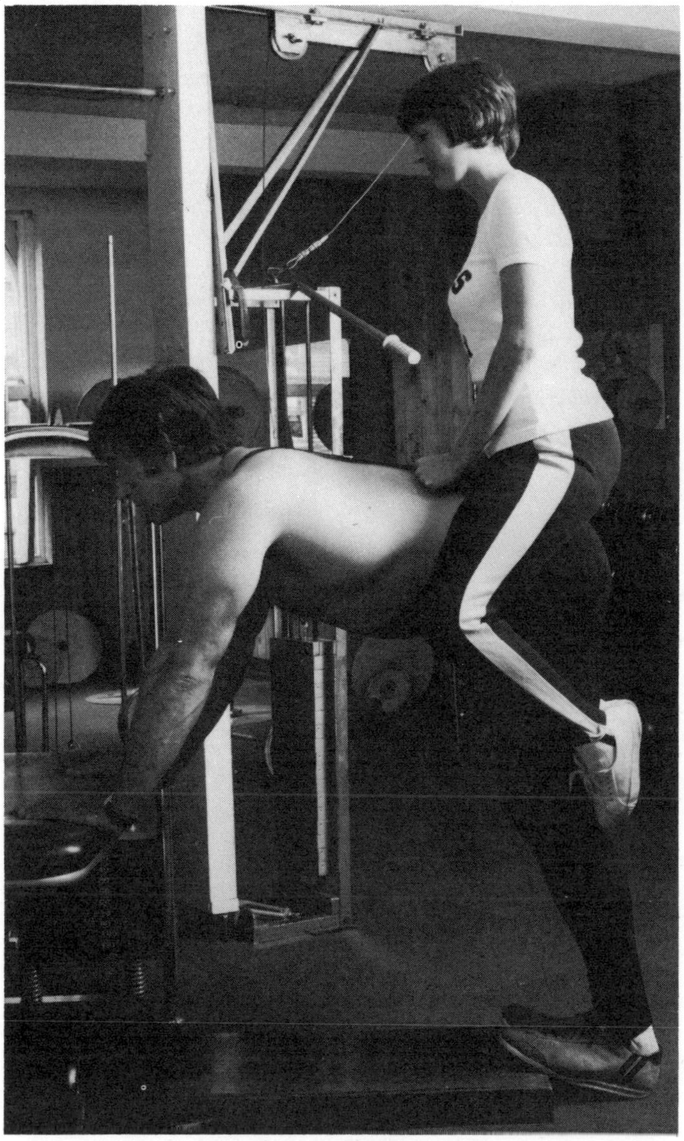

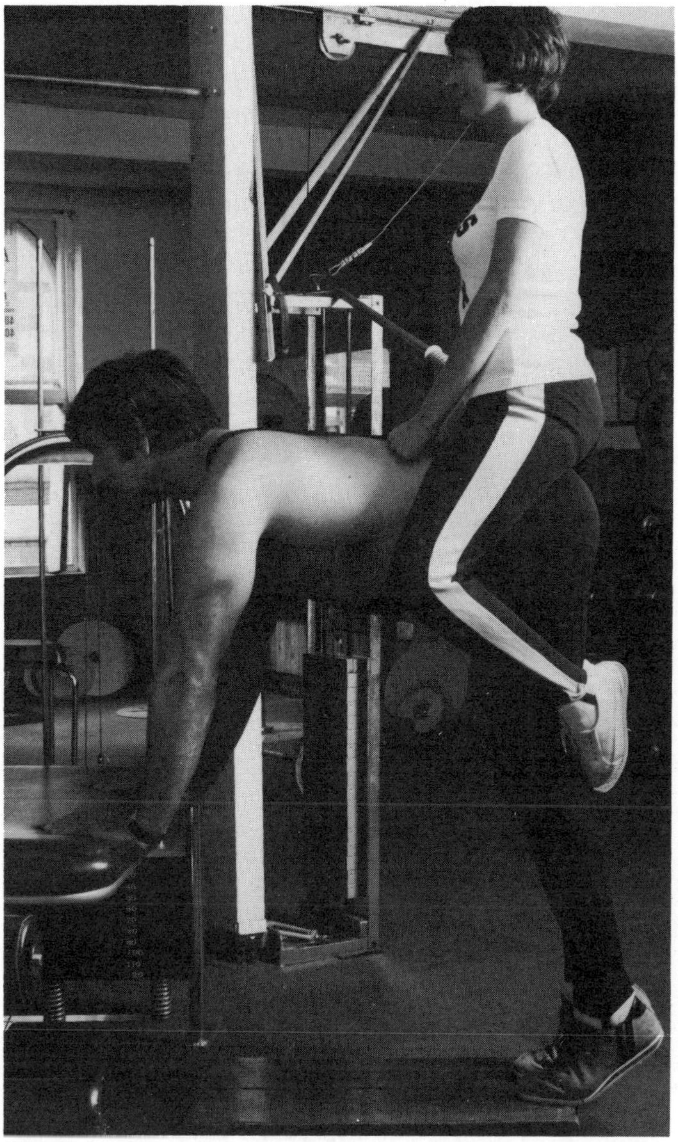

Donkey Calf Raise

For this one you must have a training partner. His job is to sit on your back . . .

1. Bend over, resting your hands on a bench so you're in the leap frog support position. Place your toes on a two-inch block.

2. Your training partner hops onto your back.

3. Raise and lower your feet until the burning sensation begins in your calves.

Single Leg Calf Raise

1. Place your toe on a step two inches high.
2. Stand up straight, holding onto something to keep your balance.
3. Raise your heel from the floor to the toe-pointed position.
4. Return heel to floor.
5. Repeat 20 to 30 times, *until the calf muscle burns*.
NB Wrap the spare leg round the leg being used, to ensure that this is a one leg exercise.

One of my best friends, Don Lee, who used to train with me in Bristol, was a former Gloucestershire weightlifting champion. He was an insurance agent and had to get up early in the morning to be on his travels. The only calf exercise he used to do was the single leg calf raise, by the side of the gas stove, waiting for his morning kettle to boil for his tea. He had fine calf muscles. . . . You can do this anywhere, when you're standing on the escalator, leaving the tube, waiting for the bus, on the stairs at home.

Incidentally, one of the major causes of aches and pains in girls' legs when they go on holiday is revealed here. Because they're on high heels all day in their normal life, the calf muscles tend to get shortened. When they come down to flat heels, running along the beach, say, or skiing, girls get terrible aches and pains and find they can't walk properly. In fact they're experiencing a form of muscle-binding caused by fashion which has created wrong posture.

When people come to me for pre-ski training, this is one of the exercises I make them spend a great deal of time practising.

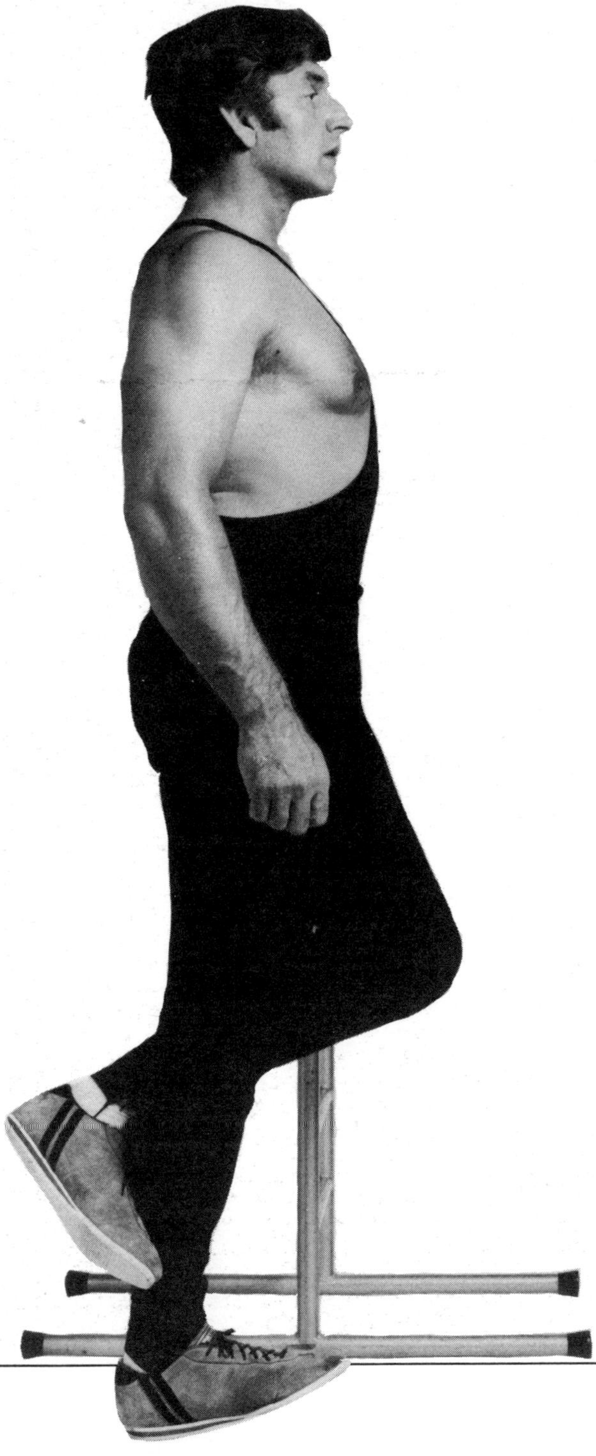

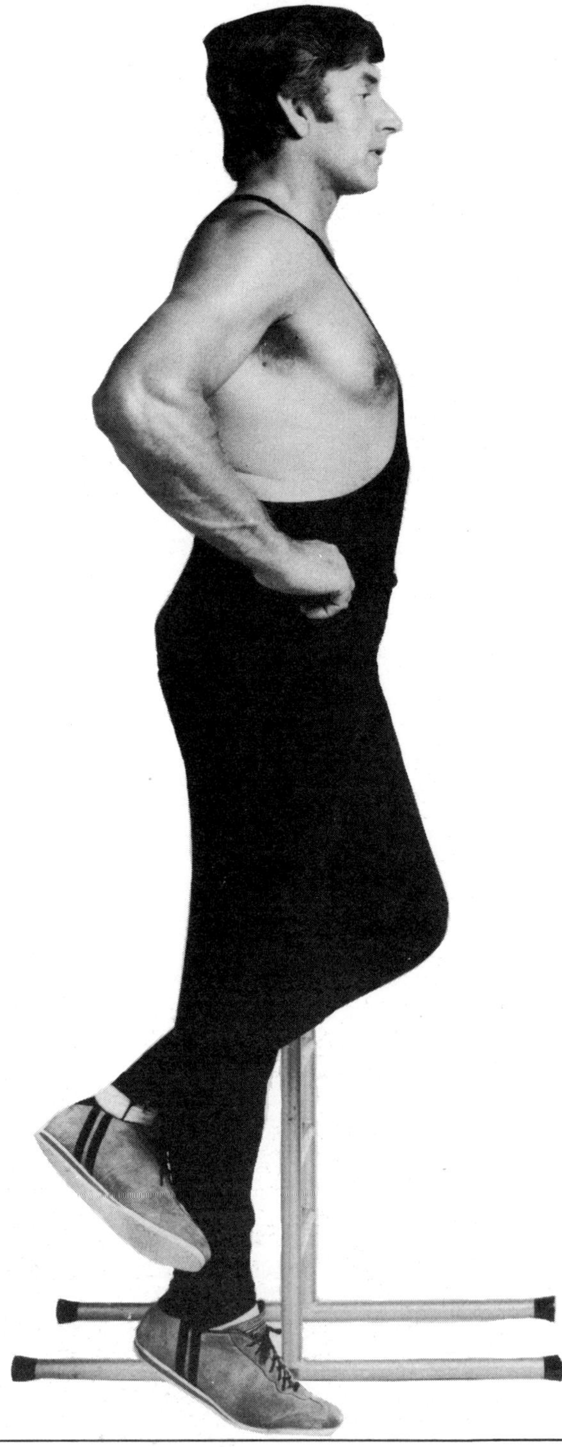

Chapter 15

WAISTING AWAY

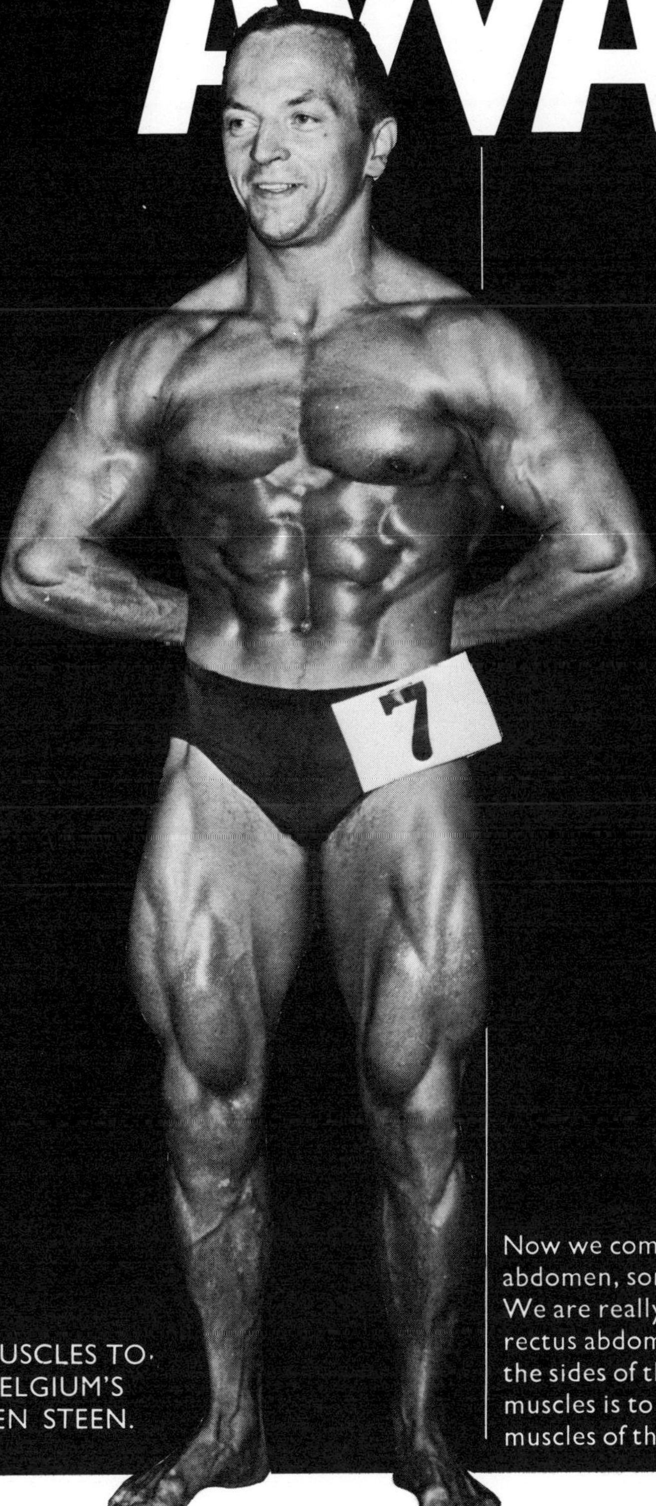

ABDOMINAL MUSCLES TO PERFECTION. BELGIUM'S PIERRE VAN DEN STEEN.

Now we come to the nice showing muscles of the abdomen, sometimes referred to as the 'washboard'. We are really concerned with the upper and lower rectus abdominus, and the oblique muscles which are on the sides of the waist. The action of the abdominal muscles is to draw the legs up to the chest; the erector muscles of the back straighten the body out.

The Sit-up

Probably the most famous of all stomach exercises, this is sometimes referred to as the Abdominal Raise. You can either do them on the floor or on an abdominal board for more serious training.

1. Lie flat on the floor. *Anchor* your feet under a piece of heavy furniture.

2. Put your hands out in front of you. Bend your knees slightly.

3. Sit up straight and try to touch your toes.

4. Repeat 20 times (5 sets).

NB Keep the tension on the abdominal muscles all the way through the exercise, and never let the muscles relax between repetitions. The way to do this is to keep your head forward.

To make the exercise more difficult without an abdominal board, start by folding your arms across your chest and when you've mastered that, clasp your hands behind your head. Then you can begin using weights.

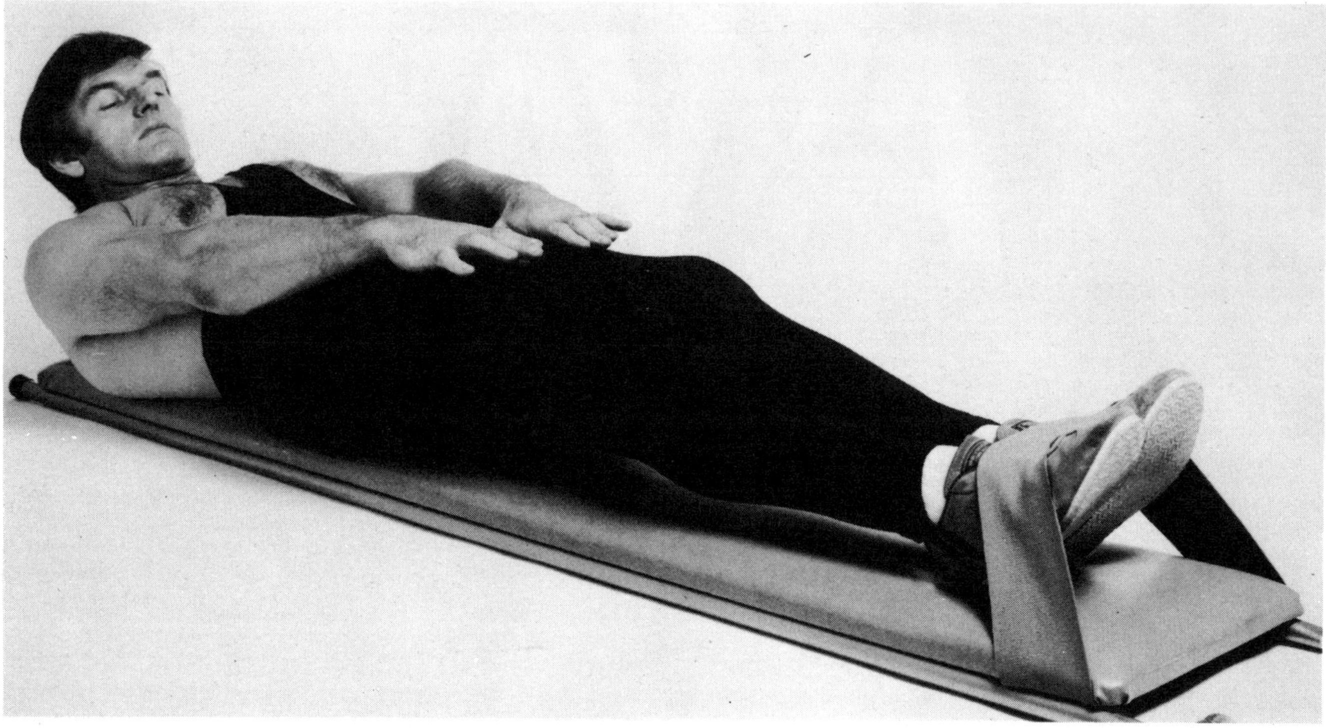

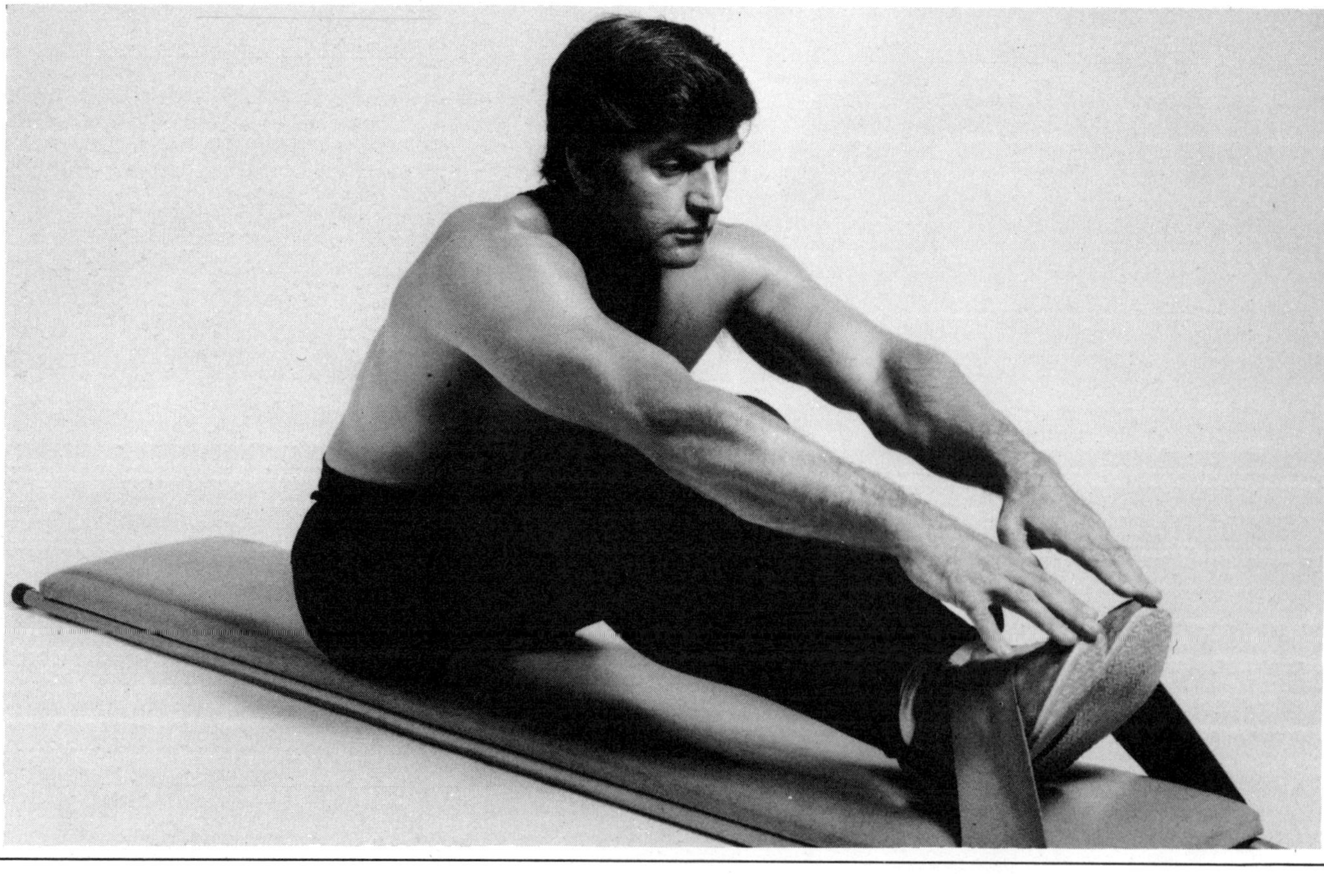

The advantage of an abdominal board with an adjustable rack is that you can raise the board to make the exercise much more difficult. In a fully equipped gymnasium you can do the exercise on a board raised to about 60 degrees. Years ago one famous body-builder did all these abdominal exercises *hanging upside down by ankle straps*. But I wouldn't wish that on you. . . .

The sit-up exercise can be done with a slight variation – a twist on the way up. You only do this when you've got to the stage when you're doing the exercise with weights, or with your hands behind the neck. As you come from the lying-down position to the sit-up, you twist your body so that your elbows touch opposite knees – left elbow touches right knee, right elbow touches left knee, and so on, alternating. This puts additional strain on the oblique muscles and makes it a very good and serious waist exercise.

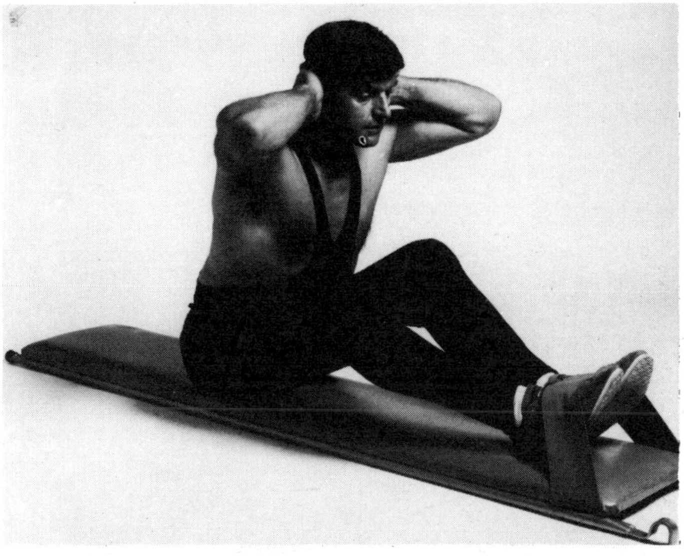

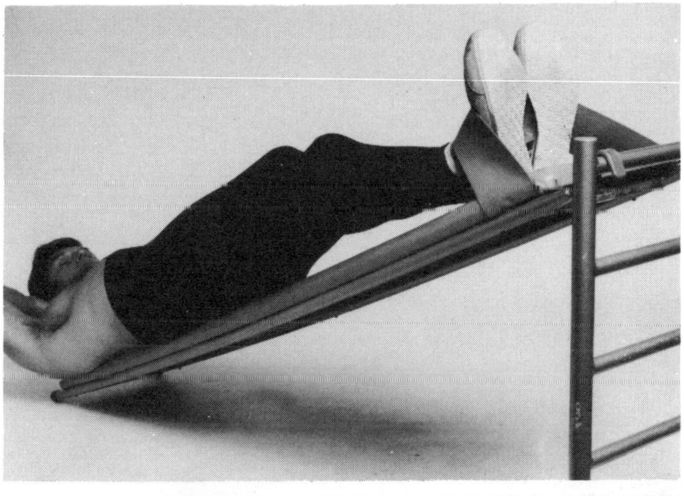

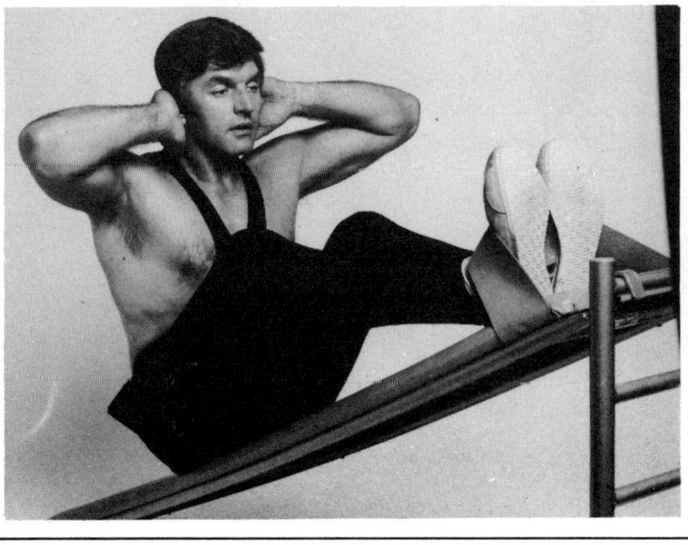

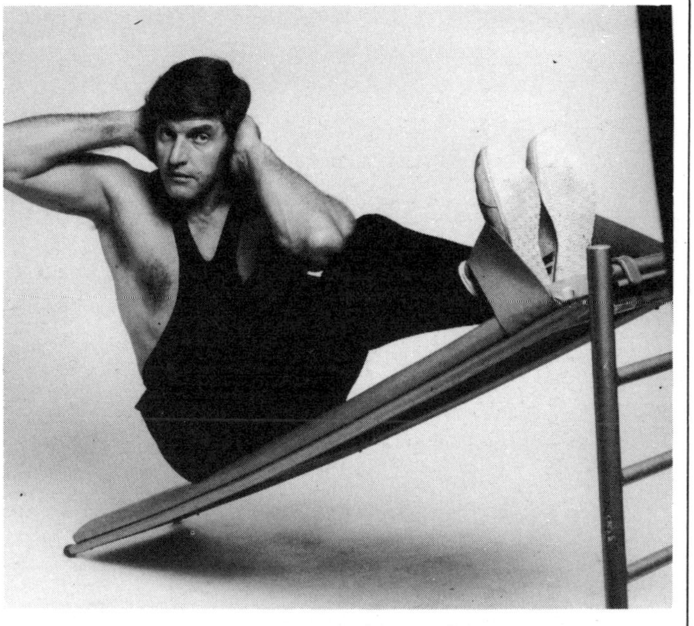

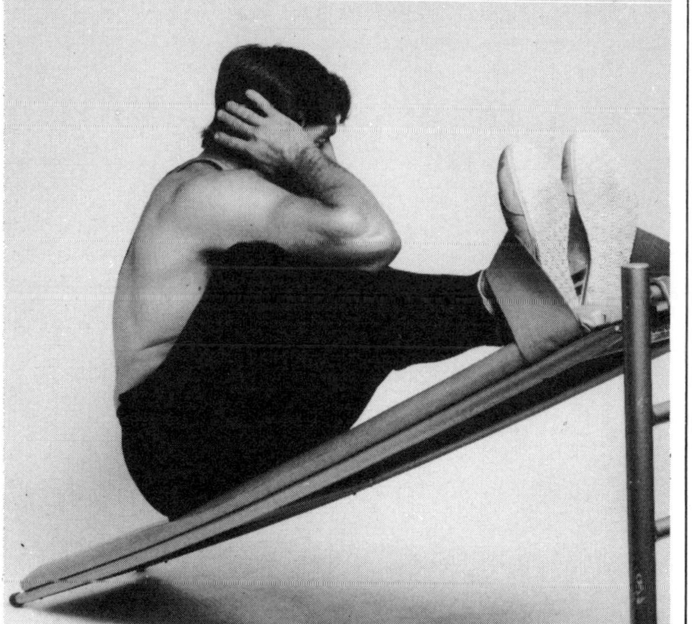

The Leg Raise

1. Lie on the floor with hands clasped under your behind to protect the coccyx.
2. Raise your legs together to about 60 degrees.
3. Lower until the heels just touch the floor but do not relax muscles.
4. Raise again. Repeat 20 times (5 sets).

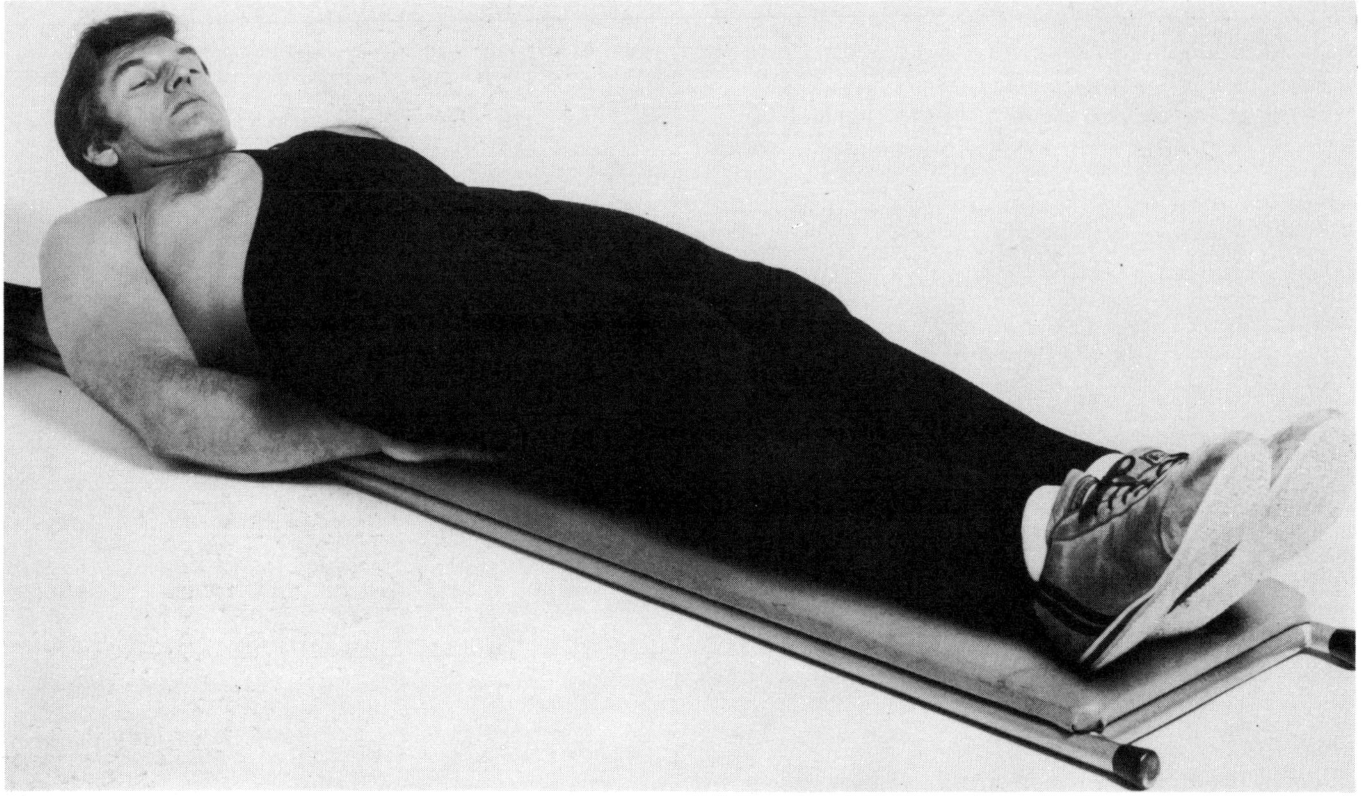

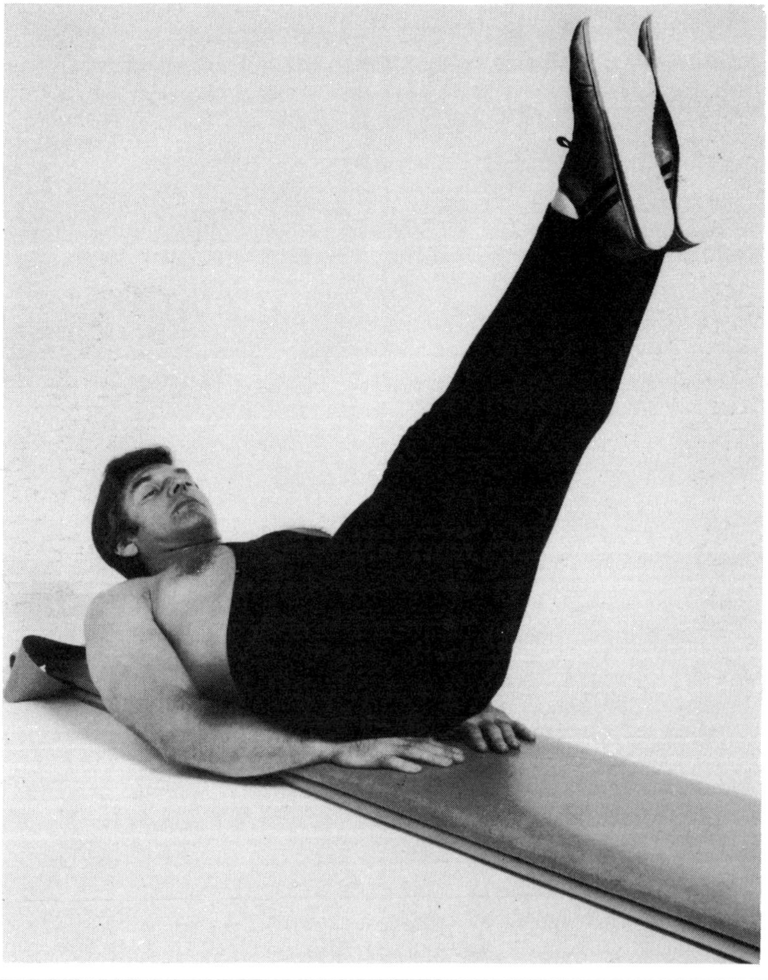

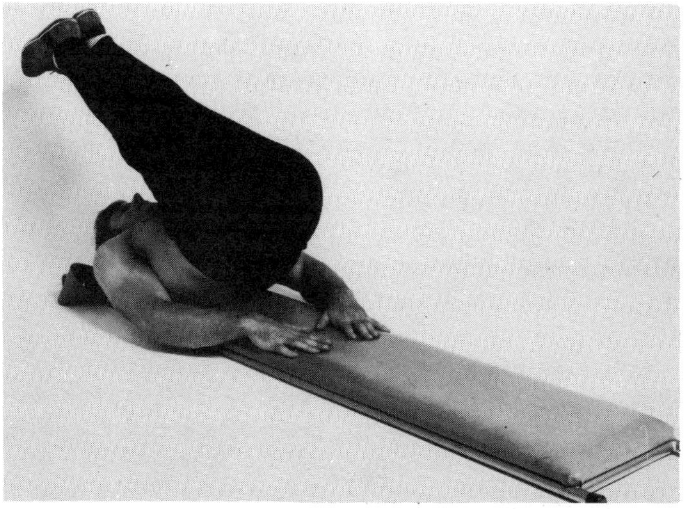

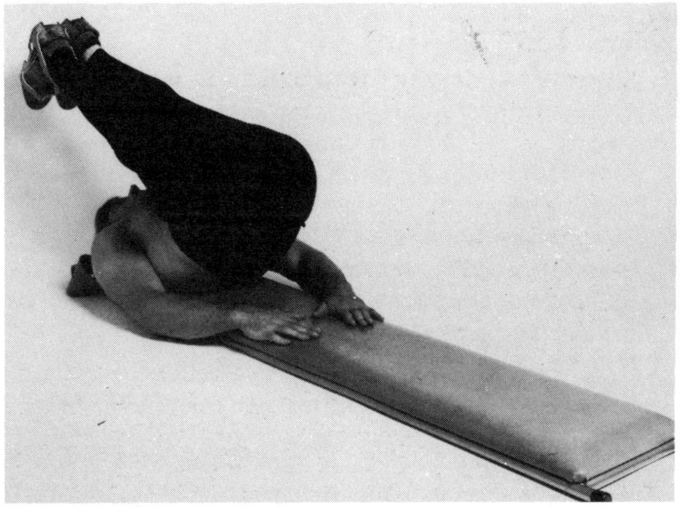

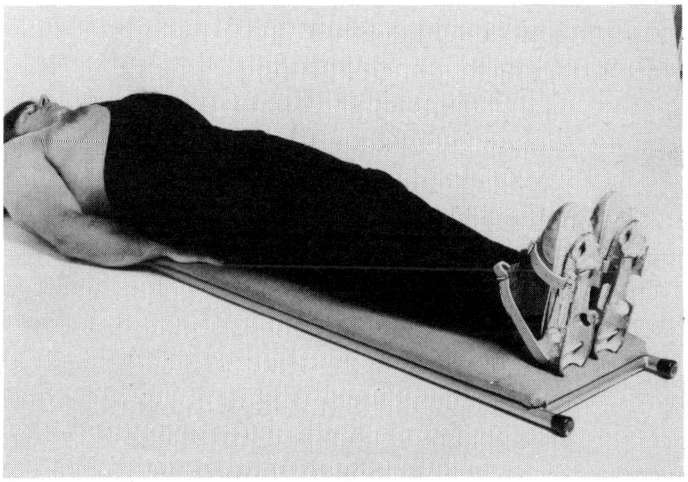

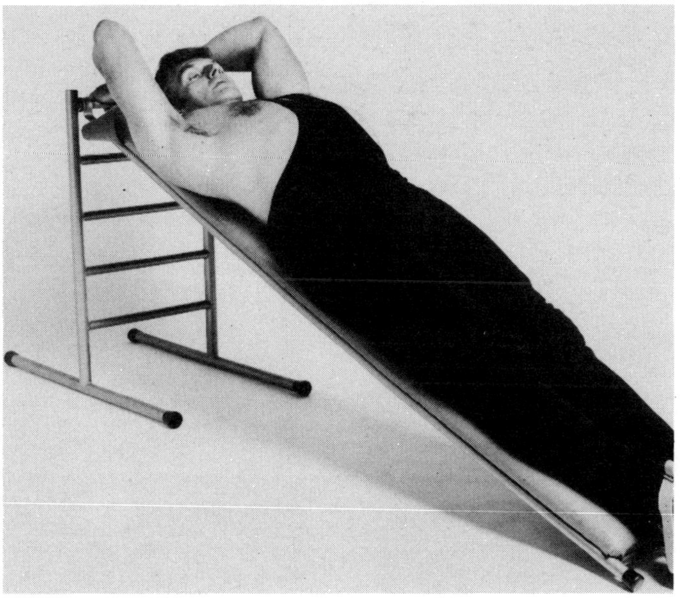

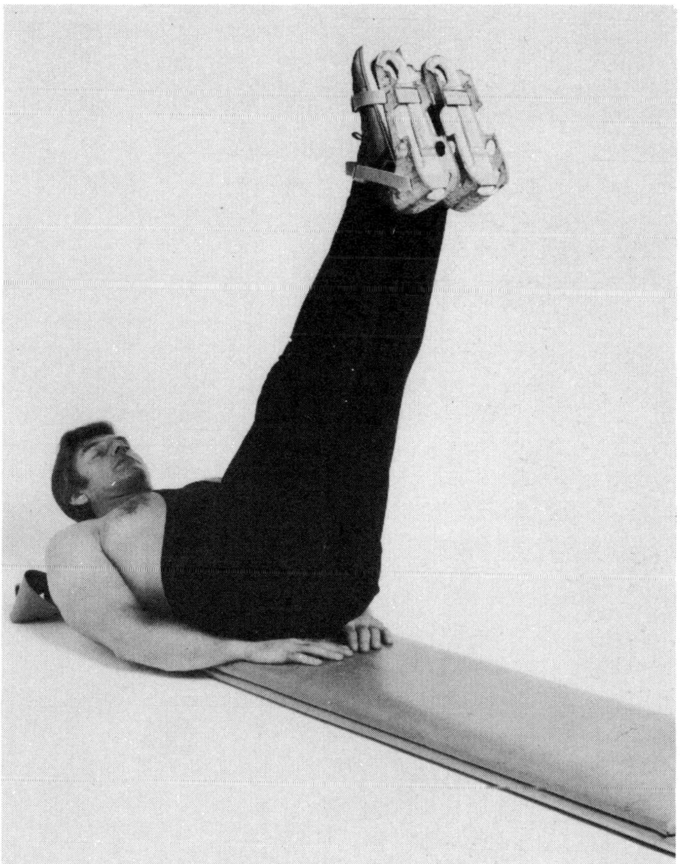

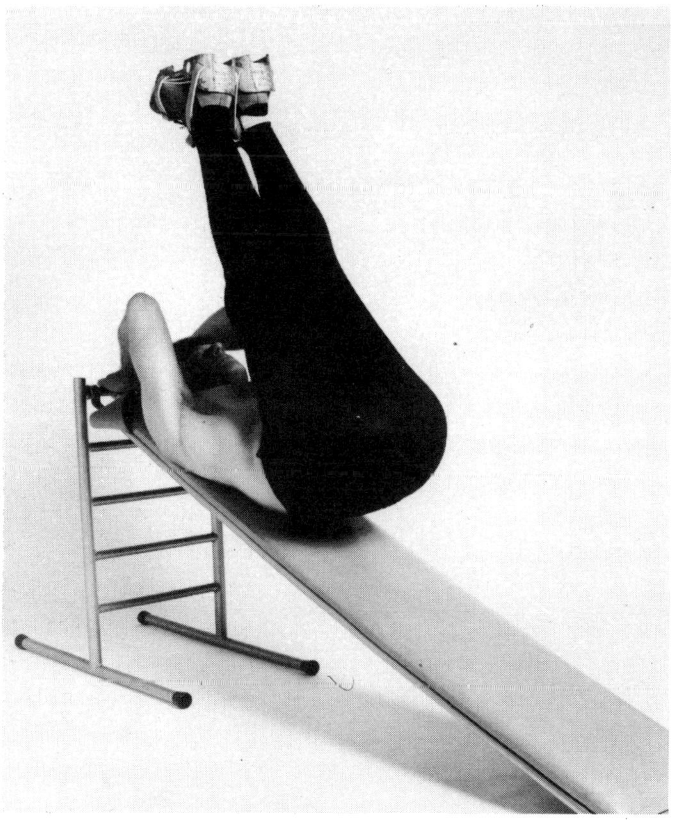

The Twist

1. Place the incline board at its steepest angle.
2. Hook your feet under the strap at the top end of the board.
3. Bend your knees quite considerably.
4. Fold your arms across your chest.
5. Sit up so your back is 10–12 inches off the board.
6. Twist as far to the right as possible, and back as far to left as possible, maintaining the lie-back position.
7. Repeat 100 times (5 sets).

Once you get used to this you can set up a sort of rocking motion, which enables you to get up into the hundreds quite quickly. But a beginner won't be able to cope – he won't be able to maintain the lie-back position essential to success. Scissors is another waist exercise which has been demonstrated in Family Exercise Programme No 1; so has the curl-up or waist-away. You can use these, too.

Finally, I feel that although the programmes we have shown in detail so far have all been geared to body development, we've said very little about fitness and cardio-vascular development, so at the end of this section, I want to include four exercises for this. Two of them you've seen already – the two hands swing (page 54) and the squat and press (page 56). The other two exercises are the power snatch and the two hands clean from the hang. They are both designed primarily to get you puffing and blowing. They're done as massive movements i.e. they affect the whole of the body system. (Occasionally I've had people in the gym who wanted a tough one exercise programme; and when set ten sets of ten power snatches, they've had to crawl away afterwards.)

When I was running *Power* magazine, back in the late 1960s, one of the most popular series of features I wrote were the interviews with top body-builders throughout the world on their training methods, dieting, and so on. I must have interviewed 15 to 20 specialists in the field, and what stood out in the interviews was that they *all* used the same abdominal exercise. It's one for which you have to have an incline board, and it's called the twist. Each and everyone of them used to do 500 at least as a warmer-up *before* they began exercising seriously. It's not quite as difficult as it sounds, but it takes a bit of getting used to. It's the best waist exercise I know, and I use it regularly.

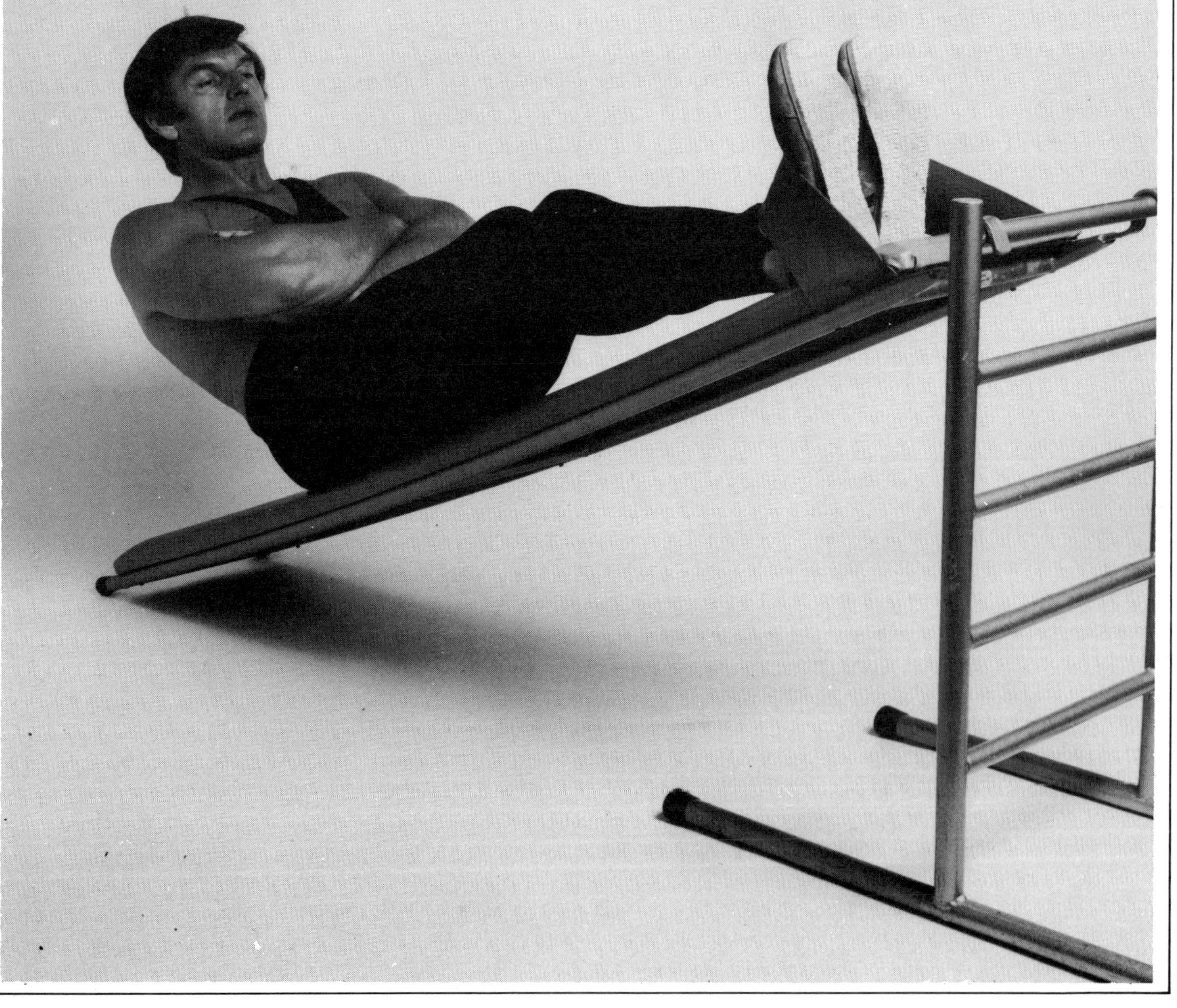

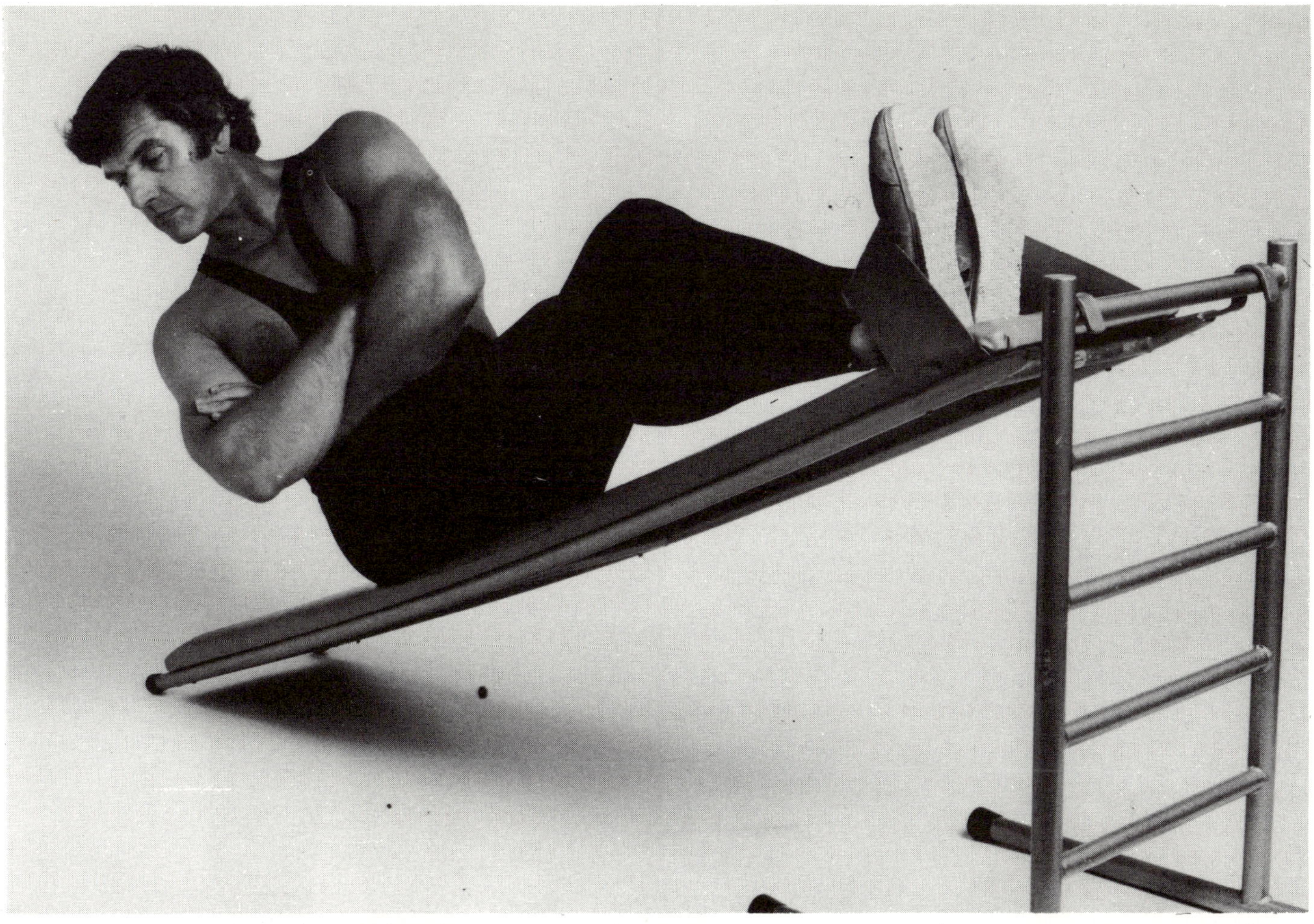

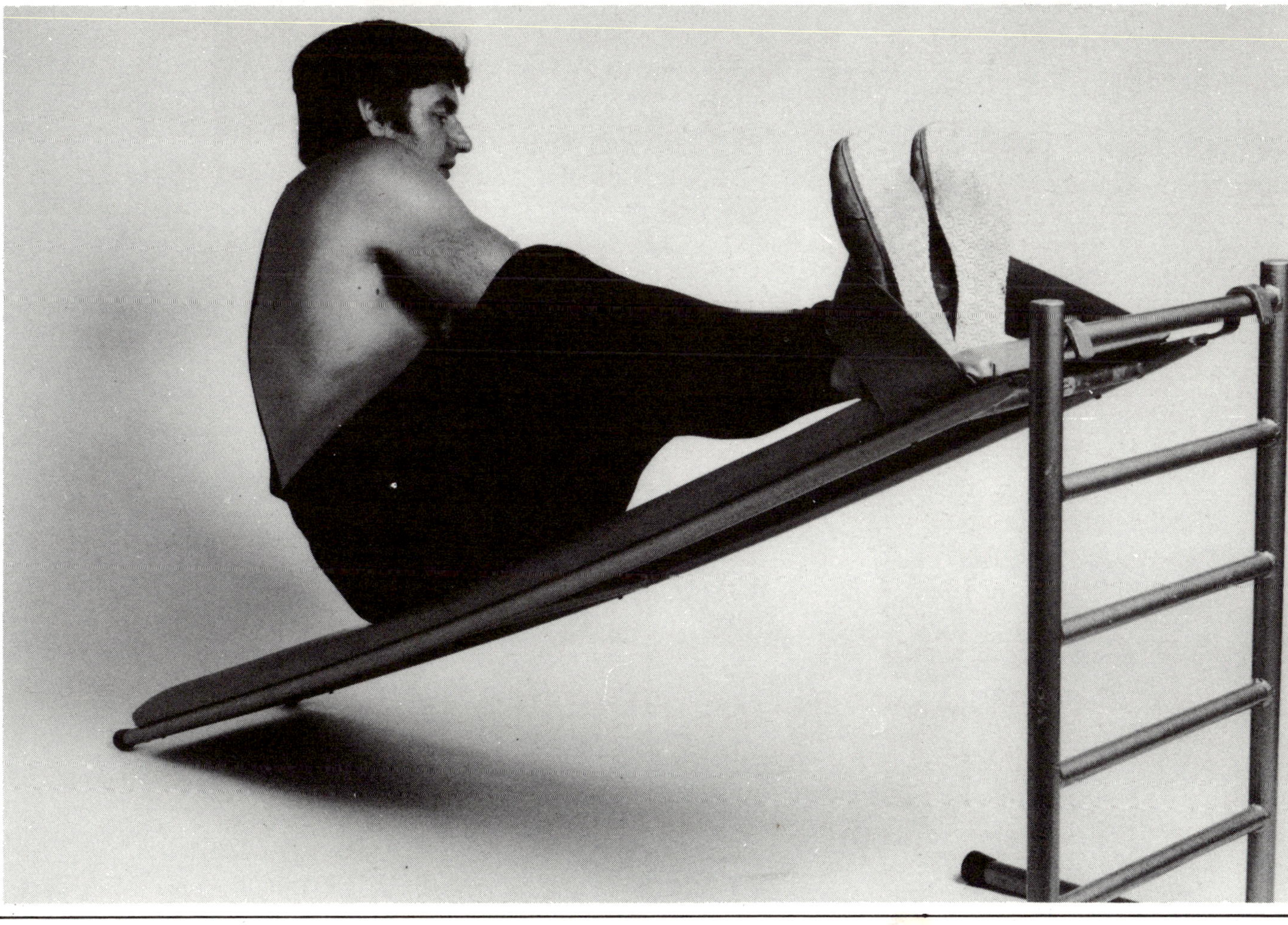

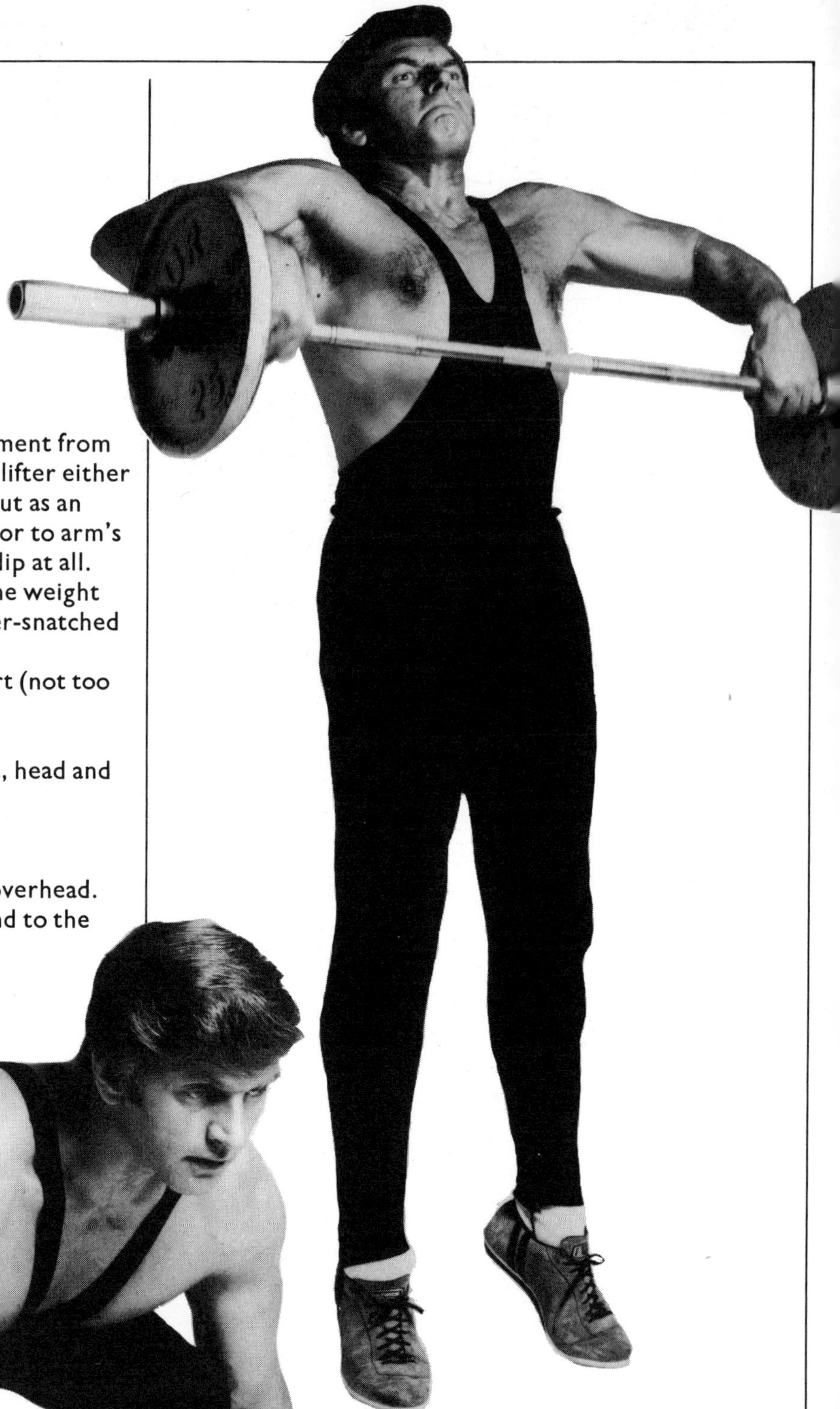

Power Snatch

The bar has to be taken in one smooth movement from the floor to arm's length. In competition the lifter either squats under the bar or he 'splits' under it. But as an exercise, the bar has to be taken from the floor to arm's length above the head with no squat and no dip at all. So of course you can't handle anything like the weight you would in competition. I've actually power-snatched over something like 220 lbs.

1. Stand at the bar, with feet about 9 ins apart (not too wide).
2. Adopt a wide hand spacing.
3. Bend down with knees bent, back straight, head and shoulders up.
4. Breathe *in*.
5. Drive with your legs.
6. Pull the bar smoothly up to arm's length overhead.
7. Lower to your chest, then to the thighs and to the floor.
8. Repeat ten times (3 sets at first, up to 6).

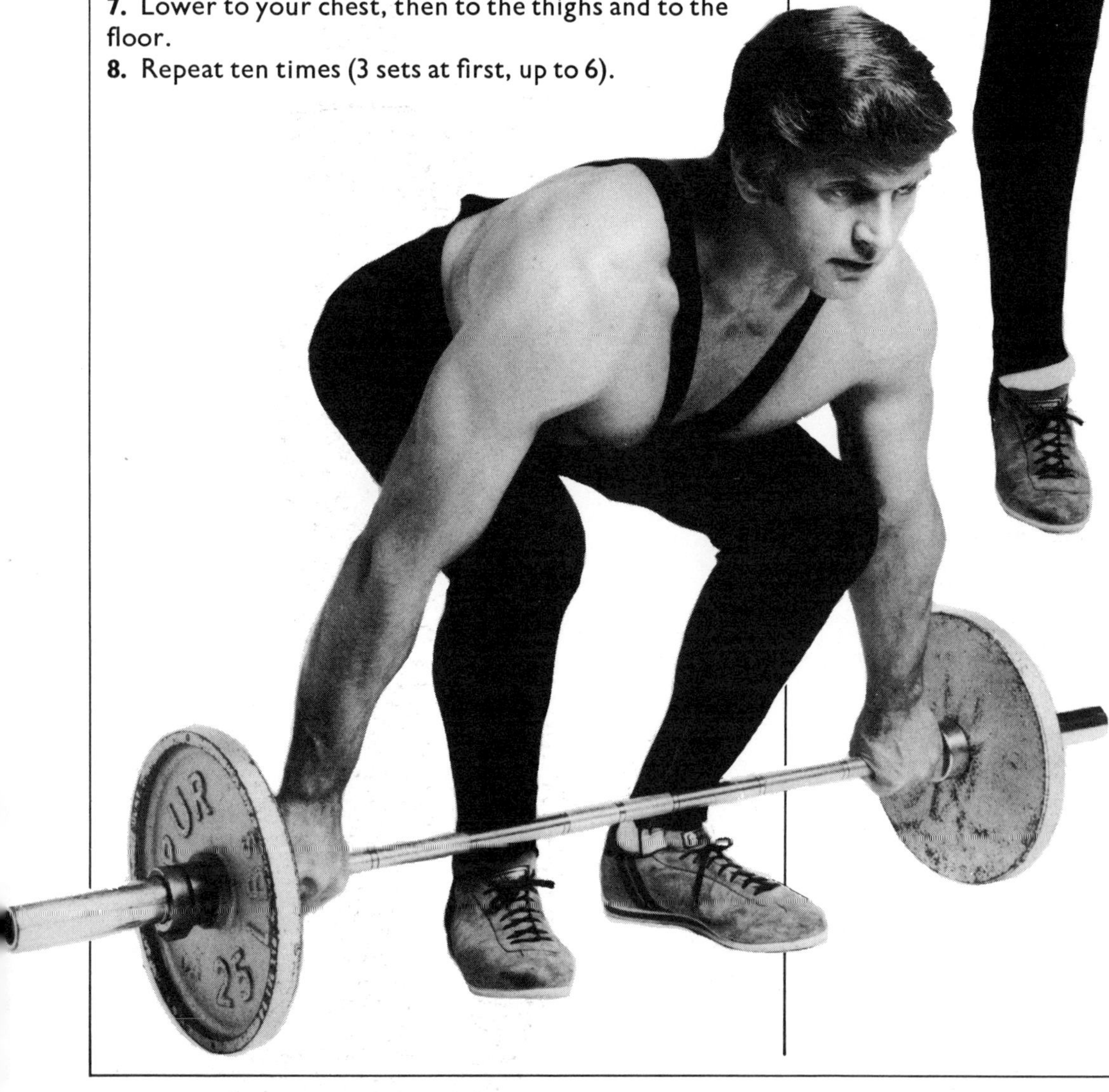

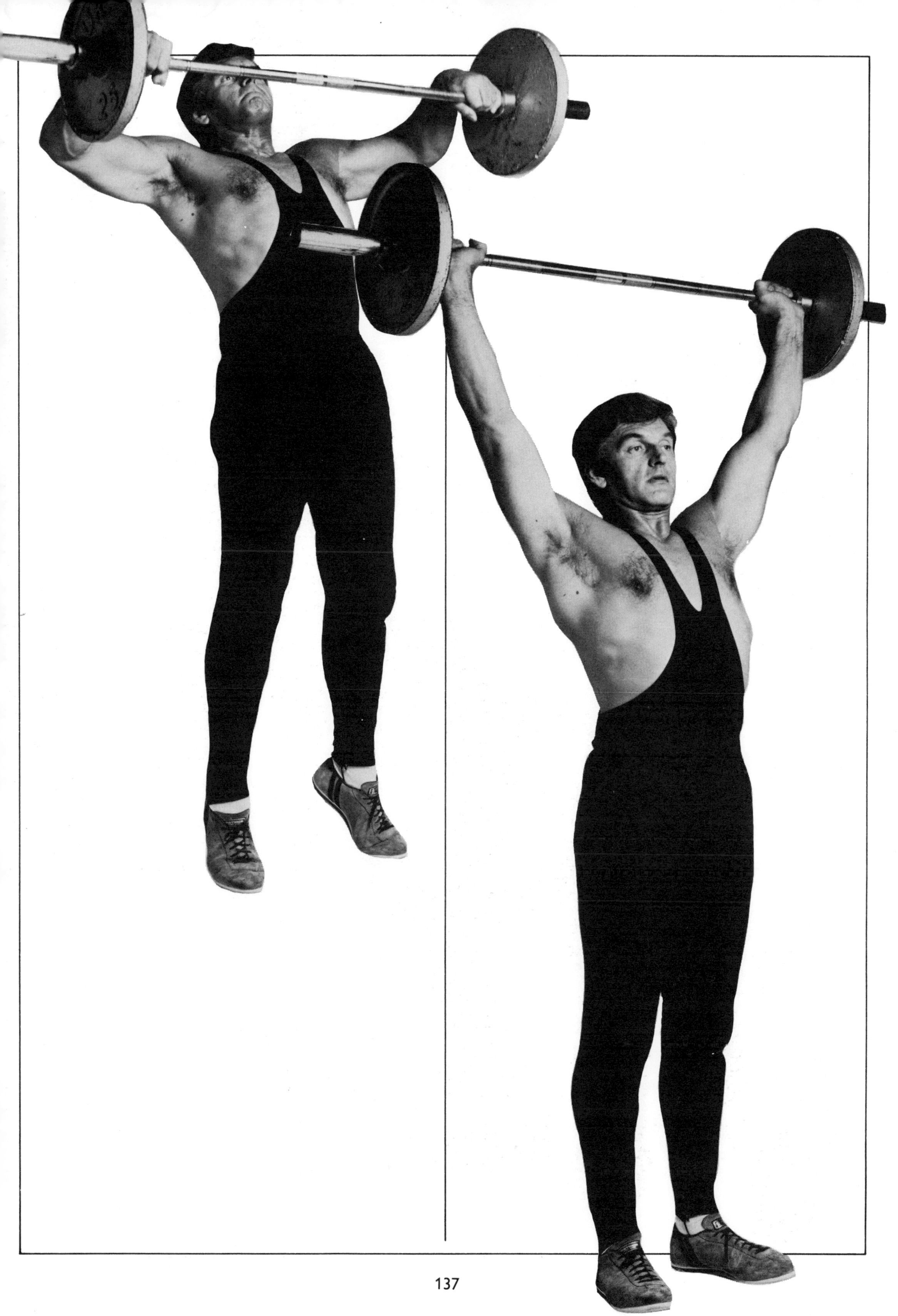

Two Hands Clean from Hang

The clean from the hang exercise differs from the simple clean in that instead of being lifted to the shoulders from the floor, the barbell is now lifted from the hang position – resting in front of the thighs. You can handle quite a bit of weight on this exercise and it should be done vigorously.

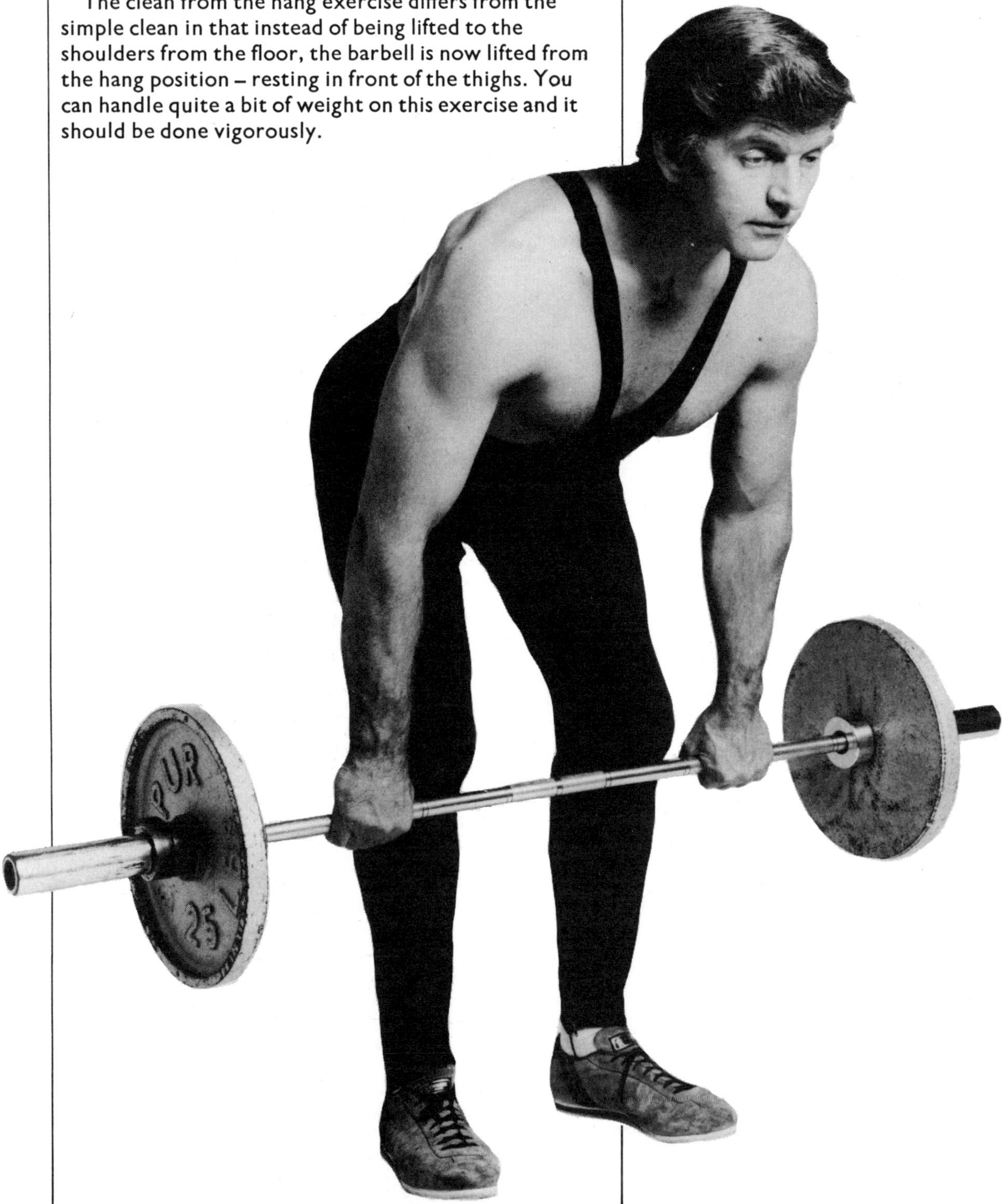

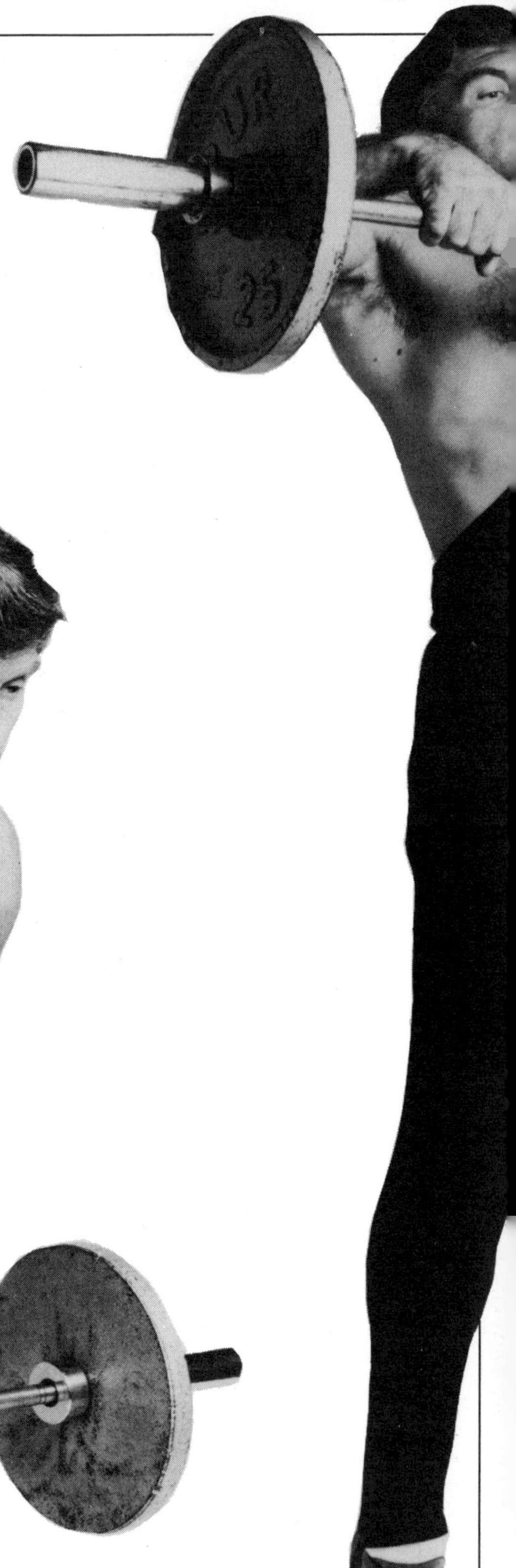

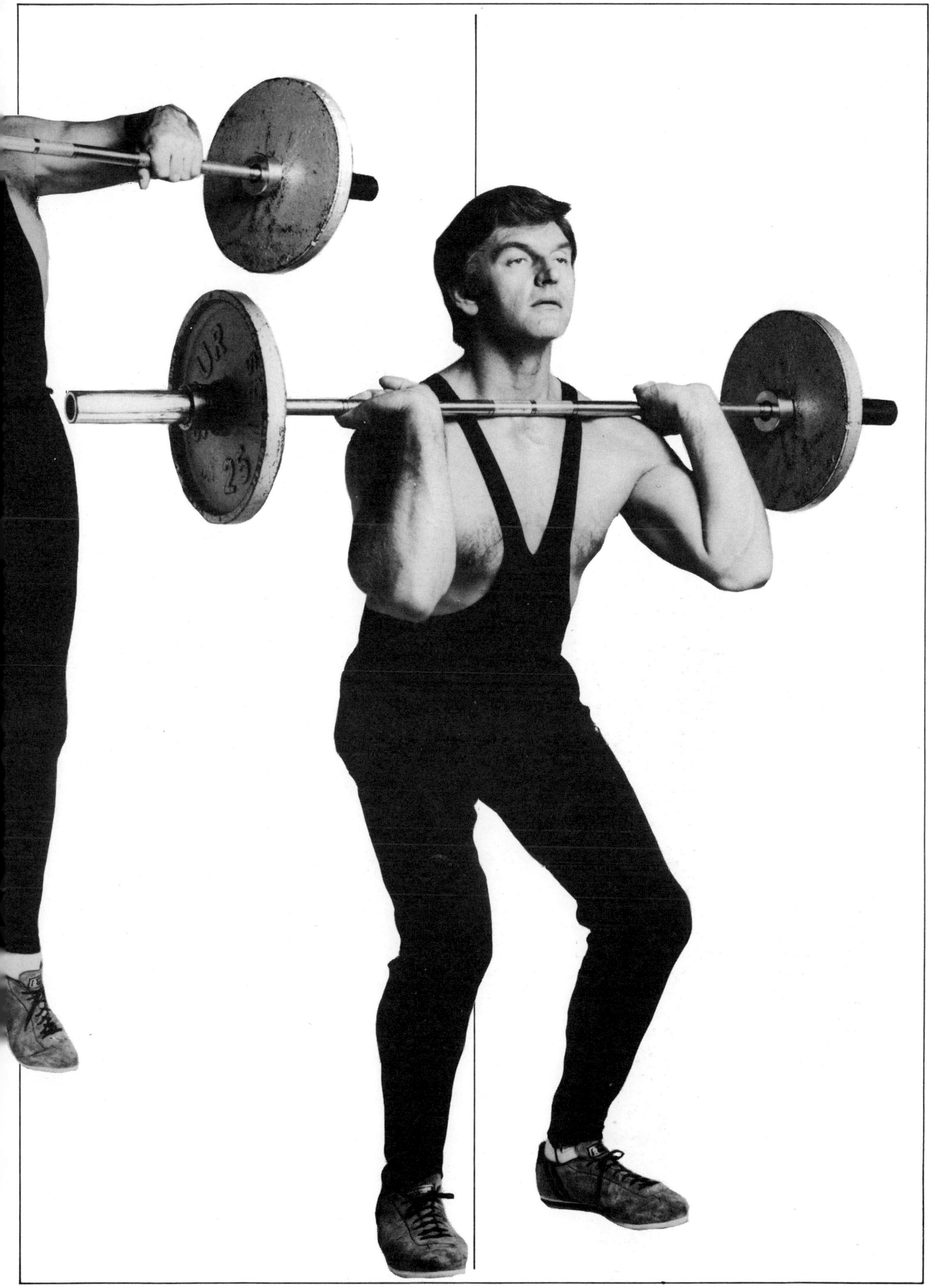

Chapter 16

HOW TO BUILD A SCHEDULE

What I've given you is not, of course, a comprehensive list of exercises. There are hundreds more exercises you can perform, and variations on each exercise. But from the basic list I have made you can select a schedule, or two schedules, or three to suit your every bodily need. I said at the beginning, but it will bear repeating, that you must get your training aims right. Fitness comes first; then strength; then mobility; and figure last. If you train in this way, I guarantee you'll make progress.

The first, family schedules, were given in Chapter Six. Now I'm assuming you're on top of those two programmes and you're getting bored. Now you want to move on to something a little more difficult, more advanced, and more beneficial. You'll have seen the various exercises laid out in sections, each dealing with a particular muscle group. Fairly obviously, I don't want you to start at the beginning and work through to number whatever-it-is. That's the way to become a candidate for the hospital bed.

The thing to do is to decide in which area of the body you want to see most progress and then to concentrate on that particular part, but without excluding the rest of the body. Balanced exercise, like balanced diet, is most important. For the first two months of your training, adopt the most general of schedules, then begin to specialise gradually as you discover, through the knowledge of yourself that the initial training will bring, where you wish to concentrate your efforts.

Picture your schedule in terms of a graph, which must be physiologically correct. The idea is to build up the exercises slowly to a peak of difficulty; relax briefly; come to another peak; and then tail off gently. The graph will look like a double-humped camel. Make up your mind which are going to be the two main exercises in your schedule; and then build around them. It's usually a good idea, if not essential, to go for a full schedule of about ten exercises.

Let me give you an example. This whole programme will take you, say 45 minutes to an hour to complete.

Training Schedule No 1

1. Leg raises (page 46). Stomach, hips, thighs.
2. Lateral raises to the side (page 51). Shoulders.
3. Press behind neck or two hands press (page 73). Shoulders, neck, arms.
4. Upright rowing (page 77). Shoulders, neck.
5. Bench press (The first 'peak' exercise) (page 96). Chest, arms, shoulders.
6. Triceps dip (page 88). Chest, arms.
7. Squat (the second 'peak' exercise) (page 122). Thighs, chest.
8. Two hands curl (page 82). Biceps.
9. Bent-over rowing (page 106). Broad back muscles.
10. Sit-up with twist (page 130). Waist

You will find, though, that as you progress in your training you tend to begin to ignore the physiologically correct method and go for the specific training that you need. In your earlier training you may well find that some muscle groups tend to lag behind others. Some people, for example, have weak chest muscles, so it would be quite in order for them to concentrate all the chest exercises in the first half of the schedule. When I go into a gymnasium it's usual for me to go straight to do bench pressing. I like bench pressing. I can lift a lot of weight this way and get a great deal of satisfaction out of it. I take light weights to begin with and I might do 15 or 20 sets until I work up to my maximum. But I certainly would not recommend this method for beginners . . .

That schedule, by the way, would be an excellent introduction to progressive weight training. Now, here's a second schedule, mainly for men who want to progress towards body-building.

Training Schedule No 2

1. Two hands clean (page 70). Whole body.
2. Two hands press (page 72). Arms, shoulders.
3. Alternate lateral raise to front (page 75). Shoulders, neck.
4. Two hands curl (page 82). Upper arm.
5. Triceps travel (page 92). Upper arm.
6. Seated dumbell curl (page 84). Upper arm.
7. Bench press (page 96). Chest, arms, shoulders.
8. Incline dumbell press (page 100). Chest, arms, shoulders.
9. Bent-over rowing (page 106). Broad back muscles.
10. Dead lift (page 110). Lower back.
11. Squats (page 122). Legs and chest.
12. Sit-ups on incline board (page 130–31). Abdomen.

Just to finish off this schedule, do some running on the spot; or if you have access to an exercise bike, then get on it and pedal like mad for a few minutes.

A woman has all the same muscles as a man – biceps and triceps and latissimus dorsi and the rest of them. More often than not a woman's skeleton is less strong than a man's – the bones are less sturdy, more brittle. A woman's clavicle is usually smaller than a man's and her upper arms are longer in relation to the rest of the body, meaning that she has less power in pushing. At the same time most girls are more supple than most boys. I'm inclined to think it's a combination of evolution and environment; but as the proprietor of a successful health studio, I have nearly as many women customers as I do men. But all of them come in for one thing – figure control.

It never ceases to amaze me that women know so little about exercising, for all their concern about their figures. They walk up the steps to my gymnasium, and the sight of the dumbells, and barbells and the weights never fails to terrify them. However, once I've explained the theory behind all this imposing apparatus, they accept the system of progressive resistance training quite readily. What worries them in the first place, of course, is that progressive resistance training will mean that they'll grow vast muscles; and as I've explained earlier in the book, that just isn't so. Once they've got hold of that idea, they think nothing of pressing and cleaning 50 or 70 or even 100 lbs of weights around the gymnasium. It's as if the weights had become part of the jargon of their new sport and ceased to concern them.

However, it is an exception to find a woman who will train with as much intensity as a man, no matter what cause. Very often both sexes will come in because they're going on holiday, say, in six weeks' time. In six weeks the average man will get himself into super trim. He'll be off the beginner stage in a fortnight, and straight into the progressive resistance training. The average girl will take three months to get bored with the initial stages, and only then she'll come and say, 'Isn't it about time I was doing something else?' This is not a bad thing. To any girl, my first piece of advice is always: don't try to do too much too soon. You can't expect to become Miss Universe next week. So more than 60 per cent of the schedules I work out for girls are hip, waist and thigh exercises, some bust exercises, and with shoulders and arms thrown in for good measure. We start with a little, gradually increasing the amount and the work load. And it works.

It's nearly always quite a job to persuade a girl that she isn't going to develop muscles. As I've explained before, girls *can* do so – look at girl swimmers, gymnasts, shot-putters and so on – but only if they train exceptionally hard *and* choose a high-protein diet to go with the training. Your muscle development, whether you're male or female, depends on how hard you train and on your protein intake. Because they will not train with sufficient intensity, and because nearly every girl I know is on a low-protein diet which would hardly keep a cat alive, there's no danger of bulging muscles.

Bust development is something else again. I can't do anything to increase the actual size of a girl's mammary gland; no-one can, unless it be done through hormone treatment or artificially by silicone injection (both of which are way outside my scope). What I can do, is to enlarge and improve the size of the pectoralis muscle, which tends to give the breast a better shape and uplift.

Training Schedule for Girls

The main areas of exercises for most girls will be hips, thighs and waist; and the schedule I'd suggest would be something like this:

1. Leg raises (page 46). Tummy, hips, thighs.
2. Half sit-up (page 46). Abdomen.
3. Waist-aways (page 47). Tummy, hips, thighs.
4. Scissors (page 47). Tummy, hips, thighs.
5. Side leg raises (page 48). Hips, thighs.
6. Hip kicks (page 48). Hips, thighs, lower back.
7. Press-ups (page 49). Bust, arms, shoulders.
8. Flyers (page 50). Bust, shoulders.
9. Free squats (page 54). Hips, thighs.

Start off by doing one set of each exercise; working up to two and then three sets. Then you'll be ready for some progressive resistance training. But you'll be fitter and trimmer than you've ever been before . . .

This is an ideal schedule for a woman who's just had a baby, or an office girl who's growing pear-shaped in her typist's chair. It's amazing how quickly you progress, doing this schedule just three times a week. It's cheap (costs you nothing), it's easy and you can do it anywhere. But you will find, as you grow interested, you'll need to progress into resistance training, making the exercises harder and yourself fitter in the process.

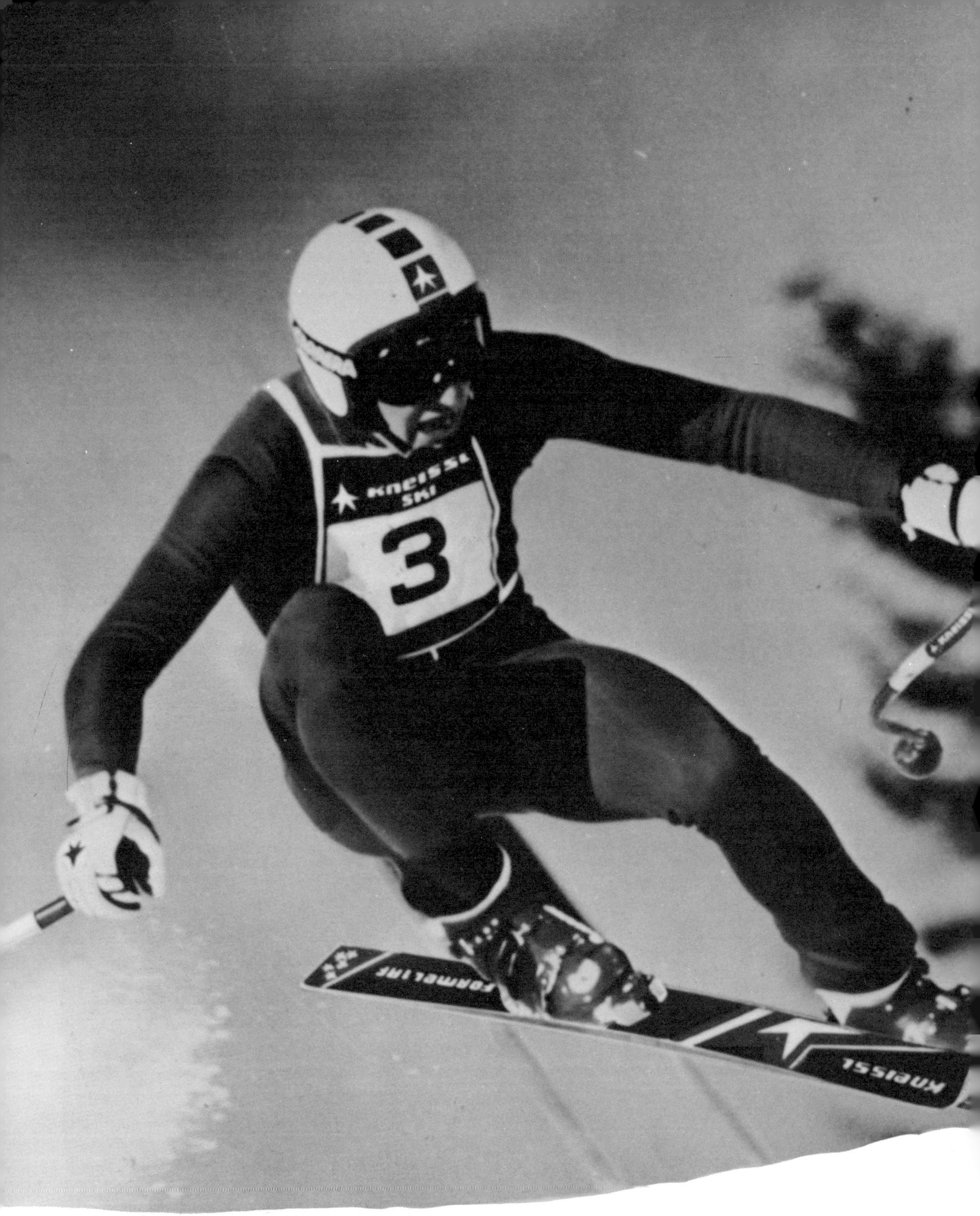
KNEISSL
SKI
3

Chapter 17

PREPARING FOR THE SKI-RUN

Skiing is undoubtedly Britain's fastest growing sport, and it's something that every physical training specialist and every health club trainer should be thinking about because they have a most important role to play in it. Every weekend, from December until May, people flock to the snow grounds, both in Britain and on the Continent, meeting the hazards that must be faced by experts and beginners alike.

Sliding downhill at anything from 20 to 100 miles an hour can have unfortunate consequences. Unexpected objects are likely to get in the way, and unguarded or inexpert movements cause a spill. When you consider that many participants are not particularly athletic normally, you can expect a higher instance of injuries here than in most other sports. Accidents are most common towards the end of the day when fatigue begins to creep in, and this is where weight training comes in. Physical conditioning for skiing can take many forms, and I have discussed this with many skiing authorities and competitors both here and abroad. Many top skiers use exercises specially designed to prepare people for the snow. The movements I'm going to show you are closely linked to skiing movements and place the body in positions not normally met in everyday life. The muscles and joints gradually strengthen and mobilise to ensure your holiday is not spoilt by unaccustomed exercise. The real difference, however, between these and the normal exercises you'll get from a ski instructor is that these are proper progressive resistance movements, which really get at the joints as well as the muscles.

Every training enthusiast knows that ski training with weights will toughen the body, give added fitness and make one a more efficient skier. It will also improve one's appearance in the latest ski fashions.

In the programme are eight specific ski training movements, some of which are used in normal weight training routines, some of which are identified with ski training only.

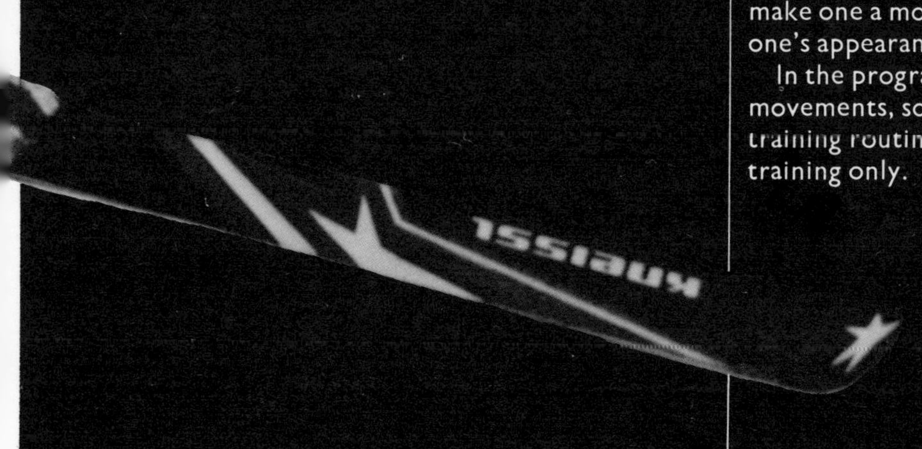

Ski Swing

(Done with two dumbells.)

1. Select two dumbells, 10–15 lbs (girls: 5–10 lbs). Stand up straight with dumbells hanging at arm's length by your side. Breathe *in*.

2. Swing the dumbells up in front of you at arm's length to just above shoulder height, keeping arms straight.

3. Keeping your head up, swing the dumbells in an arc down in front of you past your thighs to an arms straight position behind you. You should be in the half squat position.

4. Repeat 20 times (up to 3 sets).

This is a great fitness exercise, a good triceps exercise and good for stickwork. You'll find that the momentum of the dumbell does most of the work.

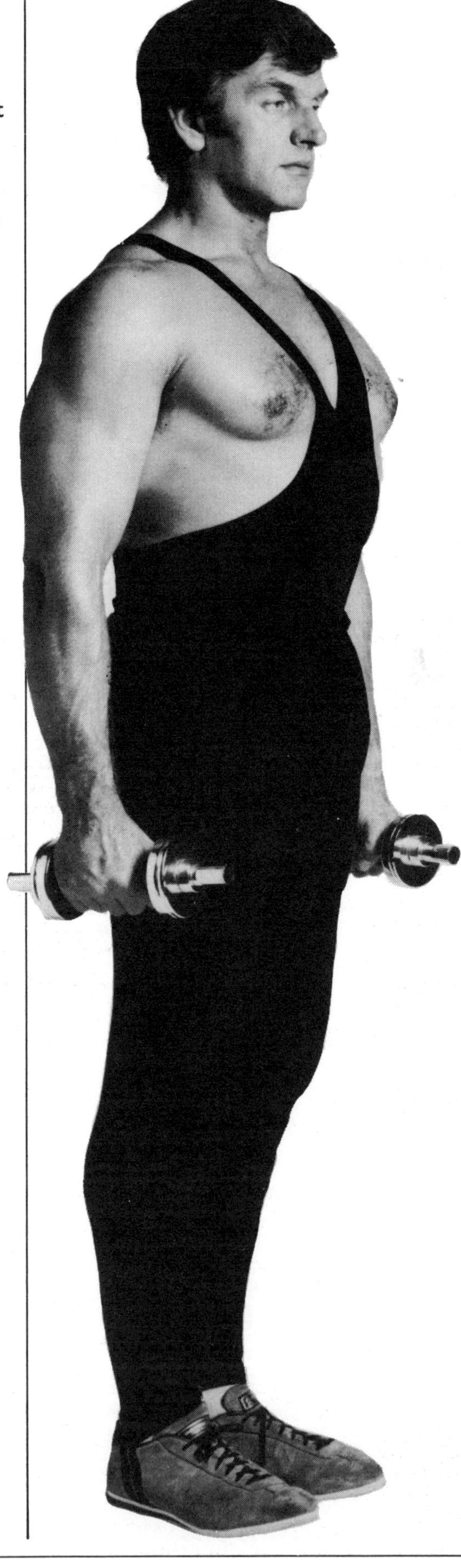

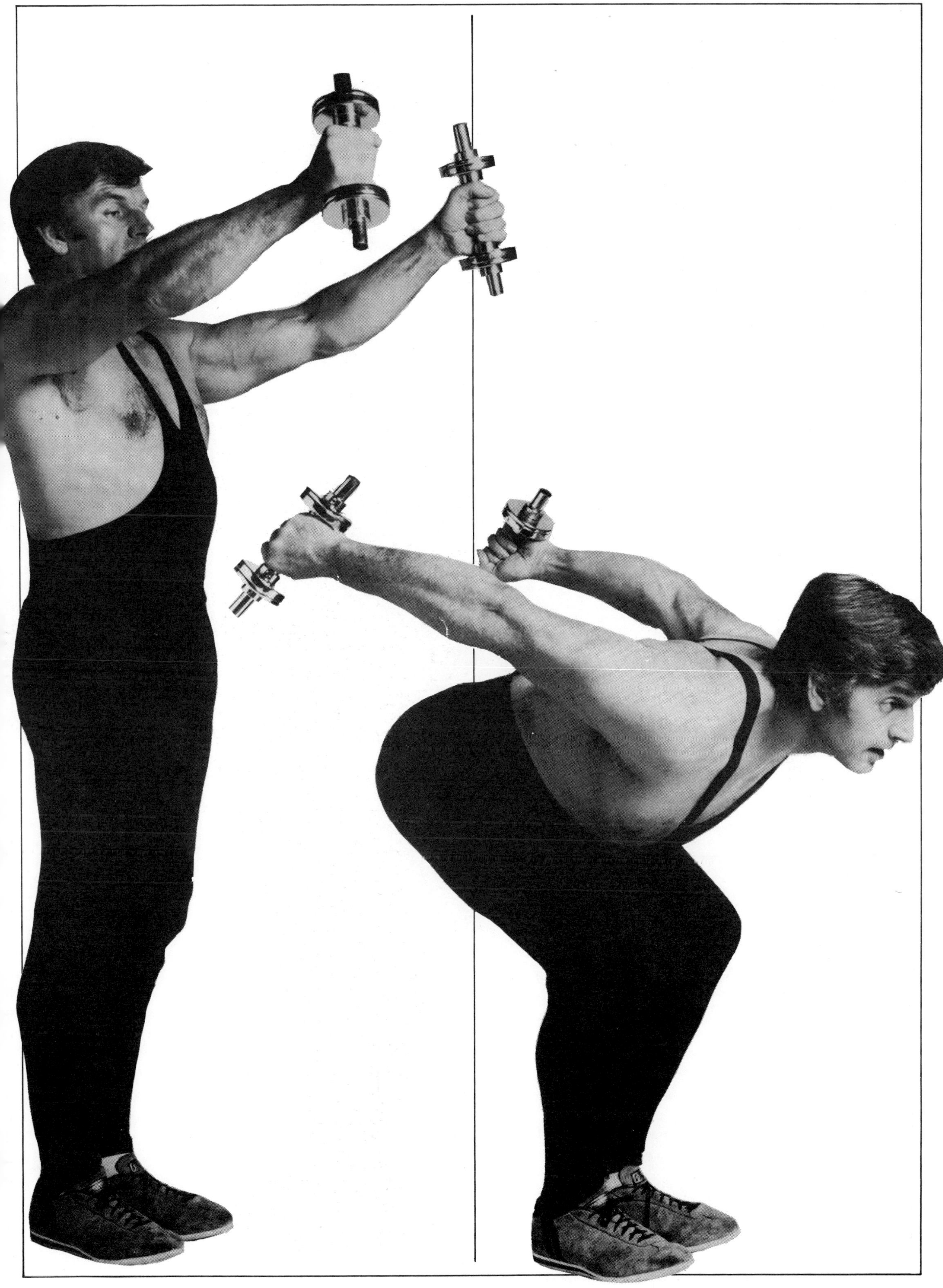

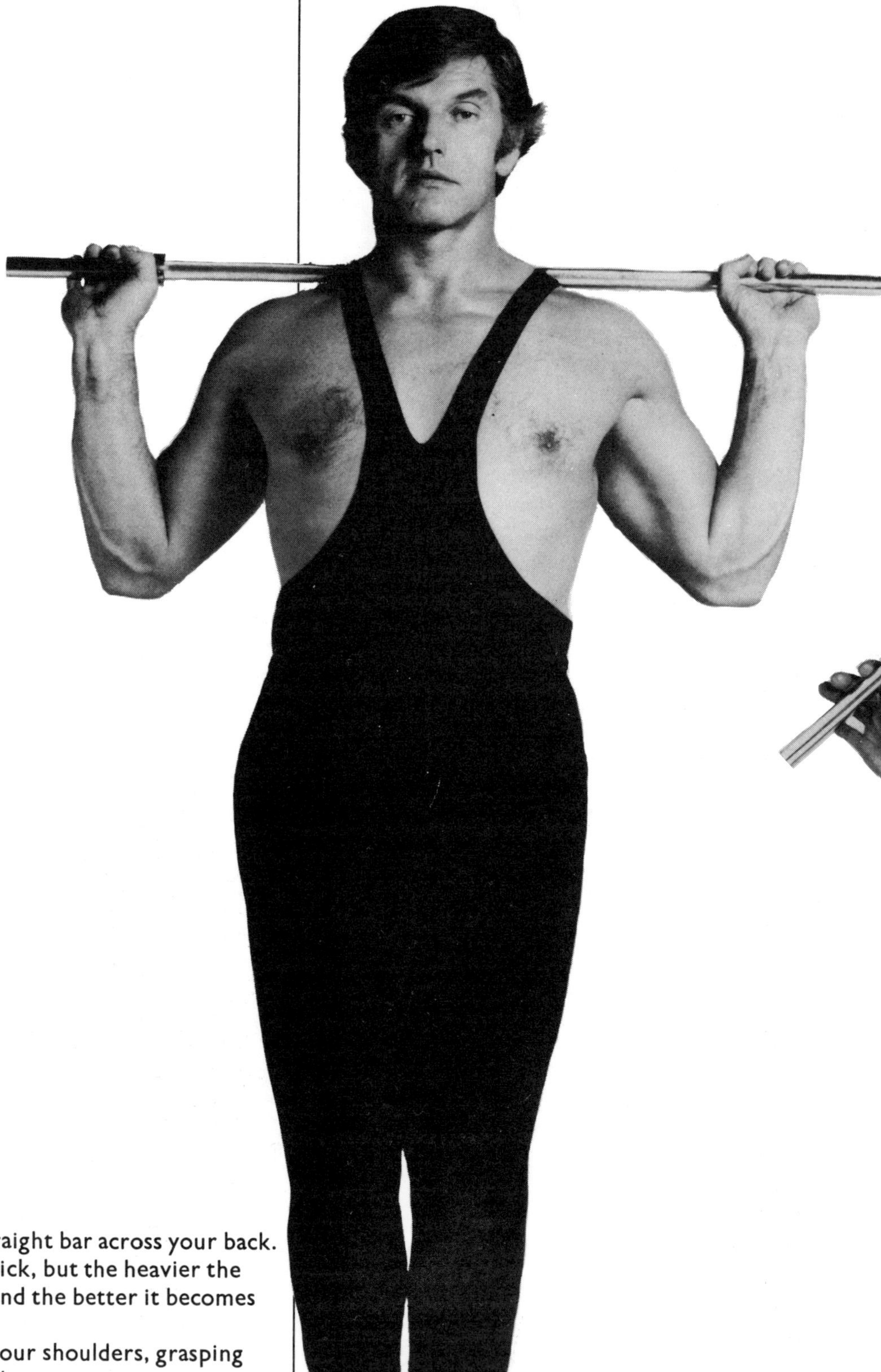

Hip Lunge

This should be done with a straight bar across your back. It can be done with a broomstick, but the heavier the bar, the more the resistance and the better it becomes as a strengthening exercise.

1. Stand with the bar across your shoulders, grasping the bar outside shoulder width.
2. Go into a side bend position, bending your knees slightly and going onto the sides of your feet.
It's important to get a side hip lunge.
3. Bend as far over as you possibly can.
4. Return to upright position.
5. Repeat 20 times on one side; repeat 20 times on other side (3 sets in all).

This is specifically a waist, back and inner thigh exercise.

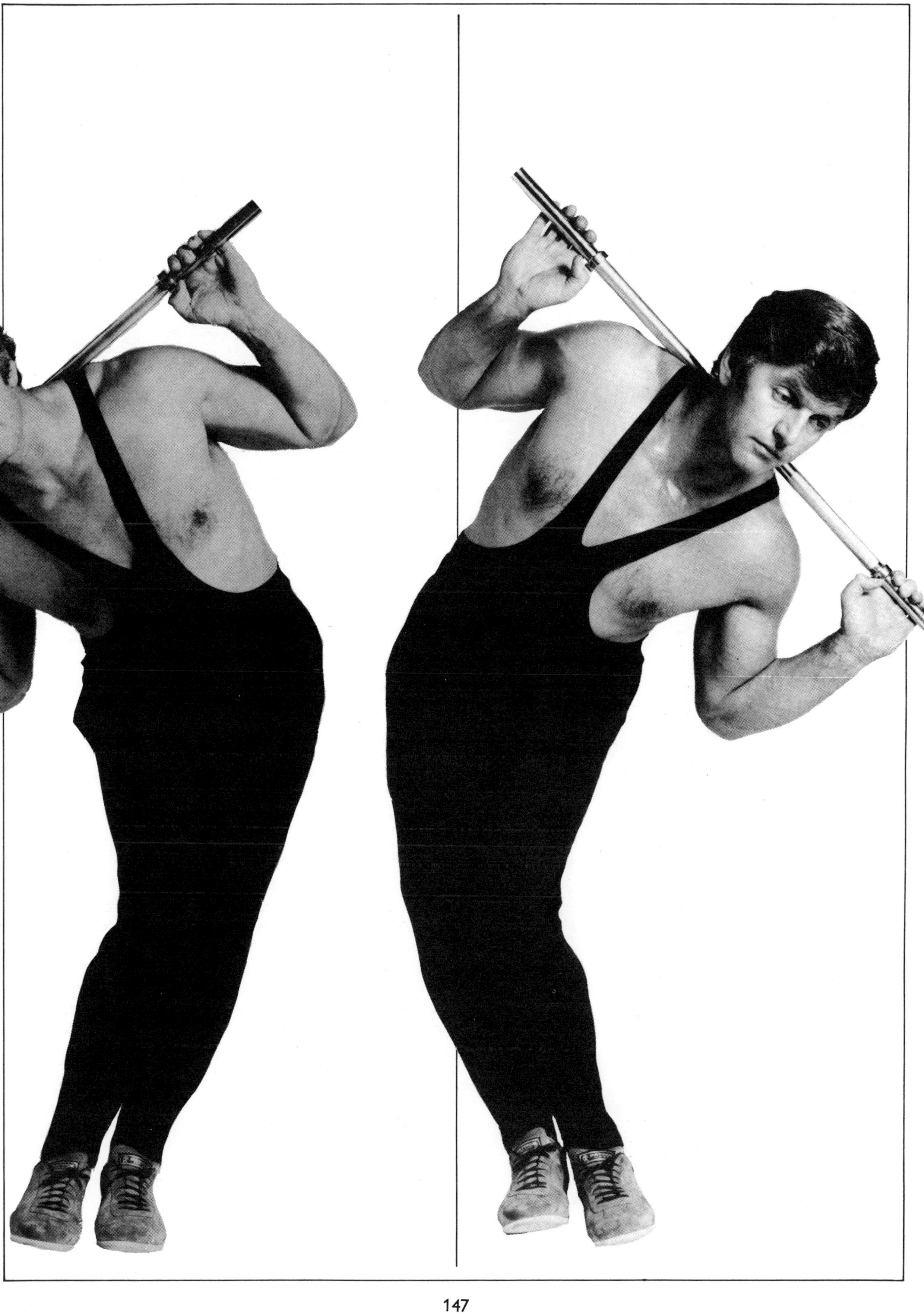

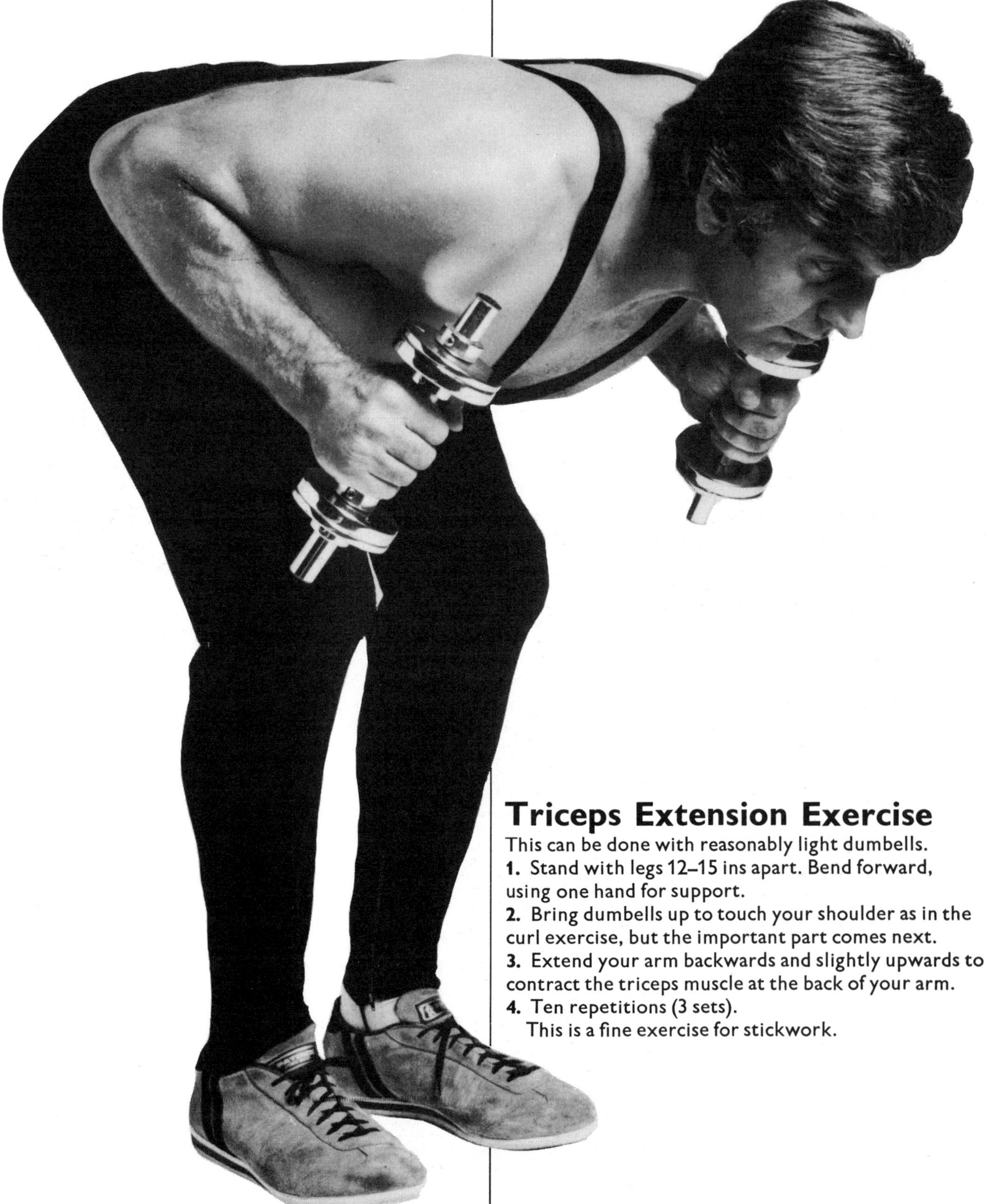

Triceps Extension Exercise

This can be done with reasonably light dumbells.

1. Stand with legs 12–15 ins apart. Bend forward, using one hand for support.

2. Bring dumbells up to touch your shoulder as in the curl exercise, but the important part comes next.

3. Extend your arm backwards and slightly upwards to contract the triceps muscle at the back of your arm.

4. Ten repetitions (3 sets).

This is a fine exercise for stickwork.

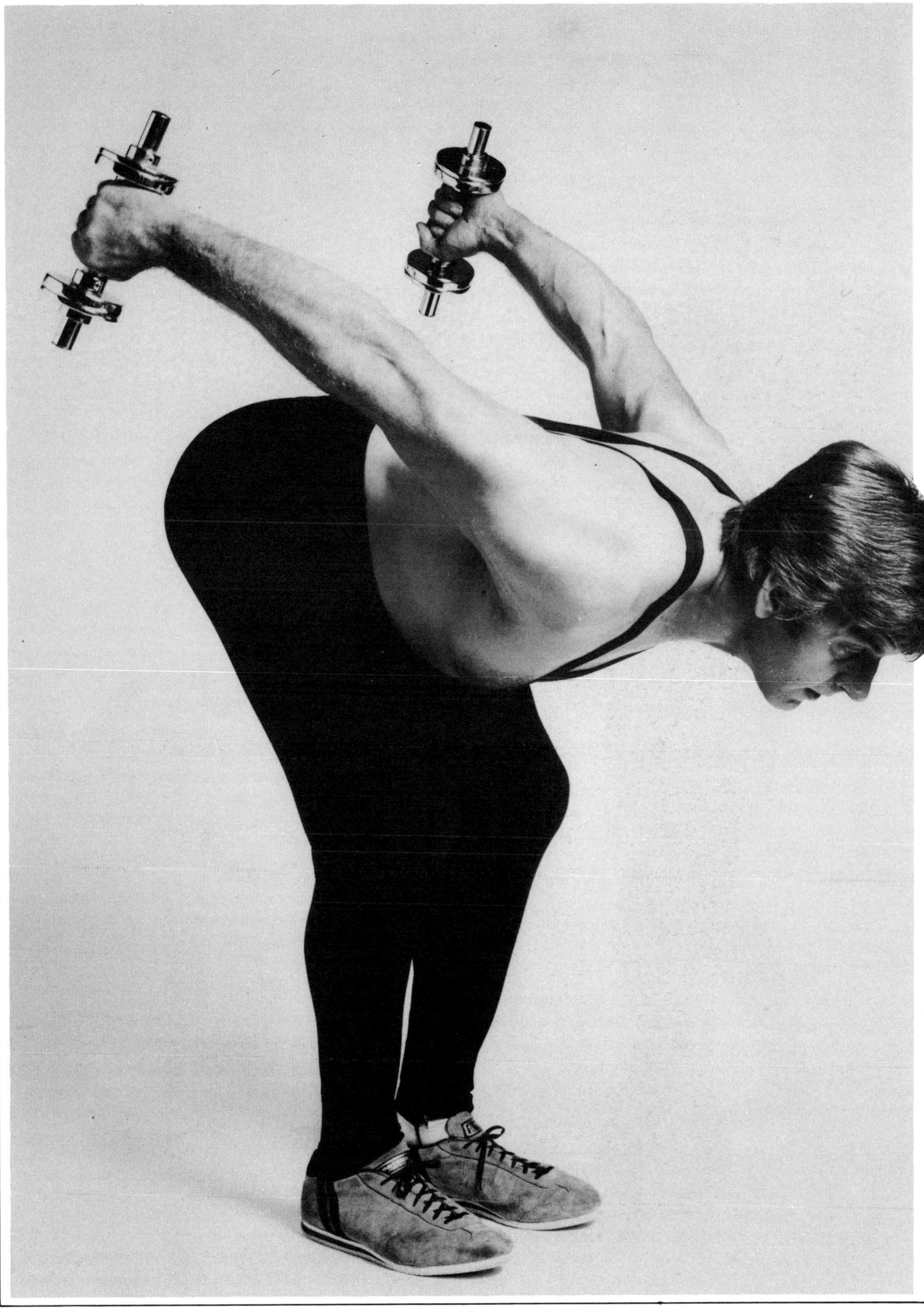

Forward Lunge

1. Stand upright, feet 15 to 20 inches apart, with the barbell across your back.
2. Take a long pace forward.
3. From this split position, bend your back forwards so your shoulders practically touch your knees.
4. Return to upright split position.
5. Repeat 20 times. Alternate with other leg forward (3 sets).

This is primarily a back exercise, not a leg exercise.

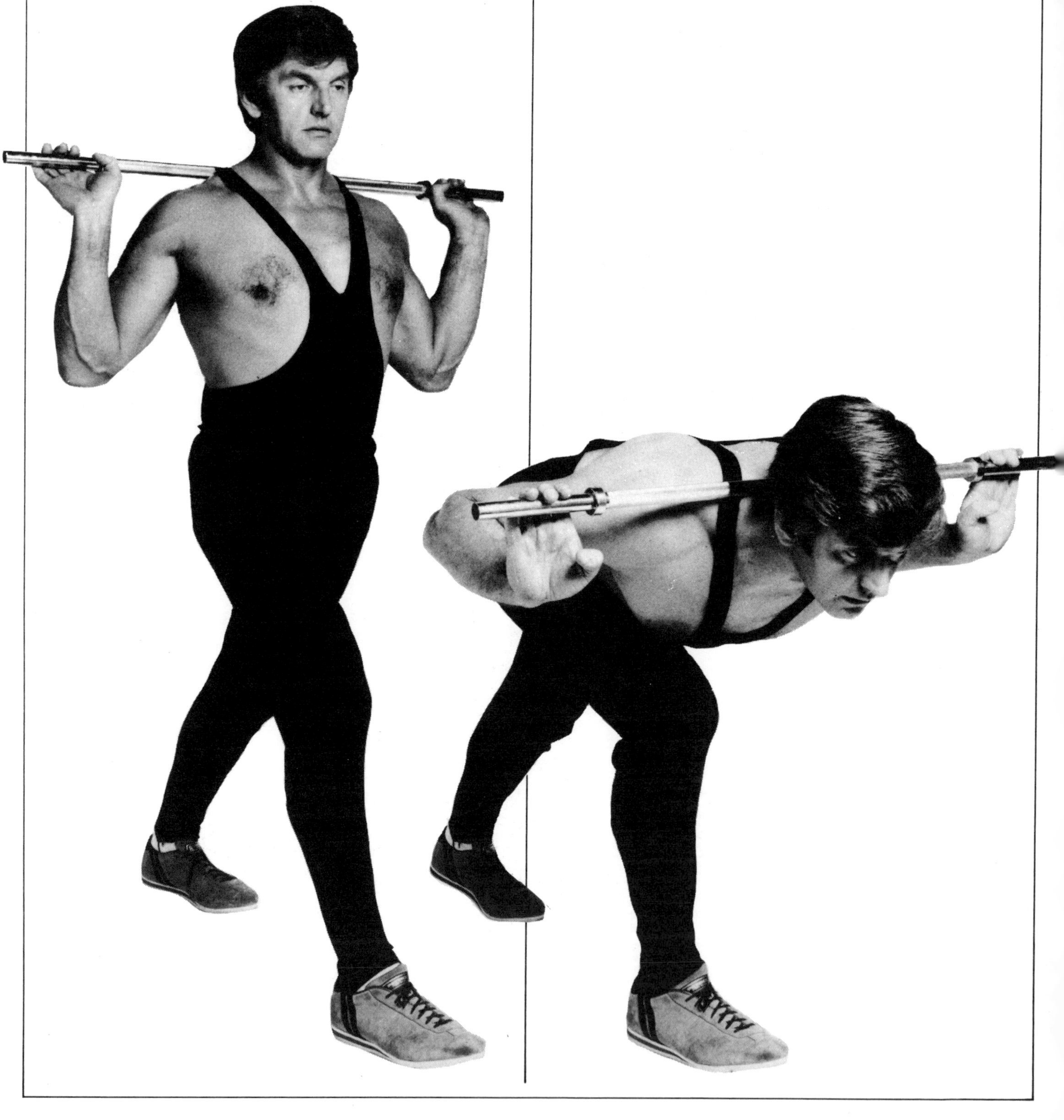

Chest Dip

To make this more effective, I would suggest you do this between the backs of two chairs, which makes it a much better work-out for the chest, arms and shoulder muscles.

1. Place the low-backed chairs back to back about two feet apart and make sure they are stable (get two people to sit on them).
2. Place your hands on the backs of the chairs and lower yourself into an incline position, so your shoulders are practically touching your hands.
3. Push back into the upright position.
4. Do 20 repetitions (3 sets).

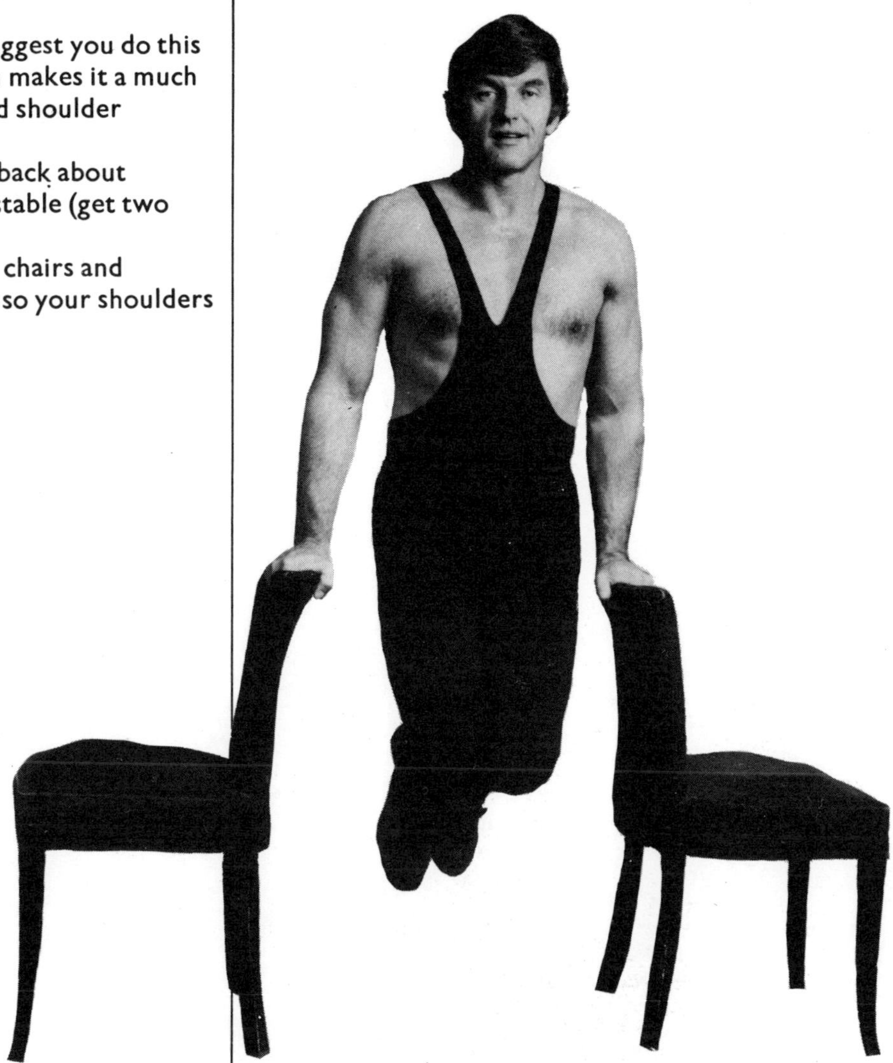

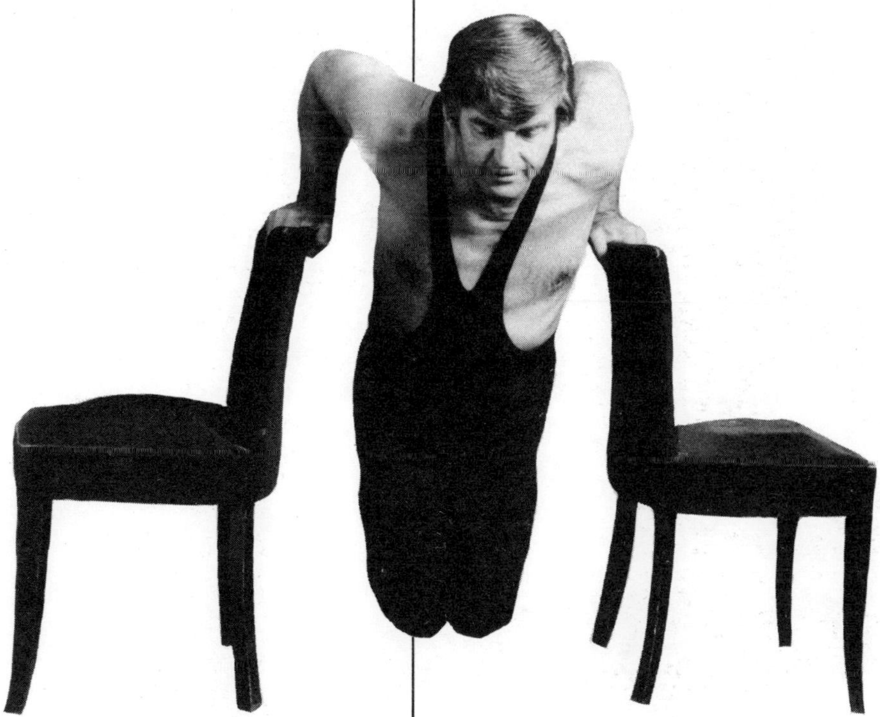

Twisting Sit-up

This is a marvellous abdominal exercise, and the way we're going to do it will also affect the external oblique muscles. If you have access to a sit-up board or incline bench, lovely. If you haven't, you'll have to do it on the floor. (You should not approach this exercise until you've done all the lesser forms of sit-up exercises previously described.)

1. Lie on the bench or floor. Hook your feet under something or get someone to hold your ankles.
2. Put a mat or cushion or some form of padding under your bottom.
3. Bending your knees slightly, you pull yourself up until your left elbow touches your right knee.
4. Return to prone position.
5. Pull yourself up until your right elbow touches your left knee.
6. Repeat 20 times (up to 5 sets).

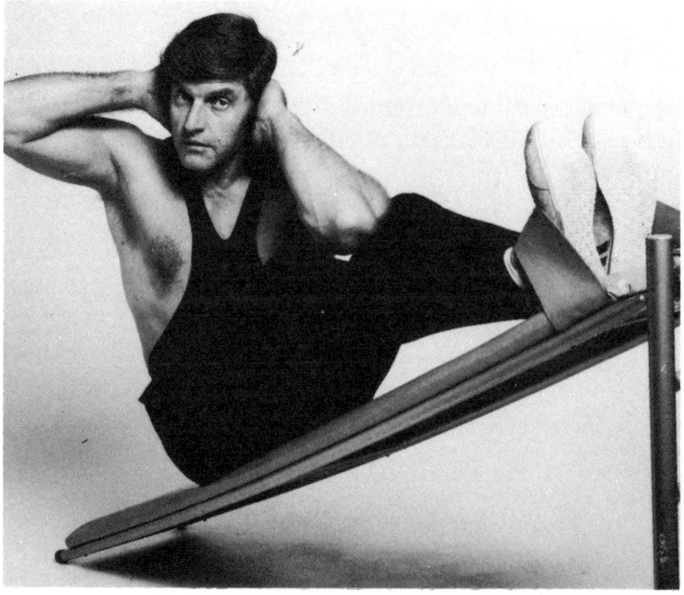

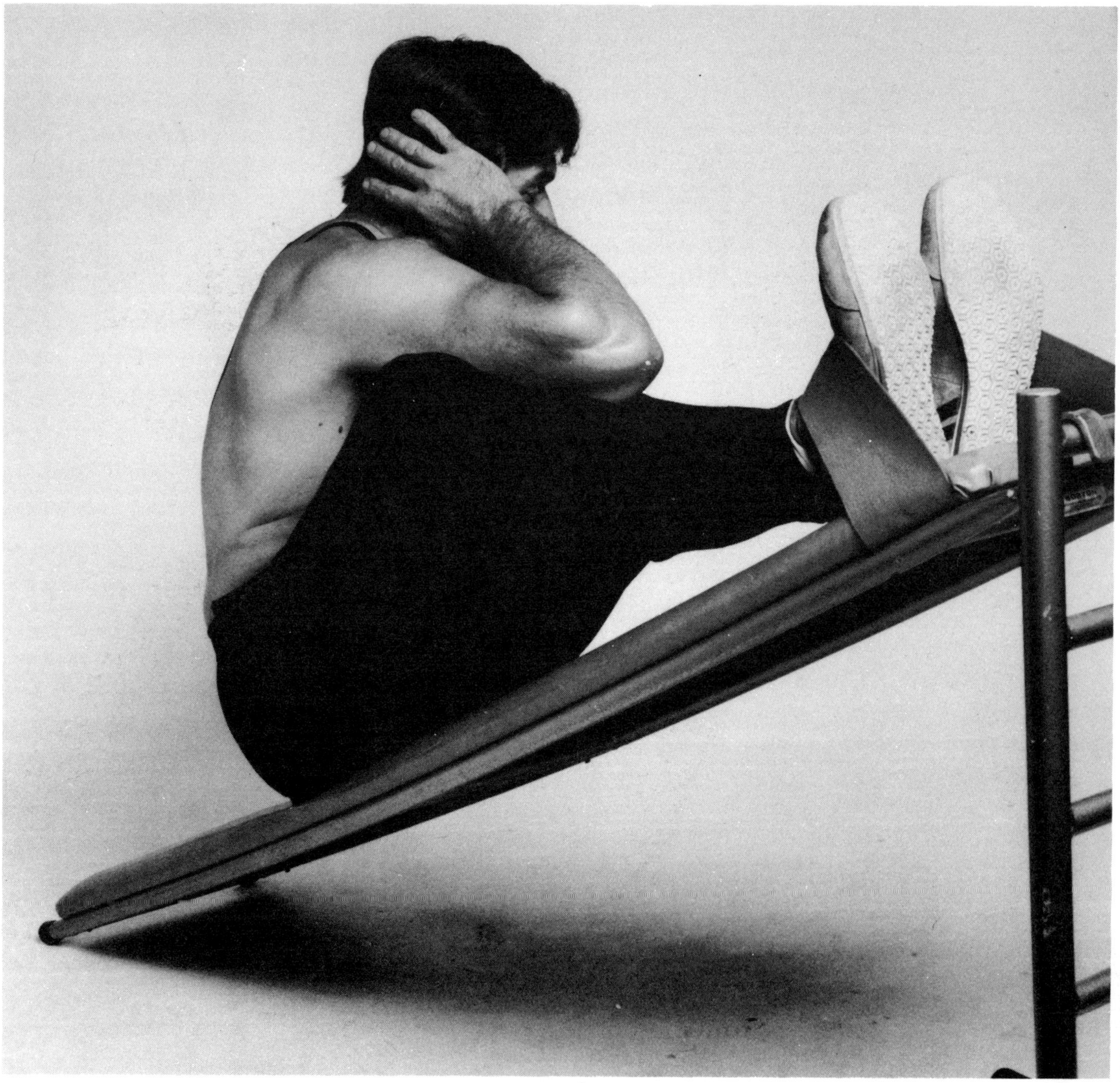

Twisting Squat

This is a peculiar exercise not seen in any other form of weight training programme.

1. Stand with barbell across your back, with all your weight on one leg. The other leg acts purely as a support.
2. Go down on the one leg into a twisting half squat.
3. Return to upright position.
4. Repeat 10 times.
5. Go onto the other leg. Repeat 10 times (3 sets).

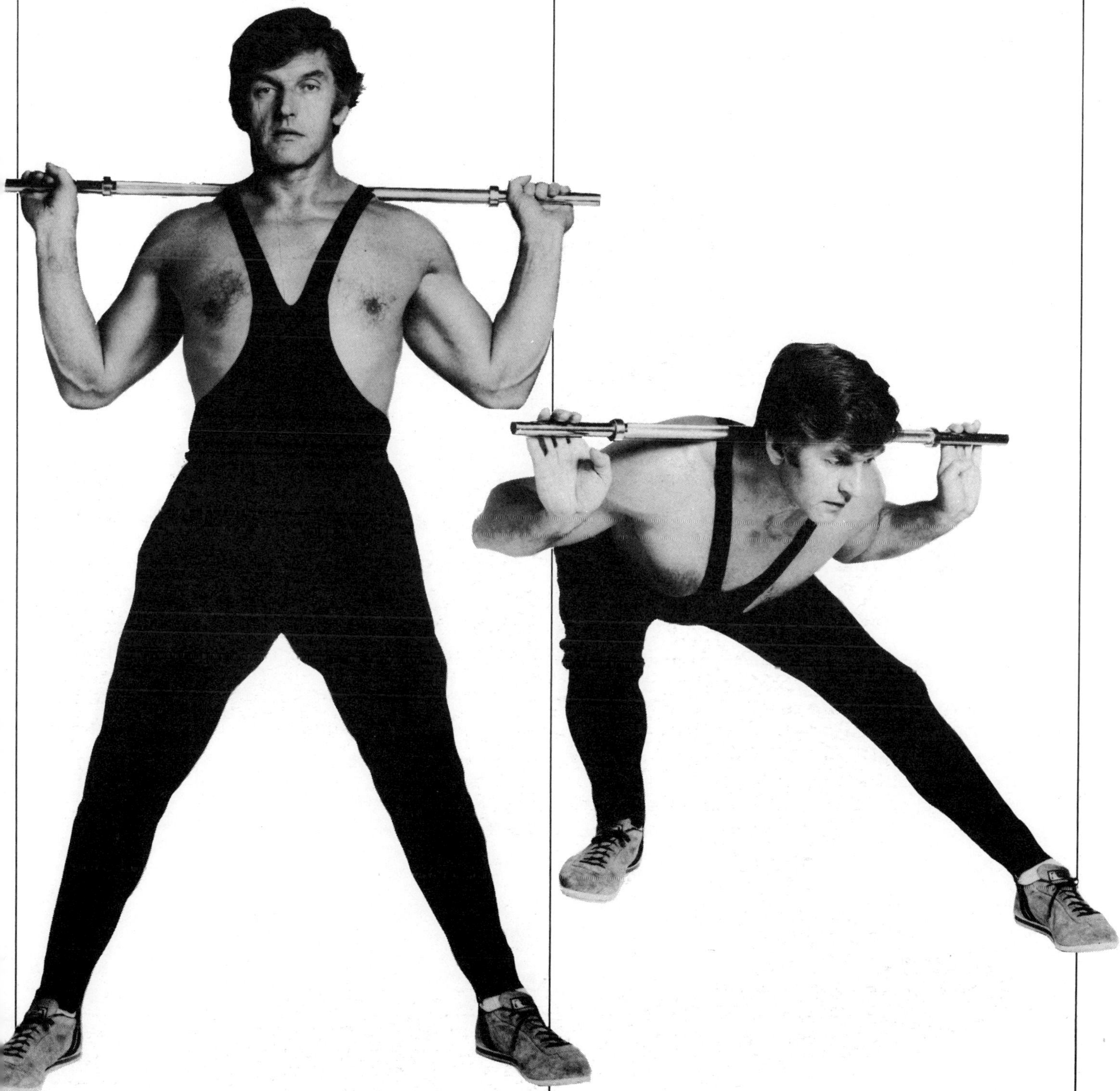

Leg Extension

You'll need the use of a leg extension machine, or an iron shoe, or at a pinch you can make your own weights by making a canvas bag filled with sand. The exercise strengthens the knee joint and is very good for the muscle on the inside of the knee, the vasta interna.

1. Sit on a high bench or a table, with the underside of your knee resting on the edge of a table, your knee bent to right angles.
2. Straighten the weighted leg as far as it will go.
3. Hold straight position and lower slowly.
4. Repeat 10 times for each leg (3 sets).

This is an exercise in which the average person can handle quite high weights – in my gymnasium I've often seen people using up to 150 lbs on the leg extension machine – so you'll soon find you'll have to increase the weight if you want to get any serious benefit out of it. If you have the necessary weights, do it as a strengthening exercise and make three sets of ten repetitions. If your weights are smaller, then increase the number of repetitions and sets if necessary.

It's vitally important, if you're going on a ski holiday, that you do some form of pre-conditioning and this routine is one of the best possible means of getting you in shape. If you follow it for a few weeks before you go, you shouldn't have to spend the better part of your holiday in your hotel bedroom nursing your various aches, pains and sprains. Remember, most injury is caused when you're overworking muscles unused to the strains you're imposing on them.

As far as other sports are concerned, you'll often hear people say, 'Oh well, I don't need special exercise, I play squash,' or tennis, or swim, or whatever. Unfortunately, there are very few sports or pastimes you can take part in that give you everything that a progressive resistance programme can. Swimming, for instance, is a grossly over-rated pastime as far as physical improvement is concerned. I have been to many swimming clubs and I wouldn't give you tuppence for some of the physiques on view.

Swimming itself is an exercise which definitely does affect most of the muscles of the body. However, the resistance involved in swimming is so low that the swimming exercise will only work the muscles over their range of movement and will not improve your physique or your figure one iota. If you swim regularly and vary the type of swimming you do then the programme is quite good for fitness training. However, most people when they decide they're going to swim to keep fit do exactly the same as the joggers do. They set themselves a certain amount of work to accomplish – say 20 lengths of the bath or three or four miles – but they don't vary the type of exercise they do. So the work-load placed on the body is not really increased – the swimmer ploughs up and down the length of the bath just as the jogger runs round and round the park.

As I have kept stressing, training, to do you any good whatsoever, must be progressive; that is, as you get fitter and stronger, so the programmes must get harder and harder. You should always be striving for improvement – to your physique, your general well being, your strength, your heart recovery rate, and so on.

Squash is another sport always quoted as being the great figure controller. Nothing could be farther from the truth. Squash is a marvellous fitness activity; you're chasing round the court, your heart is racing, you get periods ranging from doing nothing to working flat out; it improves your co-ordination and makes you sweat like mad. People often pick up squash at the same time as they take up a diet, and after three months they've lost a stone in weight. The truth is that they've lost the stone because they're on a diet and the squash itself has a relatively slight effect on their weight. Even if they've lost all they want to, they'll often find they're not the shape they want to be, because squash does not provide the sort of programme where you can control the shape and size of your body as you can with the type of exercise programmes in this book.

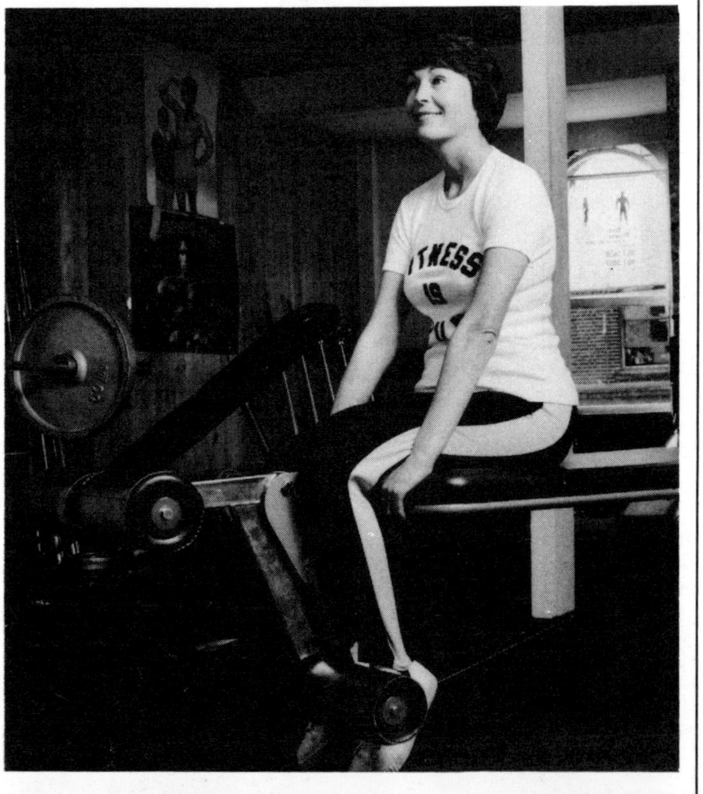

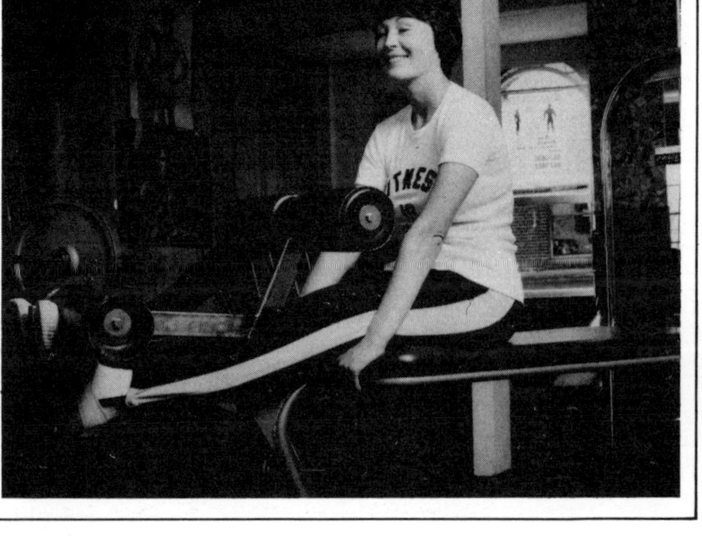

Chapter 18

TAKE IT WITH A PINCH OF (MENTAL) SALT

There are two basic components of fitness: diet and training. The greater of these is diet, but the two are complementary. No matter how hard you train you will not lose – or gain – weight unless you diet accordingly. But if you don't train, you have no control over where you shed – or gain – the weight. This is particularly true of women, who find that when they diet they lose weight downwards – i.e. the flesh comes off the face and neck first and off the hips last. Intelligently applied exercise can correct this tendency.

Fashions in dieting are constantly changing, just as they are in clothing. However, as medical knowledge advances, one hopes the changes in dietary advice are based more on facts than on arbitrary opinions and commercial and financial interests. Many of the theories popularly held in the fifties and sixties have been disproved in the seventies, and many widely believed 'truths' are being turned upside down by research. It's now thought that as many as one-third of all deaths among people over 35 could be postponed for as much as ten years if modern dietary advice were followed.

The basic reasoning is that the Western diet provides too much meat, fat, sugar and processed foods for the body to cope with adequately. It is now reckoned, for example, that a far smaller quantity of proteins is necessary for the body to function healthily. One man's fad is another man's poison, so the best advice I can give you is to shop around until you find a diet that suits you and enables you to maintain your weight at its healthiest level.

In general terms, the more natural your diet, the more healthy it will be. It's generally recognised now that heat destroys the vital goodness in natural foods; and the fewer processes food goes through before you eat it, the better it is for you. If it's natural, the fresher the better, too. Fruit and vegetables begin to deteriorate the moment they are picked or harvested. Every hour further from their natural, growing state, is another hour of loss.

My advice is to avoid excess in everything – including enthusiasm (your own and other people's). The wider your diet the more likely it is that it will be balanced, and that you'll be getting the correct doses of vitamins, proteins, carbohydrates, minerals and enzymes needed for good health. And you'll be getting them from the right sources, the food itself not the 'supplements' like vitamin and other pills which purport to supply a bodily need but in fact are more likely to unbalance the bodily chemistry and create more troubles than they cure.

In *Food For Fitness*, a recent publication containing a good deal of commonsense, an article by Dr Otto Brucker, an American nutrition researcher, makes the following point, 'A man can stay healthy with proper nutrition but without sufficient movement; he *cannot* remain healthy on any amount of exercise if nutritional elements are lacking.'

Dr Brucker attacks 'old nutritional theory' which assumed that a supply of the three basic nutritional elements – protein, fat and carbohydrates – along with certain minerals was sufficient for health, with vitamins added to the basic list. 'Countless other substances are required,' he says. 'They are called vital substances, and include not only the generally recognised vitamins and minerals, but also minerals present in the tiniest amounts (trace elements), a large group of enzymes, polyunsaturated fatty acids and aromatic substances. Some of these are necessary for good health; others *must* be present for life itself to go on.'

Manufactured nutritional products, says Dr Brucker, are marked by a lack of those vital substances. The more concentrated a product is, the fewer vital elements it will contain and the more harmful it might be. Injury to health comes mainly from manufactured nutritional products, like the purchased 'convenience' foods and drinks. Previously, the worth of a diet was measured by its calorie content. Nowadays, nutrition is based on the diet's *vitality*. The more food is left to nature, the more alive it is; the less natural, the less lifelike.

The two 'killer-foods' produced for society's consumption are white (that is, processed) sugar and refined flours from which white bread is made. Industrial sugars, which include white 'raw' brown and 'dark' varieties, cause a chain reaction of harm. They lack vital substances and act as vitamin thieves because they require vitamins (particularly B vitamins) for their digestion. In addition, they interfere with enzyme activities central to the production of energy, particularly in athletes. 'Eating these sugars drains away vital substances while adding none; it disturbs enzyme functions and in the end increases strength and energy not at all,' says Dr Brucker.

In the process of making 'white' flour, 22 nutrients are removed from the wheat that makes the bread. So-called 'enrichment' re-instates only four of these, but the food value remains almost nil because the enrichment vitamins are usually unassimilable, inorganic chemicals in unbalanced amounts and combinations. Dr Brucker concludes that white bread contains virtually no food value whatsoever; indeed it acts like glue in the intestines, severely inhibiting the absorption of food through the intestinal lining. Literally, gumming up the works, and being the main cause of the 'modern' disease – diverticulitis.

Nobody likes a good steak better than I do, and I've eaten many hundreds of portions of succulent Scotch beef in my campaigns to build my body to its peak fitness and condition. But it seems I must moderate both my claims and my appetite. For now meat is being seen as yet another danger food. Although meat is indeed the high-quality supplier of proteins we believe it to be, modern research now tells us that the body will function at its best on *less than half* the current recommended daily protein intake. It's now believed that a meat-heavy diet causes bone decay (bone atrophy or osteoporosis). One experiment on 20 professional footballers over 18 years found 100 per cent instances of ankle arthrosis *and* 97.5 per cent arthrosis of the knee among heavy meat-eaters.

The basic minerals potassium and magnesium are both in short supply in an everyday diet rich in meat, eggs, cheese, fat, sugar and grains. Meat-eating also hinders the absorption of magnesium, a shortage of which leads to arteriosclerosis, high blood pressure, migraine, eclampsia, leaching of calcium from teeth and bones, liver damage and disturbances of the neuro-muscular vessel system.

It used to be thought that protein derived from meat and animal products such as milk and eggs was superior in value to vegetable proteins, which could not do the same job. But now it is reckoned that man cannot obtain the proper nutritional value from cooked meat, because the heating necessary in the cooking destroys the vital substances; or from milk proteins, which are similarly damaged by the pasteurisation process, or by cooking. But uncooked vegetables and fruits, supplemented by whole grains and cereals, can supply all man's protein needs.

Physiologically, man is not a carnivore (meat-eater). Carnivores, omnivores (mixed meat and vegetable diet) and frugivores (fruit-eaters) in the animal kingdom are set apart by peculiarities in tooth structure and intestinal tract which correspond to the problems of eating and digesting the characteristic food of the animal's diet. Meat decays quickly in the warmth of the intestinal tract. Thus carnivores have an intestinal tube only three times the length of their body. Their stomachs manufacture abundant hydrochloric acid, suitable for digesting bone and flesh. Herbivores (like cattle) have several stomachs and an intestinal tract ten times the length of their body. Their alkaline saliva contains ptyalin for the digestion of starches. Grains don't decay as rapidly as meat, so they don't form the toxins of decomposition in the long intestinal tract. The digestive tract of a frugivore is 12 times the length of its body. So is man's.

Carnivores' teeth are made for stabbing, ripping and tearing; herbivores have grass-cutting and grinding teeth with broad, flat molars; and frugivores have pre-molars and molars suited to cracking nuts and grinding fruit and vegetables. On both these counts, then, man is made to eat fruit.

Now, a few words about slimming. In the first place, don't be misled by what you 'ought' to weigh. Tables of height/weight relationship may have their claims to 'scientific' analysis; but all they are at best is a statement of averages. It is odd that the individualists of the western world like to have their 'norms' dictated to them, in fitness if not in other things. Perhaps it's a sign of the mystique that is maintained about fitness. If you're trying to lose weight and at the same time maintain your fitness, the best programme is a gradual one of moderate calorie restriction. If you lose weight at more than one third of a pound a day, you're liable to lose muscular strength and fitness.

It's true that with almost any serious reducing diet you'll lose four to five pounds in the first two or three days. But that's not fat but water. It's after that first loss that the steady one-third of a pound loss should be aimed at. Any reducing diet inevitably results in some carbohydrate restriction.

Try to combine calorie restriction with increased exercise. For example, if you weigh 170 lbs and want to lose 10 lbs, cut your calories and exercise a bit more. You probably need to consume around 3,000 calories a day to maintain your current weight, so cut it to 2,000 calories (not a starvation diet by any means). If you exercise for an extra half an hour a day (or run five miles) that's another 500 calories per day lost. The total 1,500 calorie deficit will put you right on the goal of a loss of one third of a pound per day.

Basically, then, my recipe for eating for fitness, goes like this:

1. Balance your diet.

2. Eat as much fresh fruit and vegetables as you can. Don't overcook vegetables.

3. Use wholemeal flour, and bread made from it.

4. Avoid white flour and things made from it.

5. Avoid white (refined) sugar and things made from it. Use honey instead.

6. Avoid all 'convenience' foods containing white flour, white sugar and synthetic additives and preservatives.

7. Don't eat meat at more than one meal a day.

8. And finally, take all you read with a (mental) pinch of salt.

So, let's summarise.

First: *get your priorities right.* I can't stress enough that you train for fitness *first.* You train to improve your heart recovery rate and your respiration. You train to improve your strength and mobility and suppleness and lastly you train for your figure – for cosmetic reasons.

Second: make sure you're in a healthy state to start with. If you're at all concerned about operations you might have had, possible heart or respiration problems, high or low blood pressure, or anything at all, *consult your doctor* before indulging in any exercise programme of any sort. Get a complete check-up.

Third: make certain that you keep nice and warm while you're exercising. There are different psychologies of exercising and one school says you don't wear very much and watch yourself all the time in a mirror. That way goes the theory, you can see what's wrong and instinctively work harder at putting it right. I feel that when you're exercising, your body functions much better when it's warm. There's no point in wasting a lot of energy merely getting warm. I always like people to perspire well during their programmes. Wear track suits, with tee-shirts as undergarments.

Fourth: diet is obviously of paramount importance. Irrespective of your training aims, you must make certain that your diet is adequate for them. If you want to gain weight, you should be on a high protein, high calorie diet, If you want to lose weight, your diet should be fairly high in protein but low in calories. In both cases, you exercise the areas you want to improve. Diet and exercise work together. PS Don't get too faddy. I've no time for the eccentric diet – eggs all day, nothing but grapes, and so on. Beware the fads. It's amazing what you can do by being sensible.

Fifth: don't try to accomplish too much too quickly, either by exercise or diet. Take a few exercises and work them through properly, rather than dabbling at a number of exercises. A lot of a few exercises is better than a little of a lot of exercises.

Sixth: don't worry about doing too much. For example, many girls worry about developing unsightly muscles. The only problem is in the first couple of weeks when many people may put themselves off exercising by getting stiff and sore. Once you've got over that period, the biggest problem is persuading you to do sufficient exercising. Your body can cope with enormous amounts of work – far more than you'd ever expect.

Seventh: don't be frightened of weights. They're the be-all and end-all of healthy exercise and, used judiciously, will give you everything you want. You'll find it fun, and as you progress, you'll want to do more and more.

The information I've given in this book is probably adequate for all but a tiny fraction of readers – that 0.01 per cent who take a fanatical interest in weightlifting and body-building, specialist athletes and coaches for whom this book is not technical enough. The ordinary reader can find everything he or she needs to progress from the raw beginner to quite an advanced state of fitness.

As for me, well, I'll be around for a long time yet. My various activities keep me fit and in training all the time, and I still find it interesting and rewarding – and fun. As for the future, well, who knows? I've spent part of this year in America, attending seminars and conventions in connection with science fiction. As Darth Vader, I'm in constant demand over there – and there are more *Star Wars* pictures to come. I've done two marvellous series with the BBC – the Strong Man in *Horseman Riding By*, and the very expensive production of *As You Like It*, in which I play the part of Charles the Wrestler. I was very worried going into my first Shakespearean part in the company of such fine actors as Richard Pascoe and James Bolam, Helen Mirren and Angharad Rees but they were all marvellous and helped me a great deal.

One of the more interesting aspects of the play as far as I was concerned was that I had to choreograph the fight between Orlando (Brian Stirner) and Charles the Wrestler, which Orlando has to win. Brian is about six feet tall and weighs ten and a half stone, and beside me that was patently absurd. The first problem was that in those days they used to wrestle Cumberland style, a most uninteresting style of wrestling as far as spectacle is concerned, and even more stupid when we compared Brian's 147 lbs with my 250 lbs. The only solution was for me to be thrown out of the ring and be injured, and we developed quite a nice little sequence on those lines. But I got cold feet and began to worry about authenticity; so we found an expert on Cumberland style to coach us in all the correct falls. But the producer didn't like it, so we went back to my original in which Brian threw me through a wooden barrier round the ring.

My part in *Horseman Riding By* was a perfect example of typecasting – acting the part of a fairground strongman billed as the strongest man in the world, bending iron bars crooked and horseshoes straight; and I hope there are plenty more where that came from. And now I've just come back from yet another tour as Green Cross Man, and I hope that goes on for a very long time too.

When I was last in America I went to see George Lucas at his home in San Anselmo, and he filled me in on *Star Wars* plans for the future. In fact in the sequence of events the first *Star Wars* film was number four, and *Star Wars Two* we're working on this year is actually *Star Wars Five*. *One*, *Two* and *Three* are still to come, and episodes six to twelve. Actually George's dream is for a complete 24-hour showing of *Star Wars* . . . so although Darth Vader will no doubt die in an episode sometime in the future, I hope it's a long time yet.

With it all, and with my family, I'm going to have fun – and keep fit.

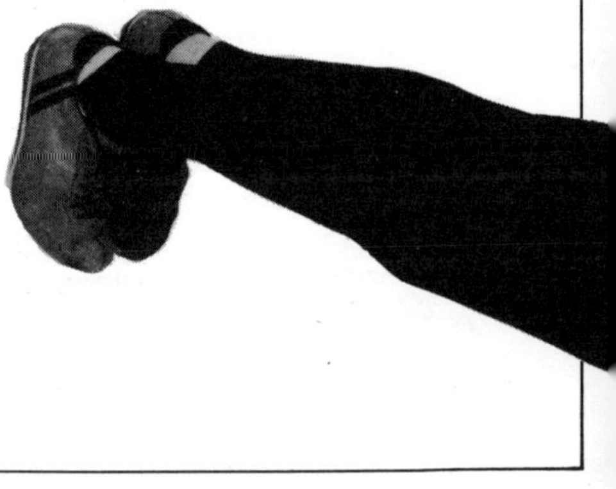

The Dave Prowse Ten Day Diet

BREAKFAST:	½ grapefruit (or unsweetened grapefruit juice) 2 eggs any style and bacon, minimum 2 slices, maximum 12. Coffee but no milk, cream or sugar (use artificial sweetener if you must) or tea with lemon.
LUNCH:	½ grapefruit. Meat, any style, any amount. Salad, dressed without sugar, as much as you can eat. Black coffee.
DINNER:	½ grapefruit. Meat, any style with gravy if it is not thickened with flour, or fish if you like. Any amount of any green, yellow or red (except beetroot) vegetables. Salad as above, as much as you want. Black coffee. If you are a bedtime snacker, tomato juice or skim milk.

NO fruit except for the grapefruit.

NO puddings, rice, potatoes, bread, pasta (in fact no starches, they form liquids which in turn form fat).

NO skipping anything, the bacon at breakfast or the salad at lunch or dinner. It's the combination that burns the fat.

NO eating between meals.

YOU MUST begin each meal with grapefruit which acts as a catalyst to start the fat burning.

YOU MUST cut down on coffee to one cup a meal. Coffee affects the insulin balance needed for the burning up process.

YOU CAN drink, but as sugar is forbidden, try to stick to dry wines or spirits, straight or with soda.

YOU CAN have your eggs fried in butter and your vegetables swimming in it, for fat does not form fat, in fact fat burns up fat.

YOU CAN eat as much as you want. You should eat until you are full.

YOU SHOULD restrict your fluid consumption as much as possible.

It's comparatively painless. AND IT WORKS. But then as with all diets, if in doubt, consult your doctor before embarking on the regime.
REMEMBER: For the first four days, your scales will show no change, then on the fifth day, you should find that you have lost five pounds. After that you lose a pound a day until the tenth day.
Determined dieters, who persevere beyond that, will find they will lose 1½ lbs every other day.

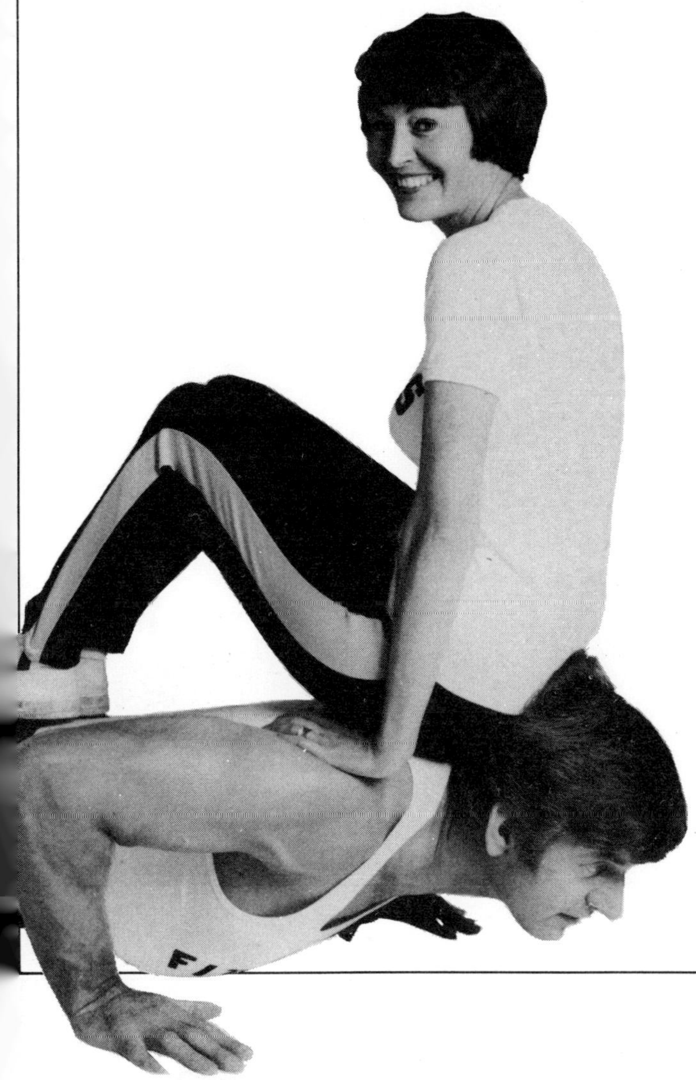

Photographic Acknowledgements:

We would like to thank the following sources:

Derek Rowe, *2, 17*
Courtesy Ogilvy, *6*
Benson and Mather, *Strength Athlete* and *Health and Strength, 15*
George Kirkley, *Strength Athlete, 18, 66*
Ian Blantern, *22*
Hammer Films, *28, 31*
Hawk Films, *31*
Twentieth Century Fox, *33*
Ian Cooke, *34*
BBC Radio Times Hulton Library, *35*
Max Factor, *36*
BBC Radio Times Hulton Library, *39*
Dave Webster, *64*
Santi Chakraborty, *94, 104*

Back cover photographs:
Ian Cooke, Hammer Films and Brian Moody, Scope Features